BASIC CLINICAL PARASITOLOGY

FIFTH EDITION

BASIC CLINICAL PARASITOLOGY

HAROLD W. BROWN

M.D., Sc.D., Dr. P.H., L.H.D. (Hon.), LL.D. (Hon.)
Professor Emeritus of Parasitology
Columbia University College of Physicians and Surgeons
Former Parasitologist, Presbyterian Hospital
New York, New York

FRANKLIN A. NEVA

M.D., M.A. (Hon.)
Chief, Laboratory of Parasitic Diseases and Head
 Section of Clinical Parasitology
National Institutes of Health
Bethesda, Maryland
Former John Laporte Given Professor of Tropical Public Health
Harvard School of Public Health
Boston, Massachusetts

 APPLETON-CENTURY-CROFTS/Norwalk, Connecticut

Copyright © 1983 by APPLETON-CENTURY-CROFTS
A Publishing Division of Prentice-Hall, Inc.

83 84 85 86 87 / 10 9 8 7 6 5 4 3 2 1

Prentice-Hall International, Inc., London
Prentice-Hall of Australia, Pty. Ltd., Sydney
Prentice-Hall of India Private Limited, New Delhi
Prentice-Hall of Japan, Inc., Tokyo
Prentice-Hall of Southeast Asia (Pte.) Ltd., Singapore
Whitehall Books Ltd., Wellington, New Zealand
Editora Prentice-Hall Do Brasil LTDA., Rio de Janeiro

Library of Congress Cataloging in Publication Data

Brown, Harold W.
    Basic clinical parasitology.

    Bibliography: p.
    Includes index.
    1. Medical parasitology. I. Neva, Franklin A.
II. Title.   [DNLM: 1. Parasites.   2. Parasitic
diseases.   WC 695 B878b]
RC119.B695   1983   616.9'6   82-16423
ISBN 0-8385-0551-1

Design: Jean M. Sabato
Production: Judith Warm Steinig

Thou shall have a place also without the camp
whither thou shall go forth abroad.
And thou shalt have a paddle upon thy weapon
and it shall be where thou wilt ease thyself abroad,
thou shalt dig therewith and shall turn back
and cover that which cometh from thee.

Deuteronomy, Chapter 23: 12, 13

CONTENTS

ARTHROPODA

TECHNICAL METHODS

PREFACE

The fifth edition has been extensively revised and rewritten to include recent important additions in knowledge. The needs of medical and graduate students, busy physicians, and laboratory technologists have dictated the selection of subject matter and the placing of emphasis upon the medical aspects of parasitology, such as pathology, symptomatology, diagnosis, treatment, and prevention. Therefore, discussion of the morphologic and biologic characteristics of the various parasites has been restricted to those that are essential for diagnosis. In the chapter on diagnostic methods, only those technical methods that are commonly used by students or hospital laboratory technologists are given. As parasitic diseases are largely preventable, pictorial life cycles have been included to make clear their vulnerable sites. The Medical Letter, Vol. 20, No. 4 (Issue 499), 1978, published by the Medical Letter, Inc., 56 Harrison Street, New Rochelle, N. Y. 10801, was most useful in preparing the chemotherapy sections.

Drs. Irving G. Kagan and Myron G. Schultz of the Center for Disease Control (CDC) were helpful in providing latest information on serologic tests and certain drugs for treatment, respectively, available at CDC. Mr. Armand Miranda and Miss Meredith Behr were of great assistance in photographing the pictorial material. Dr. Kathleen L. Hussey and Dr. Roger Williams contributed advice and drawings. These colleagues of over 35 years have given extensive help and friendly criticism. We are grateful to the many investigators in the field of parasitology, whose original contributions have provided the material for this book, and to Appleton-Century-Crofts for guidance throughout publication. Finally, it is our pleasant duty to acknowledge our indebtedness to David Belding, who prepared the first edition of *Basic Clinical Parasitology*.

Following are selected references of textbooks and journals on parasitology and tropical medicine to which the student is referred for a more thorough study. One journal, the monthly annotated bibliography, *Tropical Disease Bulletin*, deserves special mention for its invaluable abstracts of current literature on tropical diseases.

GENERAL REFERENCES FOR PREFACE

Other Parasitology Textbooks:

Faust, Beaver, and Jung: Animal Agents and Vectors of Human Disease. 4th ed. Philadelphia, Lea & Febiger, 1975.

Faust, Russell, and Jung: Craig and Faust's Clinical Parasitology. 8th ed. Philadelphia, Lea & Febiger, 1970.

Beck and Davies: Medical Parasitology. 3rd ed. St. Louis, Mosby, 1981.

Hunter, Frye and Swartzwelder: A Manual of Tropical Medicine. 5th ed., Philadelphia, Saunders, 1976.

Manson-Bahr: Manson's Tropical Diseases, 17th ed., Baltimore, Williams and Wilkins, 1972.

Markell and Voge: Medical Parasitology, 4th ed. Philadelphia, Saunders, 1976.

Noble and Noble: Parasitology, The biology of Animal Parasites, 4th ed., Philadelphia, Lea & Febiger, 1976.

Specialty Books with Coverage of Parasitic Disease:

Beeson and McDermott: Textbook of Medicine, 14th ed., Philadelphia, Saunders, 1975. (Vol. 1)

Binford and Connor: Pathology of Tropical and Extraordinary Diseases, Washington, D. C. Armed Forces Inst. of Pathology, 1976. 2 vols.

Goodman and Gilman: The Pharmacological Basis of Therapeutics, 5th ed. New York, Macmillan, 1975.

Ash and Orihel: Atlas of Human Parasitology. Chicago, American Society of Clinical Pathologists. 1980.

Marcial-Rojas and Moreno: Pathology of Protozoal and Helminthic Diseases, Baltimore, Williams and Wilkins, 1971.

Kean, Mott and Russell: Tropical Medicine and Parasitology—Classic Investigations. Ithaca. Cornell University Press, 1978 (2 vols.)

Von Brand: Biochemistry and Physiology of Endoparasites. New York, Elsevier. 1979.

Trowell and Jelliffe: Diseases of Children in the Subtropics and Tropics, 2nd ed. London, Edward Arnold, Ltd. and Baltimore, Williams and Wilkins, 1970.

Reeder and Palmer: The Radiology of Tropical Diseases Baltimore, Williams and Wilkins, 1981.

Beeson and Bass: The Eosinophil, Vol. 14. Major Problems in Internal Medicine, Philadelphia Saunders 1977.

Dawes: Advances in Parasitology, New York, Academic Press, Annual volumes beginning in 1963.

ACKNOWLEDGMENTS

Life cycle plate figures are original or from the following various sources.

Figure 4-3, Winterbottom's sign, after Koch, from Strong: Stitt's *Diagnosis, Prevention and Treatment of Tropical Diseases*, 7th Edition, courtesy of the McGraw-Hill Book Co. Figure 4-3, later stage of sleeping sickness, and Figure 13-2, severe cirrhosis, courtesy of Dr. E. R. Kellersberger. Figure 4-4, megacolon, courtesy of Dr. F. Köberle, published in *Journal of Tropical Medicine and Hygiene*, 61, 1958. Figure 4-4, primitive house, Chile, courtesy of Dr. R. Donckaster. Figure 6-2, clinical figures from S. E. Gould, *Trichinosis*, 1st edition, courtesy of Charles C Thomas, Publisher. Figure 6-4, rectal prolapse, and Figure 6-13, pinworm and perianal region, courtesy of Dr. Ralph Platou, Department of Pediatrics, Tulane Medical School. Figure 6-9, adult hookworms, and Figure 46, adult pinworms, from *Helmintologia Humana*, 1949, Habana, Cuba, courtesy of Drs. Pedro Kouri and José G. Basnuevo. Figure 6-9, cardiac enlargement, from A. W. Hill and J. Andrews, courtesy of *American Journal of Tropical Medicine*. Figure 6-13, Scotch tape swab technic, adapted from Brooke, Donaldson, and Mitchell, 1949. Figure 7-4, developmental stages of filaria in mosquito, courtesy of E. Francis, *Filariasis in Southern United States*, Government Printing Office, 1919. Figure 9-3, coracidium, procercoid, plerocercoid, scolex from the film, *The Life Cycle of Diphyllobothrium latum*, U.S. Public Health Service, 1950. Figure 10-6, brain containing cysts, Figure 13-2, liver pathology, and Figure 16-2, lesions, from J. E. Ash and S. Spitz, *Pathology of Tropical Diseases*, courtesy of The Armed Forces Institute of Pathology, Washington, D.C. Figure 10-6, cysts in muscles, from H. B. Dixon and W. H. Hargreaves, 1944, *Quarterly Journal of Medicine*.

Figure 12-2, family picture, courtesy of Drs. E. H. Sadun and C. Maiphoom, *American Journal of Tropical Medicine and Hygiene*, 1953; water nuts from E. C. Faust, *Human Helminthology*, 3rd edition, courtesy of Lea & Febiger, metacercaria, from C. H. Barlow, *American Journal of Hygiene*, Monographic Series, 1925. Figure 13-8, lesions on child, courtesy of Michigan Department of Health, from 1939 Progress Report of the Division of Water Itch Control, Stream Control Commission. Figure 15-3, head lesions and nit, from McCarthy, *Diseases of the Hair*, The C. V. Mosby Company; body louse lesions after J. B. and

B. Shelmire, from G. C. Andrews, *Diseases of the Skin*, 4th edition, courtesy of W. B. Saunders Co. Figure 15–3, nymphal stages, and Figure 15–6, egg, larva, and pupa from *Arthropods of Medical Importance*, Naval Medical School. Figure 15–9, bites, from B. W. Becker and M. E. Obermayer, *Modern Dermatology and Syphilology*, courtesy of J. B. Lippincott Co., Philadelphia.

Figure 15–2, adult and pupa, and Figure 16–2, female depositing eggs, from Metcalf, Flint and Metcalf, *Destructive and Useful Insects*, 4th edition, courtesy of McGraw-Hill Book Company. Figure 16–2, adult, from N. I. H. Bulletin No. 171, 1938. Figure 16–4, life cycle figures, from H. E. Ewing, *Journal of Parasitology*, 1944; lesions from Dr. G. W. Wharton, chigger attached from Dr. C. B. Philip, chigger bite, all courtesy of Dr. R. W. Williams, Columbia University. Figure 16–5, life cycle stages and skin burrow, from K. Mellanby, *Scabies*, courtesy of Oxford University Press; lesions from O. S. Ormsby and H. Montgomery, *Diseases of the Skin*, 7th edition, courtesy of Lea & Febiger Co.

Color plates of malaria from A. Wilcox, *Manual for the Microscopical Diagnosis of Malaria in Man*, Bulletin No. 180, N. I. H., Washington, D.C., 1943, in G. C. Shattuck, *Diseases of the Tropics*, courtesy of Appleton-Century-Crofts.

Unacknowledged figures are from earlier editions of Belding, from old pictures we have been unable to trace, or from the personal collections of H. W. Brown, K. L. Hussey, and R. W. Williams, all of Columbia University.

We have made extensive use of *The Medical Letter* in the revision of chemotherapy. It should be examined for additional details. *The Medical Letter* is published by The Medical Letter, Inc., 56 Harrison Street, New Rochelle, N.Y. 10801.

1

General Parasitology

Parasitology is the science that deals with organisms that take up their abodes, temporarily or permanently, on or within other living organisms for the purpose of procuring food, and with the relationship of these organisms to their hosts. In the restricted sense employed here the term is applied only to animal parasites belonging to the protozoa, helminths, and arthropods.

PARASITES AND PARASITISM

Parasitism includes any reciprocal association in which a species depends upon another for its existence. This association may be temporary or permanent. In *symbiosis* there is a permanent association of two organisms that cannot exist independently, in *mutualism* both organisms are benefited, and in *commensalism* one partner is benefited and the other is unaffected. The term *parasite,* however, is ordinarily applied to a weaker organism that obtains food and shelter from another organism and derives all the benefit from the association.

The harboring species, known as the *host,* may show no harmful effects or may suffer from various functional and organic disorders.

Various descriptive names denote special types or functions of parasites. An *ectoparasite* lives on the outside (infestation) and an *endoparasite* within the body of the host (infection). Parasites are termed *facultative* when they are capable of leading both a free and a parasitic existence and *obligate* when they take up a permanent residence in and are completely dependent upon the host. An *incidental* parasite is one that establishes itself in a host in which it does not ordinarily live. A *temporary* parasite is free-living during part of its existence and seeks its host intermittently to obtain nourishment. A *permanent* parasite remains on or in the body of the host from early life until maturity, sometimes for its entire life. A *pathogenic* parasite causes injury to the host by its mechanical, traumatic, or toxic activities. A *pseudoparasite* is an artifact mistaken for a parasite. A *coprozoic,* or spurious, parasite is a foreign species that has passed through the alimentary tract without infecting the host.

1

Parasites often lack the necessary organs for assimilating raw food materials and depend upon the host for predigested food. An adequate supply of moisture is assured inside the host, but during the free-living existence of the parasite inadequate moisture may either prove fatal or prevent larval development. Temperature is likewise important. Each species has an optimal temperature range for its existence and development. Both high and low temperatures are detrimental and even lethal.

Scientific Nomenclature. Animal parasites are classified according to the International Code of Zoological Nomenclature. Each parasite belongs to a phylum, class, order, family, genus, and species. At times the further divisions of suborder, superfamily, subfamily, and subspecies are employed. The family name ends in "-idae," the superfamily in "-oidea," and the subfamily in "-inae." The names are Latinized, and the scientific designation is binomial for species and trinomial for subspecies.

The law of priority obtains as to the oldest available specific name, even if only a portion of the parasite or its larva has been described. To be valid a generic name must not have been given previously to another genus of animals. The names of genera and species are printed in italics; the generic name begins with a capital and the specific name with a small letter: *Ascaris lumbricoides.*

Geographic Distribution. The endemicity of a parasite depends upon the presence and habits of a suitable host, upon easy escape from the host, and upon environmental conditions favoring survival outside the host. Parasites with simple life cycles are more likely to have a cosmopolitan distribution than those with complicated life cycles. Economic and social conditions affect the distribution of the parasites of man. Thus, irrigation projects and the use of night soil in agriculture enhance conditions for parasitic infection. Inadequate individual and community sanitation, low standards of living, and ignorance favor the spread of parasitic diseases. Such religious rites as ablution and immersion in heavily contaminated water may be responsible for their transmission. Migrations of populations have spread parasitic disease throughout the world. The importation of black people to the Western Hemisphere was accompanied by hookworm disease and schistosomiasis. Immigrants from the Baltic countries introduced the fish tapeworm into North America.

Although many important species of parasites have a worldwide distribution, tropical countries, where optimal conditions of temperature and humidity are present, are most favorable for the survival, larval development, and transmission of parasites. The short summer season in the temperate zones prevents the development of many species that require high temperatures during their larval stages. Intense dry heat or direct sunlight may destroy the larval forms. On the other hand, low temperatures arrest the development of eggs and larvae and may even destroy them. Freezing temperatures and snow force humanity to use privies and prevent general soil pollution. Moisture is essential for the development of free-living larvae, and it is also necessary for the propagation of intermediate hosts, such as arthropods, snails, and fishes. Even in the tropics dry plateaus, because of lack of humidity, are practically free from parasites except for resistant species or those that are transferred directly from host to host.

Life Cycle. Through millennia parasites have evolved a way of life, or life cycle, that involves survival and development in the external environment and in one or more hosts. This life cycle may be relatively simple or it may be incredibly complicated, with multiple morphologic forms and developmental stages. At times, generally when in the external environment, the parasite is quiescent in the form of resistant eggs or cysts; when taken up by an appropriate host it may undergo active growth and metamorphosis. As the life cycle becomes more complicated the chance of parasite survival decreases, but highly developed reproductive organs and multiplication at some stage of the parasite cycle offset the hazards of a complex life history.

The final or *definitive* host harbors the adult

or sexual stage of the parasite. Part or all of the larval or asexual stage may take place in another animal, known as an *intermediate* host, such as the snail for the schistosome. Certain species of trematodes and cestodes have two such hosts, known as primary and secondary intermediate hosts. A *paratenic* host is an animal that harbors the parasite in an arrested state of development; however, the parasite is capable of continuing its cycle in a subsequent suitable host. A human being may be a definitive host for some parasites (such as the beef and pork tapeworms), an intermediate host for others (hydatid tapeworm), or an *incidental* host. The last instance refers to the situation in which the infected individual is not necessary for the parasite's survival or development, e.g., the human being in the case of trichinosis. The human being may be the only definitive host, and thereby crucial for continuation of the cycle, or only one of several definitive hosts. Other animals that harbor the same parasite are known as *reservoir* hosts. Such reservoir hosts ensure continuity of the parasite's life cycle and act as additional sources of human infection.

From a medical standpoint, knowledge of the life cycle of a parasite is important, since it indicates how human beings become infected and the stages at which preventive measures can be most effectively applied.

PARASITIC INFECTION AND DISEASE

The transmission of parasites involves three factors: (1) a source of infection, (2) a mode of transmission, and (3) the presence of a susceptible host. The combined effect of these factors determines the prevalence of the parasite at any given time and place.

Since parasitic infections often tend to run a chronic course with few or no symptoms, an infected individual may become a carrier without showing clinical manifestations, thus serving as a potential source of infection to others. This probably represents the normal state of infection in which there is an equilibrium between the host and the parasite. Thus infection does not always result in disease.

The methods whereby parasites reach susceptible hosts from their primary sources are varied. Some parasites require only direct contact. Others with more complicated life cycles must pass through various developmental stages, either as free-living forms or in intermediate hosts, before becoming infective. Transmission is effected through direct and indirect contact, food, water, soil, vertebrate and arthropod vectors, and, rarely, from mother to offspring. The chances of infection are increased by environmental conditions favoring the extracorporeal existence of the parasite and by lack of sanitation and communal hygiene. A human being, when infected by a parasite, may serve as (1) its only host, (2) its principal host with other animals also infected, or (3) its incidental host with one or several other animals as principal hosts. In addition to the natural adaptability of the parasite in respect to its host, the ease of transmission depends upon the habits and communal associations, as well as the resistance, of the host.

Pathology and Symptomatology. Various distinctions have been made between the terms *infection* and *infestation,* although they are often used indiscriminately to denote parasitic invasion. In this textbook *infection* is applied to invasion of endoparasites and *infestation* to the external parasitism of ectoparasites, such as arthropods, or to the presence of parasites in soil or plants. Distinction between *parasitic infection* and *disease* should also be made. In the former situation the infected host suffers very little damage and no symptoms; in the latter case the infected individual develops pathologic changes and symptoms of varying degree.

The pathogenesis of disease associated with parasitic infections depends upon several general factors, such as the numbers of parasites and their tissue tropism, as well as various specific mechanisms of tissue damage. Some parasites, such as the protozoa, are capable of multiplying in the host. With the worms, which generally do not multiply in the human host, the likelihood of disease is related to worm burden or intensity of infection. After entering its host the parasite migrates to those parts of the body where conditions are suitable for temporary or permanent residence. Tissue specificity is one of the most striking characteristics of parasitic infections, but under certain conditions parasites may localize aberrantly in other organs or in a more generalized fashion. The actual mechanisms by which parasites can damage the host include (1) mechanical effects, such as pressure from an enlarging cyst or obstruction of vessels or hollow viscera, (2) invasion and destruction of host cells by the parasite itself, (3) inflammatory reaction to the parasite or parasite products, and (4) competition for host nutrients. The timing of appearance of signs and symptoms will vary with the incubation period for the particular parasite involved and the activity and the location of the parasite at various stages of its development and life cycle in the host.

Resistance and Immunity. Ability of the host to withstand infection by a parasite can be due to physicochemical barriers, factors that confer innate or natural resistance, or because of specific immunity acquired from previous infection with the parasite. Examples of the first type of resistance would be intact skin in the case of those parasites that require mucous membranes or abrasions for penetration and the chemical milieu in the upper small bowel of the definitive host for protoscolices of *Echinococcus.* Natural resistance is illustrated by the recent finding that Duffy blood group determinants on the red blood cell are closely associated with the receptor for *Plasmodium vivax* malaria. Since most West African and many American blacks lack the Duffy factor, this explains their resistance to vivax malaria. Host specificity for other intracellular parasites, such as the coccidia, may also involve cell surface receptors or other biochemical specificities that permit some and restrict other species to serve as suitable hosts. Although exact mechanisms are unknown, genetic influence over susceptibility or resistance

to various parasitic infections has been clearly demonstrated. The nature of innate resistance involved in the specificity of certain worms for a given animal host is not understood. Such natural resistance is not always complete; the parasite may remain alive, migrating in the tissues of an abnormal host, but be unable to complete its development. Factors like age and the nutritional status of the host might represent either natural or acquired resistance and can play a role as well in the severity of the disease produced. Paradoxically, with some parasitic infections, a suboptimal nutritional state actually may reduce severity of disease.

The mechanisms of immunologic response to parasitic infection and considerations that bear upon immunity to parasites, including possible vaccines, are subjects of recently expanding interest. Parasites represent a more complex and new challenge to experimental immunologists. Certain research developments coupled with failures of disease control with past methods suggest that vaccines for control of some parasitic infections are a realistic goal. Finally, there has been increasing recognition that the immune response to parasites or parasite products may have a deleterious effect in some instances upon the host and actually contribute to the disease process, i.e., produce immunopathology.

In comparison with other microorganisms, the immune responses elicited by parasites are unique in several ways. Because of their size and metabolic diversity, parasites are antigenically complex; fractionation frequently yields many distinct components. Multiplicity of antigens favors the likelihood that there will be common antigens among related forms. This likelihood makes specific diagnosis of parasitic infections by serologic tests more difficult because of cross reactions. Helminths often produce secretory and excretory products that are also antigenic. Antibodies that might neutralize a virus particle or coat a bacterium before phagocytosis are less effective in reacting with a microorganism as large as a host cell or with a worm that is centimeters in length. Parasites present an additional problem by their sojourn in the host for years. As might be expected, the immunologic consequences of persistence of foreign antigen(s) can involve the parasite as well as the host. For example, the surface of schistosomes becomes coated with blood group antigens of the host, which disguises their presence from immune surveillance of the host.

With all parasitic infections the development of humoral antibodies to components of the infecting parasite can be demonstrated by various tests: complement fixation, hemagglutination, agar-gel precipitation, and fluorescent antibody and enzyme-linked immunosorbent assay (ELISA). These antibodies, whose production is initiated by bone-marrow–derived lymphocytes called *B cells,* may be composed of different immunoglobulin classes, e.g., IgM, or IgG, or IgE. The elevation in either total IgM or IgE or an elevated level of parasite-specific IgM may be indicative of certain parasitic infections. The so-called skin-sensitizing antibodies, IgE or a subclass of IgG, which attach to basophils or tissue mast cells, release histamine and other mediators when exposed to specific antigens. This process contributes to the pathology of some parasitic infections and is also the basis for the immediately reacting skin test used in diagnosis. Another humoral component of the immune system whose activity has been demonstrated in parasitic infections is that of complement. Activation of the classical pathway with transient low complement levels has been demonstrated in malaria, for example, as has complement deposition in the kidney glomerulus in malarial nephropathy.

A variety of cell-mediated immune reactions, involving thymus-dependent or T lymphocytes are also a part of host reactions to parasitic infections. When T lymphocytes encounter an antigen to which they or their progenitors were previously exposed, they generate substances called lymphokines that, in turn, can set into motion a variety of immunologic events. Delayed hypersensitivity is one such cell-mediated reaction, of which the schistosome granuloma that develops around the parasite eggs in the tissues is an example.

In cutaneous leishmaniasis the delayed hypersensitivity reaction that develops after intracutaneous injection of leishmanial antigen is useful in diagnosis. One general test of T cell responsiveness in disease states consists of culturing lymphocytes and exposing them to specific antigens. The degree of response is assessed by the degree of proliferation or blast transformation as measured by incorporation of added radioactive thymidine. The effector substances or lymphokines produced by the T cell-antigen interaction can be shown to exhibit a wide variety of functions in vitro, including chemotaxis of granulocytes or macrophages, inhibition of macrophage migration, cytotoxic activity, and even suppression of T cell function. However, the clinical significance of many of these tests of cell-mediated immunity in terms of susceptibility to infection or outcome of disease is not always predictible.

Eosinophilia is one immunologic manifestation traditionally associated with parasitic infections. The eosinophil response often involves the tissues as well as circulating blood and is almost always related to infection with helminths rather than with protozoa. Moreover, the eosinophilia of parasitic infections is a response to tissue invasion by the parasite, not simply to their presence in the gut. Whether specific factors, such as the physicochemical nature of antigens or certain types of immune complexes, initiate eosinophilia or are simply associated with it is not known. However, it has been shown that the eosinophilic response is an immunologically mediated event requiring T cell participation. The attraction of eosinophils to local tissue sites can now be explained by the generation of eosinophil chemotactic factors by various antigen-antibody reactions, some involving the presence of complement. Finally, what purpose, if any, does the eosinophil serve? Although less active and potent than the polymorph, eosinophils do have phagocytic capacity. There is accumulating evidence that, under appropriate circumstances, eosinophils exert important cytotoxic activity on the surface of helminthic parasites.

The ultimate question is whether there is

functional immunity in parasitic infections. The answer is a qualified yes. Frequently, immunity is only partial, with reduction in intensity of infection or a milder disease the result of previous infection. The most striking evidence for immunity to parasitic infections is seen in nature, for example, immunity to malaria in adults in areas where malarial transmission is hyperendemic. In such situations the disease is seen in young children, with mild or asymptomatic infections in older children and immunity in adults. Some protozoan infections appear to exhibit a more impressive protective immunity than do helminthic infections. With parasites that undergo several stages of development in a host, there may be immunity directed to one stage of the parasite, i.e., stage-specific immunity. The immunity associated with persistence of a parasite in a host, or *premunition,* is of greater degree than residual immunity without persistence of the parasite. With parasites it may be very difficult to evaluate the relative contribution of humoral versus cell-mediated defense mechanisms to immunity, and often an interaction of both components is required. So far, immunization against parasitic diseases has not been particularly successful except in a few situations, such as cutaneous leishmaniasis and some animal helminthic infections, nor has it been of practical importance. In the chapters that follow, additional comment will be made about immune mechanisms involving the various groups and individual parasites.

Diagnosis. The clinical manifestations of parasitic diseases are so general that in most instances diagnosis based upon symptomatology alone is inadequate. Although the experienced clinician may recognize the characteristic signs and symptoms of certain parasitic diseases, the symptoms in atypical cases may be so confusing that no clear clinical picture is presented. Likewise, many infections, chiefly of helminthic origin, give few and indefinite symptoms and often are clinically indistinguishable. Final diagnosis and proper methods of treatment require the identification of the parasite in the laboratory.

Treatment. The successful treatment of the infected patient includes medical and surgical measures, adequate nutrition to build up general resistance, and specific chemotherapy. The physician should also be familiar with the patient's ability to cooperate intelligently, the sanitary environment, the epidemiology of the disease, and the best methods of controlling the spread of the infection. No efficient antiparasitic drug is entirely nontoxic to man. Successful chemotherapy depends upon the use of a drug that has a minimal toxic effect upon the tissues of the host and a lethal action upon the parasite. New chemotherapeutic agents, largely synthetic, are being constantly developed, and therapeutic methods are continually undergoing revision.

Prevention. The prevention of parasitic diseases depends upon the erection of barriers to the spread of parasites through the practical application of biologic and epidemiologic knowledge. Almost every parasite at some time in its life cycle is susceptible to special exterminative measures. Thus, barriers such as sanitary excreta disposal may be established by breaking such weak links in the life cycle as may exist at the departure of the parasite or its egg from its host, during its extracorporeal existence, or at the time of its invasion of the human host. The control of parasitic diseases includes the following procedures: (1) reduction of the sources of infection in human beings by therapeutic measures, (2) education in personal prophylaxis to prevent dissemination of infection and to reduce opportunities for exposure, (3) sanitary control of water, food, living and working conditions, and waste disposal, (4) destruction or control of reservoir hosts and vectors, and (5) erection of biologic barriers to the transmission of parasites.

The therapeutic reduction of human sources of infection is a practical measure, but usually it is not applicable to animal reservoir hosts. Education of the general public in personal prophylaxis and knowledge of the precautions necessary to escape infection and to prevent its transmission to others, including a safe water supply and thorough cooking of food, is an effective means of combating parasitic diseases. Public health education, however, is a slow process, particularly in countries with limited educational facilities. Sanitary measures of waste disposal include the establishment of sewage systems, the installation of screened sanitary latrines, and the prohibition of untreated night soil as garden fertilizer. Food handlers, who may be carriers, require careful supervision and training in personal hygiene. The reduction in number of intermediate hosts or vectors has made possible the control of many parasitic diseases. Insect vectors may be controlled by the destruction of their breeding grounds, the application of insecticides, and the protection of the susceptible host by screens and repellents. Snails, the intermediate hosts of trematodes, may be destroyed, if sufficiently segregated, by chemical and physical agents, but the destruction of such intermediate hosts as mammals and fishes is usually impractical.

TABLE 1-1. HELMINTH INFECTIONS

	Common Name of Parasite or Disease	Length of Parasite	Site in Host	Portal of Entry
NEMATHELMINTHES	ROUNDWORMS			
Necator americanus	New World or tropical hookworm Uncinariasis	To 1.1 cm	Small intestine, attached	Skin, usually feet
Ancylostoma duodenale	Old world hookworm Ancylostomiasis	To 1.3 cm		
A. braziliense	Creeping eruption, cutaneous larva migrans (hookworm larva)	To 0.3 mm (larva)	Intradermal	Skin
Ascaris lumbricoides	Large roundworm	To 35 cm	Small intestine	Mouth
Toxocara canis *T. cati*	Visceral larva migrans	0.3 mm (larva)	Liver, lung, brain, eye	Mouth
Enterobius vermicularis	Pinworm, seatworm, Oxyuris	To 1.3 cm	Large intestine, appendix	Mouth
Trichuris trichiura	Whipworm, threadworm	To 5.0 cm	Caecum, large intestine, ileum	Mouth
Trichinella spiralis	Trichinosis	To 0.4 cm	Adult: small intestine wall. Encysted larva: striated muscle	Mouth
Strongyloides stercoralis	Cochin China diarrhea (now called Vietnam diarrhea)	To 0.2 cm	In wall of small intestine	Skin

OF HUMAN BEINGS

Source of Infection, Intermediate Host or Vector	Most Common Clinical Signs or Symptoms	Laboratory Diagnosis	Therapeutic Agent	Remarks
Infective filariform larvae in soil	Anemia, growth retardation, G.I. symptoms	Eggs in stool	Pyrantel pamoate Mebendazole	Prophylaxis by excreta disposal Iron therapy important in blood regeneration
Dog and cat hookworm larvae in soil	Serpiginous skin lesions, itch	History and physical examination	Thiabendazole, or local by ointment or oral	Infection of beach bathers, plumbers "sandbox" babies
Eggs from soil or vegetables	Vague abdominal distress	Eggs in stool	Mebendazole Pyrantel pamoate Piperazine	Worms migrate into bile, pancreatic ducts and peritoneum Intestinal obstruction
Eggs from soil	Pneumonitis, eosinophilia	History and serology	Thiabendazole Diethylcarbamazine Steroids, if severe	Eosinophilia, anemia, hyperglobulinemia
Eggs in environment; autoinfection	Anal pruritus, irritability, "Mothers complex"	Eggs in perianal region Scotch tape swab	Pyrantel pamoate Mebendazole Piperazine Pyrvinium pamoate	Entire family frequently infected Personal hygiene important
Eggs from soil or vegetables	Abdominal discomfort, anemia, bloody stools	Eggs in stool	Mebendazole Hexylresorcinol enema	Frequently occurs with hookworm and Ascaris; adults seldom symptomatic
Encysted larvae in pork (rarely in bear)	Orbital edema, muscle pains, eosinophilia	Skin test, serology, muscle biopsy	Thiabendazole Steroids, if severe	Thorough cooking of pork and pork products kills encysted larvae
Larvae in soil, sometimes direct fecal contamination, autoinfection	Abdominal discomfort, diarrhea	Larvae in stool	Thiabendazole Pyrvinium pamoate	Autoinfection occurs, Exacerbated by steroids and immunosuppression

TABLE 1-1. continued

	Common Name of Parasite or Disease	Length of Parasite	Site in Host	Portal of Entry
NEMATHELMINTHES	ROUNDWORMS			
Wuchereria bancrofti	Filariasis	To 10 cm	Lymphatics	Skin
Brugia malayi	Filariasis	To 6 cm	Lymphatics	Skin
Dipetalanema perstans	Persistent filaria	To 8 cm	Body cavities	Skin
Mansonella ozzardi		To 8 cm	Body cavities	Skin
Loa loa	Eyeworm	To 7 cm	Subcutaneous	Skin
Onchocerca volvulus	River blindness	To 50 cm	Subcutaneous	Skin
Dracunculus medinensis	Fiery serpent Guinea worm	To 120 cm	Subcutaneous	Mouth
PLATYHELMINTHES	TAPEWORMS			
Taenia saginata	Beef tapeworm	To 12 meters	Small intestine	Mouth
Taenia solium	Pork tapeworm	To 7 meters	Small intestine	Mouth
T. solium (cysts)	Cysticercosis Verminous epilepsy	To 5.0 cm	Muscles, brain, eye	Mouth
Echinococcus granulosus	Hydatid cyst	To 15 cm	Liver, lungs, brain, bones	Mouth
Diphyllobothrium latum	Fish or broad tapeworm	To 10 meters	Small intestine	Mouth

Source of Infection, Intermediate Host or Vector	Most Common Clinical Signs or Symptoms	Laboratory Diagnosis	Therapeutic Agent	Remarks
Mosquitoes	Lymphangitis, fever	Blood smear, night	Diethylcarbamazine, surgery	Elephantiasis of leg, arms, scrotum, breasts
Mosquitoes	Lymphangitis, fever	Blood smear, night	Diethylcarbamazine, surgery	Elephantiasis
Culicoides (fly)	Asymptomatic	Blood smear	Diethylcarbamazine	
Culicoides (fly)	Asymptomatic(?)	Blood smear	Diethylcarbamazine	
Chrysops (fly)	Local inflammation, transient tumor	Blood smear, day	Diethylcarbamazine Surgery	Calabar swelling
Simulium (fly)	Subcutaneous nodules, loss of vision	Skin biopsy, nodule aspirate	Diethylcarbamazine Suramin	Nodules on head and body
Cyclops	Inflammation and ulcers of legs and feet	Lesions, x-ray of calcified worm	Thiabendazole Metronidazole	Boil or filter drinking water
Cysts in beef	Usually none	Segments and eggs in stool Scotch tape swab	Niclosamide° Quinacrine Paromomycin	Usually only 1 worm
Cysts in pork	Usually none	Segments and eggs in stool Scotch tape swab	Niclosamide° Quinacrine Paromomycin	Uncommon in U.S. Frequent in Latin America, India, and Africa
Eggs from feces, regurgitation of eggs	Intracranial pressure Epilepsy	Biopsy, x-ray of calcified cysts CAT scan Serology	Surgery	Uncommon in U.S. Autoinfection possible
Eggs from dog feces in soil	Pressure symptoms in various organs	Skin test, x-ray CAT scan Serology	Surgery	Uncommon in untraveled natives of U.S.
Plerocercoid in fresh-water fish	Usually none, Anemia rare in U.S.	Eggs in stool	Niclosamide Quinacrine Paromomycin	Prophylaxis by excreta disposal Cook fish well

TABLE 1-1. continued

	Common Name of Parasite or Disease	Length of Parasite	Site in Host	Portal of Entry
PLATYHELMINTH	TAPEWORMS			
Hymenolepis nana	Dwarf tapeworm	To 4 cm	Adults and cysts in small intestine	Mouth
Hymenolepis diminuta	Rat tapeworm	To 60 cm	Small intestine	Mouth
Dipylidium caninum	Dog tapeworm	15–70 cm	Small intestine	Mouth

Source of Infection, Intermediate Host or Vector	Most Common Clinical Signs or Symptoms	Laboratory Diagnosis	Therapeutic Agent	Remarks
Eggs from feces in soil Autoinfection	Abdominal discomfort	Eggs in stool	Niclosamide Paromomycin	Numerous worms, infection of children
Cysts from insects	Usually none	Eggs in stool	Niclosamide Paromomycin	Primarily a rat parasite
Flea and louse	Usually none	Eggs or egg sacks in stool	Niclosamide° Quinacrine	Usually in children

* Should not be used in pregnancy.
° See page 328.

TABLE 1-2. HELMINTH AND PROTOZOAN

	Common Name of Parasite or Disease	Length of Parasite	Site in Host	Portal of Entry
PLATYHELMINTHES	FLUKES			
Schistosoma mansoni	Schistosomiasis "Bilharzia"	To 1.4 cm	Veins of large intestine	Skin
Schistosoma haematobium	Schistosomiasis "Bilharzia"	2.0 cm	Veins of urinary bladder	Skin
Schistosoma japonicum	Schistosomiasis "Bilharzia"	2.6 cm	Veins of small intestine	Skin
Fasciolopsis buski	Intestinal fluke	2–7 cm	Small intestine	Mouth
Clonorchis sinensis	Human liver fluke	1–2.5 cm	Bile ducts	Mouth
Paragonimus westermani	Lung fluke	1.0 cm	Lungs	Mouth
PROTOZOA				
Plasmodium vivax	Benign tertian malaria	Intracellular	Liver parenchyma, red blood cells	Skin
Plasmodium falciparum	Malignant tertian malaria			
Plasmodium malariae	Quartan malaria			
Plasmodium ovale				
Leishmania donovani	Visceral leishmaniasis, kala-azar	Intracellular 2 μ	Monocytes, endothelial cells and macrophages	Skin
Leishmania tropica	Cutaneous leishmaniasis	Intracellular 2 μ	In macrophages of skin and mucosa	Skin
Leishmania braziliensis	Espundia, mucocutaneous leishmaniasis	Intracellular 2μ	In macrophages of skin and mucosa	Skin

INFECTIONS OF HUMAN BEINGS

Source of Infection, Intermediate Host or Vector	Most Common Clinical Symptoms	Laboratory Diagnosis	Therapeutic Agents	Remarks
Cercaria in fresh water, from snail	Chronic dysentery, fibrosis of liver	Eggs in stool, rectal or liver biopsy	Oxamniquine° Praziquantel° Niridazole°	Africa, South America; common in Puerto Ricans
Cercaria in fresh water, from snail	Urinary disturbances, hematuria	Eggs in urine, cystoscopy	Metrifonate° Praziquantel° Niridazole°	Africa, Middle East
Cercaria in fresh water, from snail	Dysentery, hepatic fibrosis	Eggs in stool, liver biopsy	Praziquantel°	China, Japan, Philippines, Indonesia
Water nuts and vegetables	Diarrhea, edema, abdominal pain	Eggs in stool	Praziquantel° Tetrachlorethylene	China and S.E. Asia
Fresh-water fish	Indigestion, diarrhea, hepatomegaly	Eggs in stool	Praziquantel°	Usually in Orientals
Fresh-water crustaceans (crabs)	Hemoptysis, cough, abdominal pain, fever	Eggs in sputum and stool	Bithionol° Praziquantel°	Wandering worms in brain and other organs
Anopheles mosquito Transfusions Drug addict syringe	Chill, fever, sweat, enlarged spleen	Repeated blood smears	Chloroquine Primaquine Sulfamethoxine Pyrimethamine Sulfadiazine Quinine Amodiaquine	Fever irregular in early disease; incubation long after drug suppression Drug-resistant stains
Phlebotomus (fly)	Fever, enlarged liver and spleen, leukopenia	Liver biopsy, sternal puncture, comp. fix. test, F.A.T.	Antimony sodium gluconate° Pentamidine°	Signs and symptoms resemble malaria
Phlebotomus	Chronic ulceration of exposed skin areas	Skin scrapings Biopsy and culture	Antimony sodium gluconate°	Immunity following infection
Phlebotomus	Ulceration of naso-oral region	Scrape lesions Biopsy and culture	Antimony sodium gluconate° Amphotericin B Cycloguanil pamoate	

TABLE 1-2. continued

	Common Name of Parasite or Disease	Length of Parasite	Site in Host	Portal of Entry
PROTOZOA				
Trypanosoma gambiense	African sleeping sickness	14–33 μ	Lymph glands, blood stream, brain	Skin
Trypanosoma rhodesiense				
Trypanosoma cruzi	South American trypanosomiasis	Intracellular stages Tryp. 20 μ	Tissues—heart Blood	Skin
Entamoeba histolytica	Intestinal amebiasis	15–60 μ	Lumen and wall of large intestine	Mouth
E. Histolytica	Amebic hepatitis Amebic liver abscess	Trophozoites only	Liver	Mouth
Dientamoeba fragilis		5–12 μ No cysts	Large intestine	Mouth
Balantidium coli		50–100 μ	Large intestine	Mouth
Giardia lamblia	Flagellate diarrhea	11–18 μ	Upper small intestine	Mouth
Trichomonas vaginalis		10–30 μ No cysts	Vagina, prostate	Genitalia
Toxoplasma gondii	Toxoplasmosis	4–6 μ	All organs	Mouth
Pneumocystis carinii	Interstitial plasma cell pneumonia	1.0–2.0 μ and 6–8 μ	Lungs	Respiratory
Naegleria and *Acanthameba spp.*	Meningoencephalitis	15–30 μ	Brain	Nose

Source of Infection, Intermediate Host or Vector	Most Common Clinical Symptoms	Laboratory Diagnosis	Therapeutic Agents	Remarks
Tsetse fly	Fever, rash, headache, confusion and lethargy	Blood smear, gland puncture, cerebrospinal fluid for trypanosomes	Pentamidine isethionate° Suramin° Melarsoprol° Tryparsamide°	Enlargement of posterior cervical lymph nodes, Winterbottom's sign
Kissing bug Triatomidae	Fever, spleen and liver enlarged Myocarditis	Blood smear, comp. fix., rat inoculation, F.A.T.	Bayer 2502°	Myocarditis, periorbital edema Megacolon Megaesophagus
Cysts in food and water, from feces	Mild to severe G.I. distress, dysentery	Cysts in cold stool, trophs in purged stool, serology	Diodoquin Paramomycin Dehydroemetine° Chloroquine Emetine Tetracyclines Metronidazole	Consider possibility of hepatic infection
Cysts in food and water, from feces	Enlarged tender liver, fever, leukocytosis	X-ray, serology, cysts or trophs in stool	Metronidazole Dehydroemetine° Chloroquine	Treat intestinal amebic infection
Stool (trophs)	Abdominal discomfort, diarrhea	Stool exam, trophs	Diodoquin Tetracyclines	Often asymptomatic
Stool (cyst)	Diarrhea, dysentery	Cysts and trophs in stool	Tetracyclines Diodoquin	Human and porcine sources
Cysts in food and water, from feces	Mild G.I. distress and diarrhea, weight loss	Cysts and trophs in stool	Quinacrine Metronidazole	More common in children than adults
Trophs in vaginal and prostatic secretion	Frothy vaginal discharge	Trophs in vaginal and prostatic fluid	Metronidazole	Treat both sexual partners
Congenital, Infected meat Oocysts in cat's stool	Chorioretinitis Hydrocephalus Convulsions Mimics infect. mono.	Biopsy, serology, mouse inoculation	Pyrimethamine with trisulfapyrimidines	Cerebral calcification Asymptomatic infections
Respiratory(?)	Pneumonia	Lung biopsy and special stains (?)	Pentamidine isethionate° Trimethoprim and sulfamethoxazole	Premature babies Immunosuppressed patients
Pond mud	C.N.S. symptoms		Amphotericin B	Highly toxic

° See page 328.   † Antimony sodium dimercaptosuccinate.

THE PROTOZOA

2

Parasitic Protozoa

BIOLOGY OF THE PROTOZOA

Protozoa are unicellular animals that occur singly or in colony formation. Each protozoon is a complete unit capable of performing the physiologic functions that in higher organisms are carried on by specialized cells. For the most part they are free-living, but some are parasitic, having adapted themselves to an altered existence inside the host.

Morphology. The vital functions of the protozoa are carried out by the protoplasm, a coarsely or finely granular substance, differentiated into nucleoplasm and cytoplasm. The cytoplasm often consists of a thin outer ectoplasm and a voluminous inner endoplasm, that the electron microscope has demonstrated to be very complex.

The ectoplasm functions in movement, ingestion of food, excretion, respiration, and protection. The organs of locomotion are prolongations of ectoplasm known as pseudopodia, cilia, flagella, or undulating membranes. Food may be taken in at any place in the cytoplasm or ingested at a particular point. In some species there is a definite area, the *peristome,* through which food passes directly into the *cytostome* and then through a tubelike *cytopharynx* to the endoplasm. The INFUSORIA, MASTIGOPHORA, and SPOROZOA have a cell membrane, whereas in the SARCODINA, except for the resistant cysts, there is only an ectoplastic covering.

The granular endoplasm is concerned with nutrition and, since it contains the nucleus, with reproduction. It may also contain food vacuoles, food reserves, foreign bodies, contractile vacuoles, and chromatoidal bodies. *Contractile vacuoles* function in the regulation of osmotic pressure and the elimination of waste material. In the MASTIGOPHORA there may be present a *kinetoplast* consisting of two parts, the *parabasal body* and the *blepharoplast,* from which the flagellum arises.

The nucleus is essential for maintaining and reproducing life. A nuclear membrane envelops a fine reticulum filled with nuclear sap and chromatin. In the vesicular nucleus the chromatin is concentrated in a single mass; in the granular type it is distributed diffusely.

Near the center of the nucleus is a deeply staining *karyosome,* which plays a part in promitosis. In many protozoa a *centrosome* is also present. The structure of the nucleus, particularly the arrangement of the chromatin and karyosome, helps to differentiate species. In the INFUSORIA a *macronucleus* and one or more *micronuclei* may be present. The former is believed to be concerned with the vegetative activities of the cell and the latter with the reproductive functions.

Physiology. All essential metabolic, reproductive, and protective functions are carried on either by specialized properties of the protoplasm or by structural and functional adaptations known as *organelles.*

Movement is employed to obtain food and to react to physical and chemical stimuli. It ranges from marked activity in the flagellates and ciliates to almost negligible action in the SPOROZOA, except during certain stages of their life cycles. Pseudopodia produce ameboid movements in the SARCODINA, cilia rhythmically propel the INFUSORIA, and flagella assisted by the undulating membrane permit the MASTIGOPHORA to move in all directions.

Protozoa respire either directly by taking in oxygen and expelling carbon dioxide or indirectly by using the oxygen liberated from complex substances by the action of enzymes. Because free oxygen is rarely available in the intestine and certain tissues of the host, most parasitic protozoa have an anaerobic metabolism.

Nutrition may be effected by the absorption of liquid food, the ingestion of solid particles, or by both methods. The solid material after ingestion through the ectoplasm or cytostome is surrounded by a food vacuole, where it is converted by digestive enzymes into forms suitable for assimilation. Inorganic salts, carbohydrates, fats, proteins, vitamins, and growth accessory substances are required. The undigested particles are extruded at the surface of the body or through a specialized opening, the *cytopyge.* Some species maintain a reserve food supply.

Excretion is effected through osmotic pressure, diffusion, and precipitation. The solid and liquid wastes are discharged from the general surface or at definite locations. In some species contractile vacuoles act as excretory organs.

Protozoa secrete digestive ferments, pigments, and material for the cyst wall. Pathogenic protozoa also secrete proteolytic enzymes, hemolysins, cytolysins, and various toxic and antigenic substances.

Certain protozoa at times enter an inactive cystic state, in which they secrete a resistant membranous wall and usually undergo nuclear division. In the parasitic intestinal species, encystment is usually necessary for survival outside the body and for protection against the digestive juices of the upper gastrointestinal tract. Thus, the cyst is closely associated with passage from host to host and constitutes the infectious stage of most of the parasitic amebas, ciliates, and intestinal flagellates that are transmitted through food or water. The trophozoites or vegetative forms are easily destroyed by an unfavorable environment, but the cysts show considerable resistance.

The survival of protozoa is largely due to their highly developed reproductive powers. Reproduction in the parasitic protozoa may be asexual or sexual. In the asexual or simple fission type, characteristics of the SARCODINA, INFUSORIA, and MASTIGOPHORA, the division of the nucleus may be amitotic, mitotic, or so modified that it is not characteristic of either type. Certain species may also reproduce in the encysted state, the nucleus dividing so that upon excystation each cyst may give rise to several new trophozoites. The sexual union of two cells, *syngamy,* may precede some form of division and may be temporary or permanent. Temporary union or conjugation is a rejuvenation process in some species and a reproductive process in others.

All the intestinal parasitic amebas and ciliates and most of the intestinal, luminal, and blood and tissue flagellates of humans have been cultivated on artificial noncellular mediums, usually enriched with blood, serum, and growth-accessory substances. Methods for cultivation of the parasitic SPOROZOA are more recently developed; cell culture conditions are required, and even then not all stages can be grown in vitro.

Transmission. The life cycle and transmission of the intestinal and luminal protozoa are relatively simple. The parasites pass from host to host directly or through food and water after an extracorporeal existence. In most instances the cyst, which is capable of resisting adverse environmental conditions and the digestive juices of the upper gastrointestinal tract, is the infective form. The spore containing the sporozoites is the infective form of the intestinal SPOROZOA. Its resistant covering provides greater protection than is required by the sporozoites that are passed directly from insect vectors to humans.

Most blood and tissue parasites pass an alternate existence in a vertebrate (human) and an invertebrate (arthropod) host, the latter acting as the transmitting agent or vector. Even when the life history involves two hosts, direct transmission without cyclic development may take place by contact or by biting and nonbiting insects. In indirect transmission the parasite undergoes cyclic development in a bloodsucking insect before it attains the infective stage. Temperature and humidity, by affecting the abundance of insect vectors and the developmental cycle of the parasite in the insect, are important factors in the transmission of insect-borne diseases.

Pathology and Symptomatology. Protozoa, in contrast to worms, multiply in their hosts, so disease can result from infection initiated by only a few organisms. Pathologic changes are due to invasion and destruction of cells or tissues by the parasite itself or its products. Tissue damage secondary to immune response, or immunopathology, may occur. Generalized systemic symptoms, e.g., fever, and signs like splenomegaly and lymphadenopathy are common. The early stage of infection may be subclinical, or it may be severe, leading to death or into a chronic latent stage, with relapses at times before eventual recovery.

Diagnosis. The diagnosis of some diseases, e.g., malaria or leishmaniasis, may be strongly suspected on clinical grounds from characteristic signs and symptoms. But clinical impressions should *always* be confirmed by laboratory diagnosis that identifies the parasite in intestinal contents (amebiasis) or in blood and tissues (malaria and leishmaniasis) by direct smears, concentration methods, cultures, animal inoculation, or appropriate serologic tests (toxoplasmosis).

Immunity. Immunity to each disease or group of diseases is discussed separately, but some general comments about immunity to protozoa can be made. First, there are some hosts, including human beings, that are simply refractory to infection by certain parasites. Most often such innate resistance involves parasites of heterologous species, such as specificity of coccidia for certain animals, but there are examples of natural resistance in humans to infection with parasites of humanity. Age may be a factor, with adults generally more resistant than infants or children, but differences in risk of exposure at various ages or some degree of acquired immunity are difficult to exclude in evaluating the role of age-related resistance. Natural resistance may be lowered by malnutrition, concurrent disease, or immunosuppressive drugs, but, paradoxically, some nutritional deficiencies confer protection against certain infections. Various races show different degrees of natural resistance; e.g., blacks are more resistant than whites to vivax malaria. In this instance the mechanism for natual resistance is due to the absence of a receptor, the Duffy blood-group factor, on the red cell surface that is required for parasite invasion. In most cases, however, specific causes of natural resistance are not known. Although the distinction is subtle, it may be useful to consider that what we perceive as resistance to infection is actually the absence of essential factors required in pathogenesis of infection and disease.

Protective immunity often develops to protozoan infections involving the blood and tissues, but is less effective or absent with protozoa of the intestinal tract or luminal surfaces. In the case of malaria, repeated infections are necessary before solid immunity develops among adults and older children in areas where exposure begins at an early age. The capacity of leishmanial infections to confer immunity to reinfection was the basis for the old practice in the Middle East of deliberate inoculation of children to nonfacial sites with material from lesions of active cases to protect against later disfiguring scars. With some of the intracellular protozoa, such as toxoplasma and *Trypanosoma cruzi,* an initial infection appears to confer solid immunity against subsequent reinfection. Since persistence of a few viable organisms in the tissues is a common feature of these and other intracellular protozoan parasites, the question of whether immunity is contingent upon persistent organisms, a state called *premunition,* cannot be answered. On the other hand, there is little or no evidence of lasting immunity after infection with the intestinal protozoa and with trichomonas, as repeated infections can occur.

Although many of the protozoan infections confer little in the way of protective immunity, all of them generally elicit an antibody response that can be detected by a variety of serologic tests. Such tests may be useful in diagnosis of certain protozoan infections (see Chapter 18 for details). There is evidence that in certain protozoan infections, the immunologic response of the host may have an adverse influence or even contribute to the disease process.

One such response is called *immunosuppression,* a state in which some elements of the immune system either fail to respond or respond in a less than optimum manner. Reduced antibody response to tetanus toxoid and to Salmonella antigens has been observed in chronic malaria infection and anergy to leishmanial skin-test antigens occurs in certain types of leishmaniasis. An example of another type of adverse immune response is malarial nephrosis, a form of immunopathology resulting from deposition of immune complexes in the kidney as a result of chronic malaria.

Prevention. The usual methods of reducing the sources of infection, blocking the channels of transmission, and protecting the susceptible host are employed. Each important disease presents problems that call for special methods. In general, the prevention of intestinal protozoan and helminth infections is largely a problem of sanitation and hygiene, and that of the blood and tissue protozoan infections the control of the insect vector.

REFERENCES

Kreier: Parasitic Protozoa, (4 volumes) New York, Academic Press, 1977.
Levine: Protozoan Parasites of Domestic Animals and Man. Minneapolis, Burgess, 1961.

3

Intestinal and Luminal Protozoa

AMEBAS

Members of this group of protozoa, which includes many free-living and parasitic amebas, are probably the most primitive of animal forms. Presumably, they are the close relatives of humanity's ancestors, many phyla removed, which lived in the mud millions of years ago. They are the conservative side of the protozoa family—not changing or participating in the evolution and ascent of humanity.

At least six species of amebas belonging to four genera have been definitely established as parasites of man: (1) *Entamoeba histolytica,* (2) *E. coli,* (3) *E. gingivalis,* (4) *Dientamoeba fragilis,* (5) *Endolimax nana,* and (6) *Iodamoeba bütschlii.* *All* live in the large intestine, except *E. gingivalis,* which is found in the mouth. Only one species, *E. histolytica,* is an important pathogenic parasite of humans. The differential characteristics of the six species parasitic in man are given in Table 3-1 and are represented graphically in Figure 3-1. Certain free-living protozoa (*Naegleria* and *Acanthameba*

spp.) are accidental parasites of human beings.

Commensal Amebas of Human Beings

The identification of *E. histolytica* requires differentiation from other parasitic species, of which only *Dientamoeba fragilis* is credited with possessing any pathogenicity. *E. polecki,* a rare incidental parasite of man, and the free-living *E. moshkovskii* and the reptilian *E. invadens,* which may be fecal contaminants, closely resemble *E. histolytica* morphologically.

D. fragilis is a small parasitic ameboflagellate of the intestinal tract that is found only as a trophozoite. It differs from the other intestinal amebas in that it generally has two nuclei, and by the fact that it resembles trichomonads antigenically and ultrastructurally. *D. fragilis* can be recognized only in fresh liquid or soft stools. Identification is based on its small size, two nuclei, circular appearance at rest, rapid action of the multiple leaf-shaped pseudopodia that give it a stellate appearance, and its explosive disintegration in water. Some of

23

TABLE 3-1
DIFFERENTIAL CHARACTERISTICS OF AMEBAS LIVING IN MAN

Characteristics	Entamoeba histolytica	Entamoeba coli	Entamoeba gingivalis	Endolimax nana	Iodamoeba bütschlii	Dientamoeba fragilis
TROPHOZOITE						
Size (microns)						
Average	20	25	15	8	11	9
Range	10–60	10–50	5–35	6–15	6–20	5–12
Inclusions						
RBC	Present	Absent	Present at times	Absent	Absent	Usually absent
Bacteria and other material	Absent in fresh specimens	Present, abundant	Present, abundant	Present	Present	Present
Vacuoles	Scanty	Numerous	Numerous	Numerous	Numerous	Numerous
Pseudopodia	Blade or finger-shaped, hyaline, formed rapidly	Blunt, usually granular, formed slowly	Usually blunt, hyaline, often formed rapidly	Blunt, hyaline, usually formed slowly	Blunt or fingerlike, hyaline, formed slowly	Leaflike, hyaline, formed rapidly, multiple
Motility	Active progression in definite direction	Sluggish, usually not progressive	Moderately active, progressive	Sluggish, moderately progressive	Sluggish, slightly progressive	Active, progressive
CYST						
Size (microns)						
Average	Variable	17	No cysts demonstrated	9	10	No cysts demonstrated
Range	5–20	10–33		5–14	5–18	
Glycogen in young cysts (iodine treated)	Diffuse, mahogany brown	Large mass, ill-defined, dark brown		Usually absent, diffuse, ill-defined, brownish	Usually present, large mass, compact, dark brown	
Chromatoid bodies	Often present, large bars or thick rodlike masses	Sometimes present, splinterlike with square or pointed ends		Occasionally small spherical or elongated granules	Usually absent, small granules	
Nuclei (no.)	1–4, rarely more	1–8, rarely more		1–4, rarely more	1, rarely 2	

24

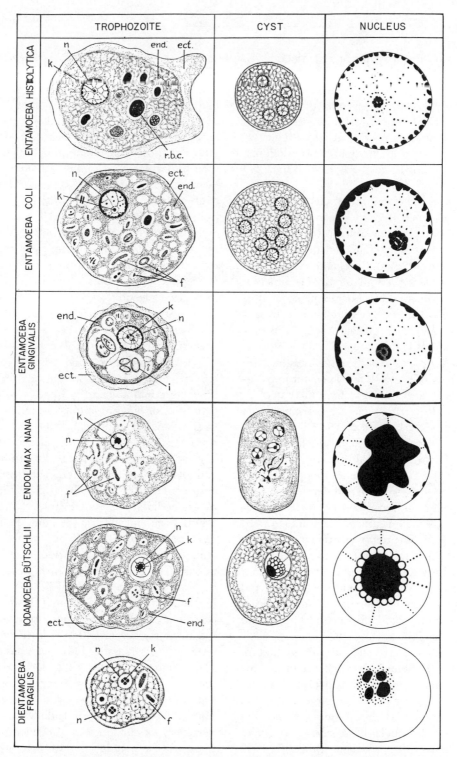

Figure 3-1. Comparative morphology of the amebas of man and schematic representation of their nuclei. Trophozoites and cysts of *Entamoeba histolytica, E. coli,* and *E. gingivalis* and of *Endolimax nana, Iodamoeba bütschlii,* and *Dientamoeba fragilis.*

ect., ectoplasm; end., endoplasm; f, food vacuoles; i, inclusion nuclei; k, karyosome; n, nucleus; r.b.c., red blood cells.

these organisms may ingest red blood cells. The incidence of *D. fragilis* is variable, averaging about 4 percent. In some individuals it produces a moderate, persistent diarrhea and gastrointestinal symptoms, but in most persons there is no apparent harmful effect. Therapy consists of diiodohydroxyquin (Diodoquin), 650 mg t.i.d. for 10 days, or tetracycline, 250 mg q.i.d. for 7 days.

Endolimax nana, an intestinal commensal, has a prevalence of 10 to 20 percent throughout the world. It is identified by its small size, sluggish movements, characteristic nuclei, and quadrinucleated cyst of irregular shape.

Iodamoeba bütschlii is an intestinal commensal with a prevalence of about 8 percent. It is identified by the characteristic nucleus, irregular shape, and large glycogen body of its uninucleated cyst.

E. coli is a parasite of the large intestine with a frequency of up to 10 to 30 percent in populations. Its life cycle is similar to that of *E. histolytica.* It is of medical importance only because it may be mistaken for *E. histolytica.* Certain differential characteristics from *E. histolytica* (Table 3-1) should be emphasized. *E. coli* has (1) a more granular endoplasm containing ingested bacteria and debris (it rarely, if ever, contains red blood cells), (2) a narrower, less differentiated ectoplasm, (3) broader and blunter pseudopodia, (4) more sluggish indeterminate movements, (5) heavier, irregular peripheral chromatin and a large eccentric karyosome in the nucleus, and (6) larger cysts with more granular cytoplasm, slender, splinterlike chromatoidal bodies, and as many as eight nuclei.

E. gingivalis is a nonpathogenic inhabitant of the mouth, being present chiefly in the tartar of the teeth and gingival pockets. Its most striking characteristic is the large number of food vacuoles and dark-staining bodies derived from the nuclei of degenerated cells in the cytoplasm. Its prevalence ranges from 10 percent in persons with healthy mouths to 95 percent in those with diseased teeth and gums.

Entamoeba histolytica

Diseases. Amebiasis, amebic dysentery, amebic hepatitis.

In 1875 Lösch discovered *E. histolytica* in the feces of a Russian with severe dysentery; he also experimentally produced intestinal lesions in a dog. However, the association of the parasite with dysentery was not definitely established until the investigations of Kartulis in 1887. In 1901 Councilman and Lafleur made their important study of the pathology of amebic dysentery and hepatic abscess. Schaudinn, of spirochete fame, differentiated *E. histolytica* from *E. coli* in 1903. In 1913 Walker and Sellards definitely established the pathogenicity of *E. histolytica* by feeding cysts to volunteers, thus furnishing the basis of our present concept of its host–parasite relation in respect to clinical infection.

Morphology and Physiology. E. histolytica may be observed in the feces as (A) trophozoite, (B) precyst, and (C) cyst (Table 3-1, Fig. 3-2).

The trophozoite or active vegetative *E. histolytica* (Fig. 3-2) is distinguished from the other intestinal amebas by morphologic characteristics of diagnostic importance. It ranges in size from 10 to 60 μ, but the majority are from 15 to 30 μ. The wide, clear, refractile, hyaline ectoplasm, sharply separated from the endoplasm, constitutes about one-third of the entire animal. The thin, fingerlike ectoplasmic pseudopodia are extended rapidly. The finely granular endoplasm usually contains no bacteria or foreign particles but sometimes includes red blood cells in various stages of disintegration. The single eccentric nucleus may be faintly discerned as a finely granular ring in the unstained ameba. Hematoxylin staining reveals a clearly defined nuclear membrane, the inner surface of which is lined with uniform and closely packed fine granules of chromatin (Fig. 3-2). The small, deeply staining, centrally located karyosome consists of several granules in a halo-like capsule, from which a linin network of fine fibrils radiates toward the periphery of the nucleus. Degenerating trophozoites show sluggish motility, a fading line of demarcation between ectoplasm and endoplasm, a more granular cytoplasm, and a more distinct nucleus.

The precystic amebas (Fig. 3-2) are colorless, round or oval cells that are smaller than the trophozoite but larger than the cyst. They

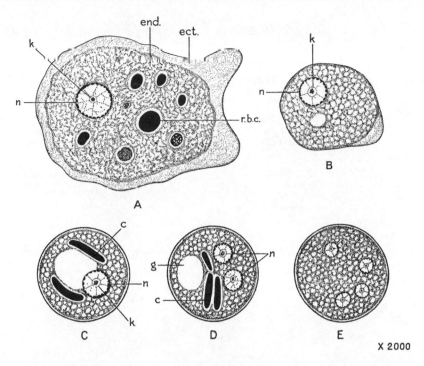

Figure 3-2. Schematic representation of *Entamoeba histolytica*. A. Trophozoite containing red blood cells undergoing digestion. B. Precystic ameba devoid of cytoplasmic inclusions. C. Young uninucleate cyst. D. Binucleate cyst. E. Mature quadrinucleate cyst.

   c, chromatoid bodies; ect., ectoplasm; end., endoplasm; g, glycogen vacuole; k, karyosome; n, nucleus; r.b.c., red blood cells.

are devoid of food inclusions. Pseudopodial action is sluggish, and there is no progressive movement.

The cysts (Fig. 3-2; see also Fig. 17-6) are round or oval, slightly asymmetrical hyaline bodies, 10 to 20 μ in diameter, with a smooth, refractile, nonstaining wall about 0.5 μ thick. The cytoplasm of the young cysts contains vacuoles with glycogen and dark-staining, refractive, sausage-shaped bars with rounded ends. These chromatoid bodies, which are reported to contain ribonucleic and deoxyribonucleic acid and phosphates, tend to disappear as the cyst matures, so that they may be absent in about half of the cysts. Both types of cytoplasmic inclusions are believed to represent stored food. The immature cyst has a single nucleus, about one-third of its diameter, while the mature infective cyst contains four smaller nuclei, rarely more. Thus, cysts containing from one to four nuclei may be passed in the feces. *E. hartmanni,* morphologically

identical with *E. histolytica* and previously called the small race ameba (cysts 5 to 8 μ and trophozoites 6 to 10 μ), are nonpathogenic.

The habitat of *E. histolytica* trophozoites is the wall and lumen of the colon, especially in the cecal and sigmoidorectal regions. They multiply by binary fission, the nucleus dividing by a modified mitosis. Reproduction also takes place via cyst formation, since eight amebulae are produced by the metacystic amebas after excystation (Fig. 3-3). Encystment is essential for transmission, since only the mature cyst is infectious. *E. histolytica* has traditionally been considered an anaerobe because it grows best under reduced oxygen tension. Yet, the parasite readily consumes oxygen when it is provided even though it has no mitochondria, cytochromes, or functional tricarboxylic acid cycle. Iron-sulfur proteins are important electron carriers in the respiratory chain. Of the carbohydrates only D-glucose and D-galactose are oxidized, various alcohols

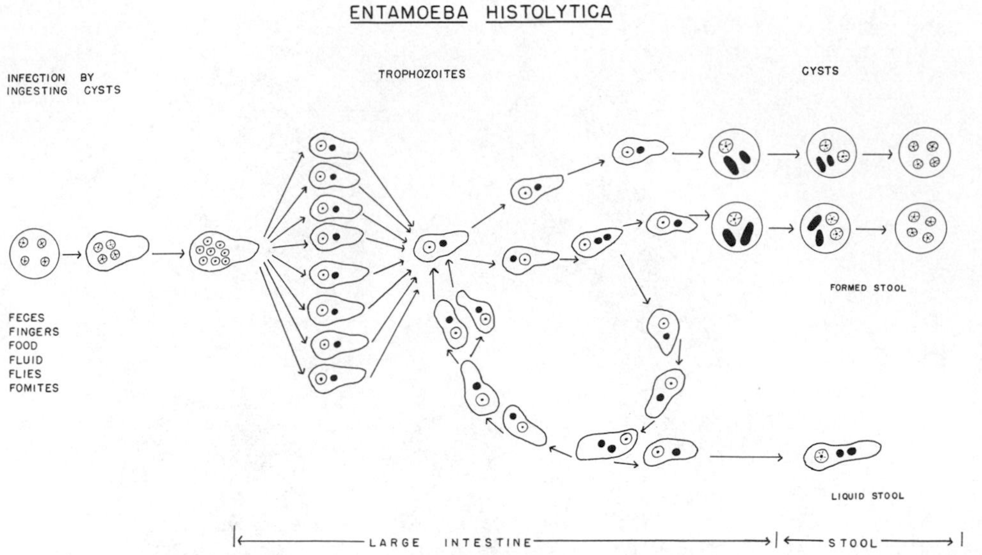

ENTAMOEBA HISTOLYTICA

Figure 3-3. Life cycle of *Entamoeba histolytica.*

can serve as substrates but L-serine is the only amino acid that elicits oxygen consumption. Several types of membrane-bound phosphatases are present. Waste products in soluble or granular form are eliminated in excretory vacuoles at the surface, while undigested particles are egested through cytoplasmic protuberances.

The ameba absorbs nourishment from the tissues dissolved by its cytolytic enzymes and ingests red blood cells and fragments of tissues through pseudopodial encirclement. It can ingest bacterial and other particulate elements from the intestinal contents. In vitro culture of *E. histolytica* originally required one or more associated bacteria as well as other nutrients, but methods and media have been developed for growing the amebae without bacteria or other living organisms, i.e., axenically. This usual dependence upon bacterial flora for growth helps explain the mechanism of various broad-spectrum antibiotics for the treatment of amebiasis by their effect upon the gut flora. The axenic culture technique for *E. histolytica* requires a period of adaptation and is still somewhat capricious, but it has made it possible to grow the organism in a semidefined medium for metabolic and biochemical stud-

ies, to test the effects of drugs and to produce antigens for immunologic and diagnostic tests. As a rule, optimum growth occurs at 35 to 37 C, at pH 7.0, and under reduced O_2 tension. Culture of amebas directly from fecal specimens for diagnostic purposes is possible, but the patients' or some other bacterial flora must be added to the culture. Such procedures are generally not available in most diagnostic laboratories.

Trophozoites are more easily destroyed than are cysts; they survive up to 5 hours at 37 C and 96 hours at 5 C. In contrast, the resistant cysts can survive for 2 days at 37 C and up to 60 days at 0 C. They can withstand freezing temperatures, but survival decreases rapidly at very low and elevated temperatures, e.g., 7 hours at −28 C and only 5 minutes at 50 C.

Strains. Except for *E. hartmanni,* which was once considered a small race ameba and is now recognized as a distinct species, different strains of *E. histolytica* cannot be differentiated on the basis of morphology. Some strains of *E. histolytica,* however, such as Laredo, are nonpathogenic for humans. They can be differentiated from pathogenic strains by certain physiologic differences, such as the ability to grow at reduced temperature, and by biochemical differences, such as genome size, DNA base ratio content, and DNA homology. Another marker that has been claimed for pathogenic strains of amebae is the presence of a variant isoenzyme: phosphoglucomutase. Although strains of *E. histolytica* probably vary considerably in their capacity to produce human disease, there are no simple in vivo methods to test virulence. The direct intracecal inoculation of rats is one method that has been used. The production of abscesses after inoculation into the liver of newborn hamsters appears to be a very sensitive indicator of virulence, but this technique requires axenically grown amebas. The virulence of amebal strains may be related to surface properties of the organism as evidenced by agglutinability with the lectin, con A, and the lack of electrophoretic surface charge. Amebae have also been found to harbor viruses, in the manner of bacteriophages, but these amebal viruses have not been linked to virulence and their role in the biology of amebas is not clear. There are many unknown factors that determine pathogenicity of *E. histolytica,* such as the intestinal flora and diet, as well as virulence of strains. In their classic studies in 1913 Walker and Sellards administered massive numbers of *E. histolytica* cysts to human volunteers. While all subjects became infected, only some developed acute dysentery. As few as 10 cysts have been shown to produce infection.

Life Cycle. The life history of *E. histolytica* is comparatively simple. The resistant infective cysts, formed in the lumen of the large intestine, pass out in the feces, and are immediately infective (Fig. 3-3). Few if any cysts are voided in acute dysentery, but they predominate in chronic infections and carriers. Human beings are the principal host and source of infection; other mammals are a negligible source. Spontaneous natural infections with amebas indistinguishable from *E. histolytica* have been reported in monkeys, dogs, hogs, and rats, and experimental infections have been established in kittens, puppies, monkeys, and laboratory rodents. On ingestion only the mature cysts, which are resistant to the acidic digestive juices of the stomach, pass to the lower part of the small intestine. Here, under the influence of the neutral or alkaline digestive juices and the activity of the ameba, the cyst wall disintegrates, liberating a four-nucleated metacystic ameba that ultimately divides into eight small trophozoites. These small immature amebas move downward to the large intestine. Intestinal stasis often enables the amebas to establish a site of infection in the cecal region of the colon, but they may be swept along to the sigmoidorectal region or even out of the body. The chances of establishing a foothold in the intestinal epithelium are reduced when the organisms are few, the volume of food large, or there is intestinal hypermotility. Thus, the massive and frequent doses acquired in endemic areas are of epidemiologic importance.

Epidemiology. The actual incidence of amebiasis throughout the world, especially in the temperate zone, remains unknown. Surveys indicate that the incidence of infection throughout the world varies from 0.2 to 50 percent and is directly correlated with sanitary conditions, which are especially poor in tropical and subtropical areas. However, it is present in cold Alaska, Canada, and the Soviet Union. It may have been the cause of Tolstoi's lifelong dysentery. It can be endemic in civilian and military groups and is particularly prevalent in mental hospitals, children's homes, and prisons. The lower economic classes show a high incidence, probably because of malnutrition, overcrowding, and insanitary environment. The infection rate in the United States is estimated to be 3 percent, most of which is asymptomatic or mildly symptomatic.

The main source of infection is the cyst-passing chronic patient or asymptomatic carrier. Acutely ill patients are not important, since they pass the noninfective trophozoite, and reservoir hosts play a negligible role. Cysts reach humans through water and vegetables contaminated with infective feces, through food contaminated by flies or the hands of infected food handlers, or by direct transmission by cyst carriers. Examination for fingerprints on pats of butter served at home or in public finds evidence of the amount of contact human hands have with our food. Likewise, artistically arranged fruit salads can only result from human hand contact. Circumstantial evidence overwhelmingly incriminates water as a vehicle of transmission. In 1933 two Chicago, Illinois, hotels experienced inadvertent connections between their water supply and sewage, which resulted in 1400 clinical infections and more than 100 deaths from amebiasis. Wells and springs, which in small rural communities are often exposed to contamination with local sewage, may serve to spread the infection. Contaminated food is the most satisfactory explanation for the widespread distribution of amebic infection. Vegetables and fruits may be contaminated by night soil or polluted water, and other foods and utensils by flies and food handlers. Viable cysts have been recovered from the vomitus, feces, and bodies of flies. Small epidemics in the tropics have been attributed to flies or other insects, particularly in military or civilian camps. The connection between food handlers and infected food is difficult to prove. Infection may be transmitted by direct contact where there is close association in home and institutional groups under insanitary and unhygienic conditions. Intrafamilial transmission in the average home environment in the United States is minimal. However, an infected mother who prepares her family's food is a potential source of infection. There appears to be a correlation between the presence of *E. histolytica, E. nana, G. lamblia,* and viral infectious hepatitis in missionaries abroad. The embedded mucosal sites of *Trichuris* may serve as portals of entry for *E. histolytica.* The carrier is a potential danger, and the detection and treatment of this person are of epidemiologic importance. Surveys to detect the numerous carriers are economically impracticable, but known convalescent patients and carriers should be treated.

Pathology. The lesions produced by *E. histolytica* are primarily intestinal and secondarily extraintestinal. The intestinal lesions, except for a few in the terminal portion of the ileum, are confined to the large intestine. The most frequent primary sites are the cecal and sig-

moidorectal regions, where the colonic flow is slow. Less frequently, the site is the ascending colon, rectum, sigmoid, or appendix. As the infection progresses, additional colonic sites of invasion develop. Extraintestinal invasion may occur in patients with clinical dysentery or in those with mild or latent infections. As would be expected, the liver is most frequently involved, but nearly every organ of the body may be affected.

The pathogenic activities of *E. histolytica* depend upon (1) the resistance of the host, (2) the virulence and invasiveness of the amebic strain, and (3) the conditions in the intestinal tract. Resistance depends on innate immunity, the state of nutrition, and freedom from infectious and debilitating diseases. There is considerable evidence that virulence varies with the strain. In culture it declines, but it may be restored or enhanced by serial passage in animals. Virulence, invasiveness, the number of the amebas, and local conditions in the intestinal tract—where invasion is facilitated by a carbohydrate diet, physical or chemical injury of the mucosa, stasis, and particularly the bacterial flora—are important in determining the extent of the intestinal ulceration. The importance of concomitant bacteria in producing pathogenic infections has been demonstrated repeatedly in both animals and humans. Germ-free guinea pigs fail to develop lesions, while a high percentage of control animals show ulcerations. The associated bacteria may stimulate the invasive powers of the ameba or produce favorable conditions for invasion.

The early lesion is a tiny area of necrosis in the superficial mucosa or a small nodular elevation with a minute opening that leads to a flask-shaped cavity containing cytolyzed cells, mucus, and amebas. In the infected individuals who develop acute or chronic dysentery, there is rapid lateral and downward extension of the ulcerative processes to both the superficial and deep layers of the intestine. The lesions vary from small, punctate, crateriform ulcers, distributed over the mucosa like craters in a bombed field, to large, irregular ulcers with undermined edges and necrotic gelatinous bases, often covered with a yellow, puru-

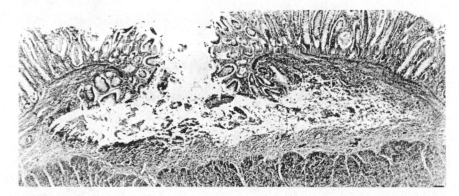

Figure 3-4. *Entamoeba histolytica* in the large intestine, characteristic flask-shaped ulcer.

lent, leathery membrane, and even to large areas of necrosis, which at times encircle the bowel. The typical flasklike primary ulcer has a crateriform appearance, with a wide base and narrow opening with irregular, slightly elevated, overhanging edges (Fig. 3-4). As the process invades the submucosa and extends laterally along the axis of the intestine, the dissolution of the tissues may become so extensive that communicating sinuses produce honeycombed areas beneath apparently intact mucosa that may eventually slough off, exposing large necrotic areas. Destruction of tissue is followed by regenerative proliferation of connective tissue, which, in cases of extensive damage, may ultimately cause a fibrous thickening of the intestinal wall.

The histologic changes include histolysis, thrombosis of the capillaries, petechial hemorrhages, round-cell infiltration, and necrosis. The process is regenerative rather than inflammatory. Signs of inflammation other than hyperemia and edema are usually absent unless secondary bacterial infection supervenes. Red blood cells are abundant because of the destruction of small blood vessels. The amebas may be found in the floor of the ulcer, particularly at the base of the intestinal glands, or scattered through the tissues (Fig. 3-5). Extensive ulceration is invariably accompanied by secondary bacterial infection, which tends to confuse the histologic picture as well as to intensify the destructive process.

The complications of intestinal amebiasis include appendictis, intestinal perforation, hemorrhage, stricture, granulomas, and pseudopolyposes. In amebic appendicitis, the appendix is nongangrenous, slightly thickened,

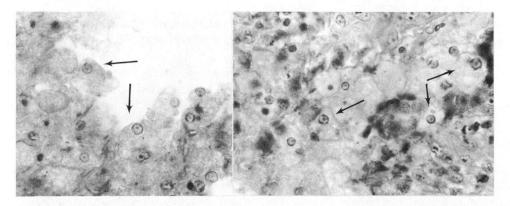

Figure 3-5. *Entamoeba histolytica* in intestinal mucosa. Arrows indicate trophozoites with characteristic nuclei.

and has irregular superficial ulcers in the mucosa. Amebic appendicitis contraindicates surgical interference without antiamebic treatment. Intestinal perforations occur most frequently in the cecum, and the erosion of a large blood vessel may produce a massive hemorrhage. Strictures are usually confined to the cecum or sigmoid and occasionally the rectum, but complete stenosis is rare. Amebic granulomas (ameboma) are firm, painful, movable, nodular, inflammatory thickenings of the intestinal wall around an ulcer, occurring most commonly in the cecum or sigmoid in a small percentage of infections. Histologically they show collagen, fibroblasts, and chronic inflammatory and granulation elements. They may be confused with neoplastic growths or tuberculous or actinomycotic granulomas, but they may be diagnosed by biopsy, serologically, or by response to antiamebic treatment.

In systemic amebiasis the liver is invaded chiefly and other organs less frequently (Fig. 3-6A). Dissemination from the primary intestinal focus is chiefly by the blood stream but at times occurs by direct extension. There are authentic records of amebiasis of lung, pericardium, brain, spleen, genitalia, and skin, and more questionable reports of involvement of kidneys, urinary bladder, testes, and other tissues. The syndrome known as "diffuse amebic hepatitis," characterized by a large tender liver and once considered a phase preliminary to abscess formation, is now regarded by several investigators as not indicative solely of amebic invasion but also as representing a nonspecific reaction of the liver to the bacteria, debris, and toxic material resulting from intestinal ulceration.

The early liver abscess is a small, oval or rounded mass with a grayish brown matrix of necrosed hepatic cells. At it increases in size the center liquefies, the wall thickens, and the contents become a viscid chocolate, reddish, or cream-colored mass of autolyzed hepatic cells, red blood cells, bile, fat, and other products of tissue disintegration, interspersed with strands of connective tissue. Rarely, if ever, does calcification occur. Hepatic abscesses may be single or multiple. The condition may arise from subclinical, as well as from symptomatic, intestinal amebiasis. Amebas have been demonstrated in the stool of approximately one-third of the patients with hepatic amebiasis. Careful search would probably disclose more. Approximately 85 percent of the abscesses are confined to the right lobe of the liver, with a predilection for the posterior portion of the dome, thus causing an upward bulging of the diaphragm. Males are chiefly affected. At times there is secondary bacterial invasion. Multiple hepatic amebic abscesses are not uncommon, even in children, and left lobe involvement facilitates pericardial invasion.

Pulmonary amebiasis, although infrequent, ranks next to liver abscess in rate of occurrence. It usually results from direct extension of a hepatic abscess and less frequently from emboli. The pulmonary abscess, often secondarily infected with bacteria, appears as a pneumonic consolidation in the lower right lung. Abscess of the brain is a rare complication usually associated with hepatic and pulmonary amebiasis; splenic abscess is even more rare. Ulcerative vaginitis, cervicitis, and involvement of the penis can occur. Amebic lesions of the penis are also seen in homosexuals.

Secondary cutaneous lesions in the form of indolent indurated ulcers with overhanging edges occur in the perianal region or at the sites of intestinal or hepatic fistulas. Chronic ulcers of the rectum may cause fissures, fistulas, and anorectal abscesses.

Symptomatology. The clinical response is exceedingly variable, depending upon the location and intensity of the infection. Outright dysenteric disease develops in but a small proportion of infected individuals in the United States. Secondary bacterial invasion may account for a considerable proportion of the symptoms, which may be vague and unlocalized despite extensive lesions. Subclinical chronic infections may persist for years with or without occasional exacerbations, at times leaving in their wake an irritable colon or postdysenteric colitis (Fig. 3-7).

Asymptomatic infections are most common,

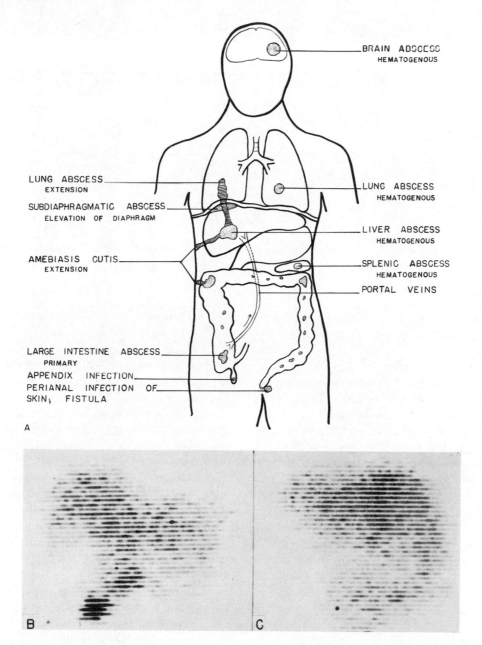

BRAIN ABSCESS
HEMATOGENOUS

LUNG ABSCESS
EXTENSION

LUNG ABSCESS
HEMATOGENOUS

SUBDIAPHRAGMATIC ABSCESS
ELEVATION OF DIAPHRAGM

LIVER ABSCESS
HEMATOGENOUS

AMEBIASIS CUTIS
EXTENSION

SPLENIC ABSCESS
HEMATOGENOUS

PORTAL VEINS

LARGE INTESTINE ABSCESS
PRIMARY

APPENDIX INFECTION

PERIANAL INFECTION OF
SKIN; FISTULA

A

B

C

Figure 3-6. Amebiasis. A. Sites of lesions. B and C. Liver abscess and photoscan of liver using Rose Bengal [131]I. B. Anterior scan, area of diminished uptake of radioactive material. C. Lateral scan shows abscess lies posteriorly. (From Schuman, Block, Eyler, DuSault: JAMA 187:709, 1964.)

especially in the temperate zone. These so-called healthy carriers may be passing millions of cysts per day, from trophozoite multiplication in the intestinal lumen. The vague abdominal discomfort, weakness, and neurasthenia reported by some patients may be related to the infection. The next stage of the infection is characterized by a syndrome that lacks specificity. These patients have moderate, though definite, malaise. Constipation

AMEBIASIS

ENTAMOEBA HISTOLYTICA

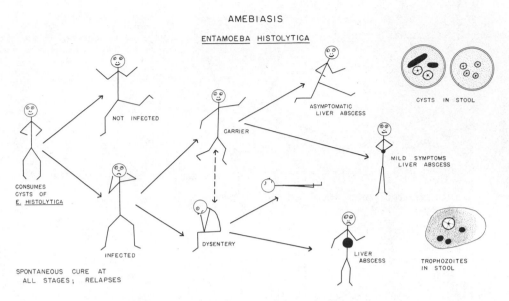

Figure 3-7. Amebiasis, courses of infection.

may alternate with mild diarrhea. Irregular colicky abdominal pain with or without local abdominal tenderness is present, indicating mucosal invasion by the parasite.

Acute intestinal amebiasis has an incubation period of from 1 to 14 weeks. There is severe dysentery with numerous small stools containing blood, mucus, and shreds of necrotic mucosa, accompanied by acute abdominal pain and tenderness, and fever of 100 to 102 F (38 to 39 C). Dehydration, toxemia, and prostration may be marked. A leukocytosis of 7000 to 20,000/mm³ without eosinophilia is not uncommon and may be a partial reflection of superimposed bacterial infection. Trophozoites of *E. histolytica* are found in the stools.

Chronic amebiasis is characterized by recurrent attacks of dysentery with intervening periods of mild or moderate gastrointestinal disturbances and constipation. Localized abdominal tenderness is present, and the liver may be enlarged. In long-standing infections, psychoneurotic disturbances may be present. This chronic debilitating disease leads to marked weight loss and cachexia. Ulcerative colitis, carcinoma of the large intestine, and diverticulitis must be considered in the differential diagnosis.

Hepatic amebiasis, which includes amebic hepatitis and abscess of the liver, is the most common and a grave complication of intestinal amebiasis. Hepatic amebiasis is due to metastasis of the infection from the intestinal mucosa by way of the portal blood stream. Amebic hepatitis is characterized by an enlarged, tender liver, with pain in the upper right hypochondrium that may radiate to the right shoulder. The signs and symptoms of amebic abscess of the liver are very similar to, though usually more severe than, those of amebic hepatitis. Leukocytosis of 10,000 to 16,000/mm³ with increased polymorphonuclear neutrophils helps distinguish it from viral hepatitis. The erythrocyte sedimentation rate may be elevated. Fever is common and chills may occur. Liver function tests are usually normal or only mildly abnormal; alkaline phosphatase is likely to be elevated. Mild jaundice is present in an occasional patient. Elevation and relative immobility of the right diaphragm and severe pain referred to the right shoulder are often present. The abscess may extend through the diaphragm into the lungs or rupture through the abdominal wall.

Hepatic amebiasis occasionally is present for a considerable time without the classic signs and symptoms and may be very difficult to diagnose, especially when it is not included in the differential diagnosis or if present in the left lobe of the liver.

Pulmonary amebiasis is characterized by chills, fever, leukocytosis, and evidence of pulmonary consolidation.

Amebic infections of the brain give the usual signs and symptoms of brain abscess or tumor. Unfortunately, these infections have only been diagnosed at autopsy.

Modern therapeutics yields a high percentage of cures, but irrespective of the type of treatment, relapses occur. Persons subject to continuous exposure in an endemic environment are frequently reinfected.

Diagnosis. The final diagnosis of amebiasis rests upon the identification of the parasite in the feces or tissues, and serologic studies. All available methods should be exhausted before accepting a clinical diagnosis. On the other hand, diagnosis by therapy must be resorted to occasionally.

The clinical diagnosis of intestinal amebiasis requires differentiation from other dysenteries and intestinal diseases, and that of hepatic abscess from viral and bacterial hepatitis, hydatid cyst, gallbladder infection, malignancy, and pulmonary disease. Clinical diagnosis is based on a history of residence in an endemic area, typical gastrointestinal and general signs and symptoms on physical examination, sigmoidoscopy, and roentgenology. With the sigmoidoscope it is possible to recognize the classic ulcerative or congestive granular petechial lesions. However, the picture is not always pathognomonic, and sigmoidoscopic diagnosis should always be supplemented by the microscopic examination of aspirated or biopsied specimens. Roentgenology is useful in detecting the shagginess of localized areas in colitis, cecal deformities, inflammatory amebomas, and strictures in intestinal amebiasis, and in defining abnormalities above and below the right diaphragm in hepatic and pulmonary abscesses (Fig. 3-6B and 3-6C). Bacillary dysentery may be distinguished by its acute onset, short incubation, fever, leukocytosis, epidemic character, lack of response to antiamebic drugs, and type of stool.

Laboratory diagnosis (see Chap. 18, for details) may be made by the microscopic identification of the parasite in the feces or tissues. Its microscopic detection depends upon the proper collection of material and the diligent examination of carefully prepared smears or sections. Diagnosis is not always easy and requires repeated examinations, especially in chronic cases. Failure may result from faulty technique, inadequate search, or confusion of *E. histolytica* with other protozoa, cells, artifacts, or macrophages.

The following schedule outlines the usual diagnostic procedures in the order in which they should be undertaken. In intestinal amebiasis no one method is superior, and the best results are obtained by their combination (Chap. 18).

Intestinal amebiasis
  Examination of feces by direct smears
    Diarrheic or fluid feces for trophozoites
      Material examined from fresh, warm feces in saline mount
      Feces obtained after magnesium sulfate or phosphosoda purge given in the morning on an empty stomach. Both formed and liquid specimens examined. (Do not purge pregnant women or patients with right lower-quadrant pain.)
      Permanent mounts with trichrome, Lawless, or iron hematoxylin stains
    Solid or formed feces for cysts (carriers or chronic patients)
      Examined in saline or iodine mounts, especially shreds of mucus or flecks of blood on formed feces
    Concentration methods (see p. 317)
  If local laboratory facilities are not available, feces may be preserved in P.V.A. or M.I.F. fixative and sent to the nearest laboratory (see p. 317)
  Sigmoidoscope examination (one-half of the patients have lesions in the sigmoido-rectal region)
    Visual for lesions
    Material aspirated with plastic tube examined immediately for trophozoites
    Biopsy specimens

Culture of stool
> Material collected through sigmoido-
> scope
> Serologic tests

Hepatic amebiasis
> Determine presence of intestinal amebiasis
> Leukocyte count
> Serologic tests; IHA, gel-diffusion, IFA, etc.
> X-ray for diaphragm levels, liver scanning,
> and ultrasound
> Liver function tests
> Aspiration of abscess if readily accessible
>> Contents examined for odor and appear-
>> ance
>> Culture for bacteria
>> Trophozoites not likely to be recovered,
>> but best obtained from abscess wall

The character of the feces in intestinal ame-biasis is sometimes of confirmatory value, par-ticularly in differentiating from bacillary dys-entery. The typical amebic stool is acidic and consists of fecal material, scanty cellular exu-date, blood, from small amounts to actual hemorrhage, with degenerated erythrocytes often in adhesive masses, few polymorphonu-clear neutrophils or epithelial cells, numerous pyknotic residues. Charcot-Leyden crystals, few bacteria, and amebas. The typical bacil-lary dysentery stool is offensive, alkaline, and consists of scant fecal material, massive cellu-lar exudate, varying amounts of blood, eryth-rocytes usually unaltered, numerous polymor-phonuclear neutrophils and epithelial cells, few pyknotic residues, no Charcot-Leyden crystals, no pathogenic amebas, numerous bacteria, and macrophages that resemble amebas.

The parasite may be identified as trophozo-ites in the liquid stools of patients with acute dysentery and in aspirated material, and as cysts in the formed stools of chronic patients and carriers. *E. histolytica* requires differentia-tion from free-living amebas contaminating feces and from *E. coli* and the other parasitic amebas of humans (Table 3.1). In fresh, warm feces the trophozoites are identified by their active, progressive, directional movements, sharply defined ectoplasm, bladelike hyaline

pseudopodia, indistinct nucleus, and partly disintegrated, ingested red blood cells. The cysts are distinguished by the presence of one to four nuclei, diffuse glycogen mass, and large chromatoidal bodies. Failure to find cysts is not conclusive evidence of the absence of infection, since their number may fluctuate from day to day, from none to 6 million per gram of feces. Positive results can only be obtained, even after four or more examina-tions, in a minority of persons who pass fewer than 100,000 cysts per day. The chances of finding cysts in infected persons by direct smears of formed stools are about 20 percent for one examination, and 50 percent for three; six or more tests may be required to establish a reliable diagnosis. When combined with con-centration methods, the chances are increased to 30 to 50 percent for one examination.

If the laboratory has experience with cul-ture methods for amebas, they may reveal presence of *E. histolytica* when direct micro-scopic exam has failed. Serologic tests for anti-bodies to *E. histolytica* by indirect hemaggluti-nation (IHA) or gel-diffusion are very helpful in diagnosis of invasive amebiasis. This is espe-cially the case in individuals from the United States who are unlikely to have had previous amebiasis but have had recent short-term ex-posure abroad. Serologic tests such as the IHA are positive in virtually all patients with ame-bic liver abscess, and in 70 to 85 percent of those with clinically recognized intestinal amebiasis. Tests remain positive for months after successful treatment. Asymptomatic in-fections or those with minimal invasion of tis-sue usually have negative serology.

Treatment. In severe dysenteric infections with fever and prostration, patients should re-main in bed and receive a bland high-protein and high-vitamin diet with adequate fluids. Sedation will ensure rest. The effect of chemo-therapy includes (1) the relief of the acute attack, (2) destruction of the trophozoites in the intestinal mucosa and lumen, and (3) con-trol of secondary bacterial infection.

For severe intestinal amebiasis, metronida-zole (Flagyl) is the drug of choice: 750 mg t.i.d. orally for 5 to 10 days. Since this drug may not always cure intestinal infections, it is recommended that a course of another luminal drug such as diiodohydroxyquin (Diodoquin), 650 mg t.i.d. orally, be given for 20 days. Metronidazole's side effects consist of headache, nausea, diarrhea, and an altered sense of smell. Since it may be carcinogenic in experimental animals and mutagenic for bacteria, metronidazole should be used only when indicated. A few patients show an intolerance to diiodohydroxyquin in the form of headache, malaise, abdominal pain, diarrhea, rash, and pruritis. Iodine sensitivity is a contraindication to the drug.

An alternative drug for amebic dysentery is emetine hydrochloride, given by deep subcutaneous or intramuscular injection, 1 mg per kilogram of body weight, not to exceed 65 mg daily, for up to 5 or 6 days, until the acute dysentery is controlled. Emetine toxicity is manifested by nausea, vomiting, diarrhea, and generalized neuromuscular weakness. More disturbing evidences of toxicity that should lead to considerations of stopping the drug are marked hypotension, tachycardia and weakness, and serious EKG abnormalities. Fortunately, most of the untoward effects are mild and may even disappear while treatment is being continued. Patients receiving emetine should be at bed rest and under close observation. The drug is contraindicated in patients with renal or cardiac disease and during pregnancy, except when severe dysentery or liver abscess is uncontrolled by other drugs. Since emetine is active only against amebas in the tissues and not in the lumen of the intestine, its use should be followed by drugs that affect luminal amebas, such as a combination of tetracycline and diiodohydroxyquin. The adult dose of tetracycline is 0.5 gm t.i.d. for 7 to 8 days.

Dehydroemetine dihydrochloride°* is less toxic than emetine and apparently equally effective, but it is only available through the Centers for Disease Control. It is also given intramuscularly or subcutaneously, 1.0 to 1.5

* Drugs marked with a raised circle (°) are listed in the last chapter of this book. The reader should consult page 328.

mg per kilogram daily for up to 5 or 6 days, and like emetine it should be followed by a standard course of therapy against luminal amebas, such as tetracycline and diiodohydroxyquin.

Moderately severe or mild intestinal infections can lead to much more serious involvement and should be treated. Drugs besides metronidazole, tetracycline, and diiodohydroxyquin can be used. One of these is Paromomycin, a poorly absorbed antibiotic with a dosage for both adults and children of 25 to 30 mg per kilogram per day in three doses for 5 to 10 days. This is usually coupled with a course of diiodohydroxyquin. Another drug is diloxanide furoate in an adult dosage of 500 mg t.i.d. for 10 days. The asymptomatic cyst passer can be treated with diiodohydroxyquin alone, in combination with tetracycline or with paromomycin, or with diloxanide furoate alone, in the dosages given above.

If the laboratory continues to report amebas in the stools after several courses of treatment as outlined above, one possibility to consider is the accuracy of the laboratory diagnostic procedures.

An erroneous notion that confuses physicians as well as students regarding treatment of cyst passers is that some special medication might be needed for the resistant cysts. However, therapy is never directed against the cystic stage of the organism, whether or not the patient is symptomatic. Treatment is directed at the actively feeding and multiplying trophozoites located at some higher level in the large intestine. Therefore, treatment of the asymptomatic cyst passer is theoretically the same as that for someone with symptomatic intestinal amebiasis, except that the latter situation generally requires more rapid and thorough treatment.

Hepatic amebiasis is best treated with metronidazole, 750 mg t.i.d. for 5 to 10 days. Although the alleviation of symptoms is rapid, the cure rate is not 100 percent. Therapeutic failures should be treated with emetine or dehydroemetine in the daily doses given above, but for a period of up to 10 days, and not to exceed total doses of 600 or 900 mg, respectively. As the emetines are not likely to cure the intestinal amebic infection, they should be combined with a course of diiodohydroxyquin alone or with one of the broad-spectrum antibiotics.

Another drug that can be used for hepatic amebiasis is chloroquine, especially if there are some reasons why metronidazole or emetine cannot be used or are unavailable. Chloroquine can also be used in combination with emetine, particularly if emetine is given for less than 10 days. Chloroquine phosphate is used at a dosage for adults of 1 gm daily for 2 days followed by 500 mg daily for 2 to 3 weeks. Toxic effects of the drug are not common, but include pruritis, skin eruptions, headache, nausea, and disturbances of visual accommodation. Chloroquine does not affect amebas in the lumen of the intestine.

Small liver abscesses usually respond well to chemotherapy. Large abscesses, depending upon their accessibility and the likelihood of their rupturing, may require either surgical drainage or closed aspiration. In either event, chemotherapy of the hepatic amebiasis is, of course, also required. Resolution of liver abscess can be followed by ultrasound and liver-scanning procedures. Moderate-sized lesions

generally resolve in 2 to 4 months, but larger abscesses may take a longer resolution time.

Prevention. Since humanity is the chief source of infection, all infections should be treated and close contacts examined. Carriers should be removed from the food-handling occupations, instructed in personal hygiene, and treated (Fig. 3-8). Effective environmental sanitation is necessary to prevent water and food contamination. Sanitary methods of sewage disposal should be instituted, latrines should be screened, and feces used as fertilizer should be stored an appropriate length of time. A properly safeguarded, filtered water supply is important, since chlorination is not wholly effective. In areas where potable water is not available, special care must be taken. Boiling water is a safe, effective method of producing pleasant-tasting drinking water. Ice should be made from boiled water. Small quantities of drinking water may be treated with iodine-compound tablets (Globaline*). Residual-free iodine, 6 to 7 ppm, is cysticidal in 10 minutes at 23 C in water below pH 7.5 in the presence of 5 ppm of urea nitrogen. Tablets that release 8 ppm iodine have been

* Globaline, Maltbie Laboratories Division, Wallace & Tiernan, Inc., Belleville, N.J.

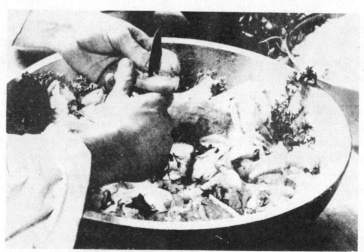

FRESH FOOD, FUSSED OVER WITH "FECALED" FINGERS

Figure 3-8. Transmission of amebiasis. (From S. A. Tydskrif vir Geneeskunde, 1944.)

compounded with an acidic excipient to reduce the pII of highly alkaline waters. Stable tablets, which are used as a disinfectant of water in canteens by the U.S. Army, contain 20 mg tetraglycine hydroperiodide, 90 mg disodium dihydrogen pyrophosphate, and 5 mg talc (Globaline).

Insects may be controlled by insecticides. Food should be screened and protected from dust contamination. Uncooked vegetables from areas where night soil is used as fertilizer should be thoroughly washed in water treated with iodine tablets or scalded at 80 C for at least 30 seconds. The public should be informed regarding methods of avoiding infection.

Free-living Amebas Causing Meningoencephalitis and Eye Disease

Several species of free-living ameboflagellates or amebas have been isolated and cultured from the spinal fluid or brain of patients who died of meningoencephalitis. Most have been due to a species of *Naegleria, N. fowleri* (Carter, 1972), which has both an ameboid and a flagellate stage, but some have been caused by species of amebas called *Hartmanella* or *Acanthameba*. In 1978, a girl who had been swimming regularly in the waters of the old Roman baths of England (Bath Spa) died of amebic meningitis. The organisms were recovered from waters of the reservoir supplying the spa. (One wonders whether imperial Romans died of a mysterious brain disease they could only blame on angry gods.) These circumstances may be the same as those in Czechoslovakia, where investigators in 1978 finally found the explanation for a swimming pool epidemic that had occurred years earlier. A pocket of water, harboring the amebas and protected from chlorine, had formed behind cracks in the pool wall.

Actually, the first cases were recognized in 1965 in Australia and Florida of the United States, but only one decade later a total of nearly 100 cases of amebic meningitis had been reported throughout the world, including many states of the United States. With *Naegle-*

ria cases, symptoms frequently developed a few days after the victim had been swimming and diving in the warm, still water of lakes, ponds, or backwater bays. The organism has been recovered from some of these waters. After entry into the nose the amebas presumably penetrate the cribiform plate and multiply along the base of the brain. Severe frontal headache, fever, and blocked nose were followed by signs of central nervous system involvement. Altered taste and smell may be present, as well as a stiff neck and Kernig's sign. The peripheral white count may be as high as 24,000, with a preponderance of neutrophils. Cells in the spinal fluid are also mainly neutrophils, as with a purulent meningitis, but there is no bacterial growth on culture. For diagnosis, the spinal fluid frequently is found to contain motile amebas that can be recovered by intracerebral inoculation of mice, or by growth on nonnutrient agar in conjunction with coliform bacteria. The clinical course is rapid, with death usually following within 4 to 5 days after onset of symptoms. At autopsy the amebas are abundant in the involved areas of the brain (Fig. 3-9) but only rarely are found in other organs. The amebas in the tissues are present only as trophozoites, without cysts being seen.

Treatment of *Naegleria* meningitis with sulfadiazine, chloroquine, emetine, metronidazole, and various antibiotics has been entirely ineffective. The only evidence of response in human infections has been with Amphotericin B, 1 mg per kilogram daily intravenously, and 0.1 to 1.0 mg intrathecally on alternate days. The addition of intravenous and intrathecal miconazole has also been recommended.

Some of the cases of amebic meningoencephalitis have been caused by members of the genus *Acanthameba,* and possibly a closely related group as well, the *Hartmanella.* Epidemiologically, the *Acanthameba* meningitis cases have also usually involved contact with soil or stagnant water, but, in contrast to the *Naegleria* cases, the clinical course is not as fulminant and sulfadiazine treatment has reportedly been effective. Another important differential feature of *Acanthameba* infections is

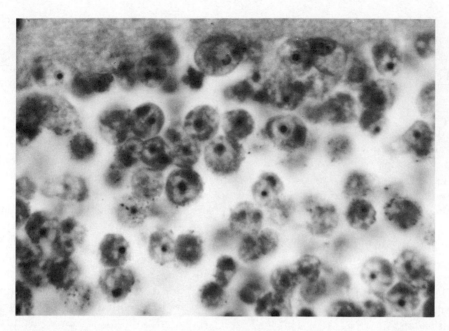

Figure 3-9. Soil amebas (*Naegleria*) showing characteristic large karyosomes and sharp cytoplasmic outlines, from olfactory trigone in 16-year-old white male. (Courtesy of Dr. Cecil G. Butt.)

that characteristic cysts with a wrinkled wall may be present in the affected tissues. The pathogenic potential of species of *Hartmanella* amebas for the human central nervous system is still somewhat uncertain. They can produce lethal meningoencephalitis when given intranasally to laboratory animals. Since they have been cultured from the upper respiratory tract of apparently normal individuals and from filtered air samples, the *Hartmanella* may represent the pathogen in those cases of amebic meningitis who have had no contact with soil or stagnant water.

Some recent reports have indicated that *Acanthameba* can also cause corneal ulceration, leading to blindness, and chronic granulomatous infections of the skin.

Since one outbreak of amebic meningoencephalitis has been traced to the use of an indoor swimming pool, measures to prevent contamination and growth of free-living amebas should be considered. Baguacil, containing 20 percent of a polymeric biguanide, is effective against *Naegleria,* bacteria, fungi, and algal growth in swimming pools.

Balantidium coli

Diseases. Balantidiasis, balantidiosis, balantidial dysentery.

Morphology and Physiology. B. coli is the largest intestinal protozoan of humans and our only pathogenic ciliate (Fig. 10). The grayish green unstained, ovoid trophozoite, averaging 60 μ (30 to 150) by 45 μ (25 to 120), is shaped like a sac (*balantidium* means "little bag") and is enclosed in a delicate protective pellicle covered with spiral longitudinal rows of cilia. The narrow triangular peristome and cytostome at the anterior end are lined with long cilia adapted for procuring food. At the posterior end is an indistinct excretory opening, the cytopyge, through which the solid waste material is discharged. Within the granular cytoplasm are two contractile vacuoles, a large, elongated, kidney-shaped macronucleus, a small subspherical micronucleus, and numerous food vacuoles. The trophozoites form a protective resistant cyst by secreting a double wall. The unstained, greenish yellow subspherical or oval cyst (Fig. 3-10), averaging about 52 to 55 μ and ranging from 45 to 65 μ,

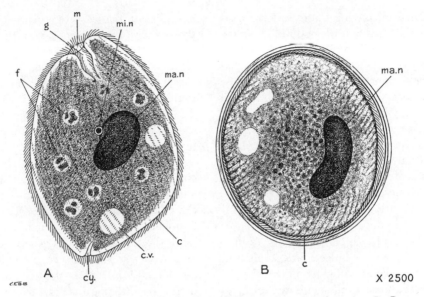

Figure 3-10. Schematic representation of *Balantidium coli*. A. Trophozoite. B. Cyst. c, cilia; cy., cytopyge; c.v., contractile vacuole; f, food vacuole; g, gullet; m, mouth; ma.n, macronucleus; mi.n, micronucleus. (Modified from Dobell and O'Connor, 1921.)

shows only the macronucleus, contractile vacuoles, and cilia.

The trophozoite lives chiefly in the lumen but also in the mucosa and submucosa of the large intestine, especially the cecal region, and in the terminal portion of the ileum. It moves actively by the rhythmic motion of its cilia. Its extreme plasticity and its rotary boring action enable it to penetrate the intestinal mucosa. Erythrocytes, leukocytes, tissue fragments, oil globules, starch granules, and other debris are carried through the cytopharynx into the endoplasm, where, enclosed in vacuoles, the materials are digested by enzymes. The trophozoite divides by transverse binary fission to form two new individuals, each containing a daughter macronucleus and micronucleus. Rapid division may produce nests of balantidia in the tissues. Trophozoites do not survive long extracorporeally, but cysts may remain viable for several weeks. *B. coli* can be cultivated on the noncellular mediums used for intestinal protozoa, but only trophozoites are formed.

Life Cycle. The life cycle of *B. coli* is similar to that of *E. histolytica*, except that there is no multiplication in the cyst. Cysts are the infective forms. When ingested by a new host, the cyst wall dissolves, and the liberated trophozoite invades and multiplies in the intestinal wall.

Epidemiology. The incidence of *B. coli* in humans is very low. On the other hand, the incidence is high in hogs (63 to 91 percent). Hogs harbor *B. coli* and *B. suis*. The former is infectious for humans, while the latter, the more common species, apparently does not infect humans. There is considerable epidemiologic evidence against the hog's being the important source of human infection. The incidence of infection in humans engaged in occupations and living in areas where closely associated with hogs is low, and humans are refractory to infection with porcine strains. During mental hospital outbreaks, people are the source of infection through hand-to-mouth transmission and food contamination.

Pathology and Symptomatology. The mucosa and submucosa of the large intestine are invaded and destroyed by the multiplying organisms. Invasion is effected by the cytolytic enzyme hyaluronidase and mechanical penetration. The multiplying parasites form nests and small abscesses that break down into oval, irregular ulcers with red, undermined edges. All degrees of severity, from simple catarrhal hyperemia to marked ulceration, occur. The individual ulcers may be discrete with normal or hyperemic intervening mucosa, or they may coalesce with communicating sinuses. In fatal cases there is multiple and diffuse ulceration and gangrene. Histologic sections show hemorrhagic areas, round-cell infiltration, abscesses, necrotic ulcers, and invading parasites, the predominating reaction being mononuclear unless secondary bacterial invasion is present (Fig. 3-11). In chronic infections during exacerbations the ulcers are small and discrete, the mucosa diffusely inflamed, and small membranous patches with raw underlying areas may be present. In moderately acute infections there may be 6 to 15 liquid stools per day, with mucus, blood, and pus. In the chronic disease there may be intermittent diarrhea alternating with constipation, tender colon, anemia, and cachexia. Many infections

are asymptomatic. Prognosis depends upon the severity of the infection and the response to treatment. It is good in asymptomatic and chronic infections. *Balantidium* very seldom successfully invades the liver; one such infection has recently been reported. The low incidence of infection and the failure of experimental infection indicates that humans have a high natural resistance.

Diagnosis. Balantidiasis may be confused clinically with other dysenteries and enteric fevers. Diagnosis depends upon the identification of trophozoites in diarrheic stools and, less frequently, of cysts in formed stools. Several stools should be examined, since the discharge of parasites is variable. In patients with sigmoidorectal infection, the sigmoidoscope is useful in obtaining material for examination.

Treatment. Treatment is oxytetracycline, 500 mg q.i.d. for 10 days, or diiodohydroxyquin, 650 mg t.i.d. for 20 days.

Prevention. The same prophylactic measures used in amebic dysentery with respect to carriers and sanitary control and water should be

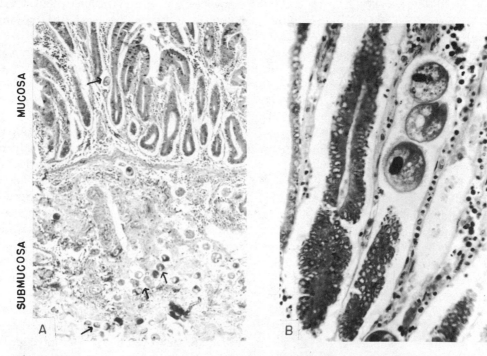

Figure 3-11. *Balantidium coli* in large intestine. A. Note that trophozoites have invaded both the mucosa and the submucosa. B. Trophozoites in mucosal crypts.

employed. Until more knowledge is available, it is well to consider the hog as a potential source of infection.

INTESTINAL AND LUMINAL FLAGELLATES OF HUMAN BEINGS

Almost every species of vertebrate can serve as host to intestinal and atrial flagellates, and a single host may harbor several species. Special organs, such as sucking disc, axostyle, and undulating membrane, have been developed to withstand the peristaltic action of the intestine. Transmission from host to host is through the formation of resistant cysts in many species, but in others infection is apparently transmitted through the less hardy trophozoites. Owing to morphologic variation, it is difficult to determine whether some species infecting humans and lower animals are identical.

Humanity is the host of seven species, including five intestinal and two atrial parasites. The five nonpathogenic cosmopolitan species are (1) *Chilomastix mesnili,* (2) *Enteromonas hominis,* (3) *Retortamonas intestinalis,* (4) *Trichomonas hominis* of the intestine, and (5) *T. tenax* of the mouth. The differential characteristics of these and the pathogenic (6) *Giardia lamblia* and (7) *T. vaginalis* are given in Figure 3-12). All have been cultivated on artificial mediums.

Giardia lamblia

Diseases. Giardiasis, lambliasis.

The trophozoite (Fig. 3-12) is a bilaterally symmetrical, pear-shaped flagellate, 12 to 15 μ, with a broad, rounded anterior and a tapering posterior extremity. The dorsal surface is convex. An ovoid, concave sucking disc occupies about three-fourths of the flat ventral surface. There are two nuclei with large central karyosomes, two axostyles, two blepharoplasts, two deeply staining bars considered to be parabasal bodies, and four pairs of flagella, although five have been demonstrated. The ellipsoidal cyst (Fig. 3-12; see also Figure 17-

3(17).), 9 to 12 μ, has a smooth, well-defined wall and contains two to four nuclei and many of the structures of the trophozoite. The flagellate inhabits the duodenum and upper jejunum and at times possibly the bile ducts and gallbladder. The lashing flagella propel the trophozoite with a rapid, jerky, twisting motion. The sucking disc enables the trophozoites to resist ordinary peristalsis. Hence, they are rarely found except in fluid stools. Food is absorbed from the intestinal contents, although the parasite may possibly obtain nourishment from the epithelial cells through its sucking disc. Multiplication occurs by mitotic division during encystment, followed by separation into daughter trophozoites after excystation. Longitudinal binary fission has been observed in trophozoites. An alkaline environment, increased by achlorhydria, and a rich carbohydrate diet favor multiplication. Under moist conditions, cysts may remain viable for months outside the host.

Humanity is the natural host of *G. lamblia,* but morphologically identical species of *Giardia* are found in a variety of animals. Transmission is through food and water contaminated by sewage, flies, or food handlers, and by hand-to-mouth. Infection is more common in children than in adults, particularly in the 6-to-10-year age group. Outbreaks of giardiasis have been described in day care centers and nurseries. There was a famous waterborne epidemic among tourists at a ski resort in Aspen, Colorado, aided by cross-contamination of the water and sewage systems. Thus, the athletic, the affluent, and the well-fed are susceptible to this infection, and abdominal discomfort, severe diarrhea, and weight loss were experienced by many; 56 of 59 passing *Giardia* experienced symptoms. Since 1970, 23 percent of nearly 1500 tourists to the Soviet Union have become ill with giardiasis, experiencing severe diarrhea—"Leningrad's curse." Infections in wilderness campers in U.S. western mountain states, as well as outbreaks traced to urban water reservoirs, have directed suspicion to wild animals as sources of *Giardia* capable of infecting humans. Large numbers of cysts are passed intermittently in the feces,

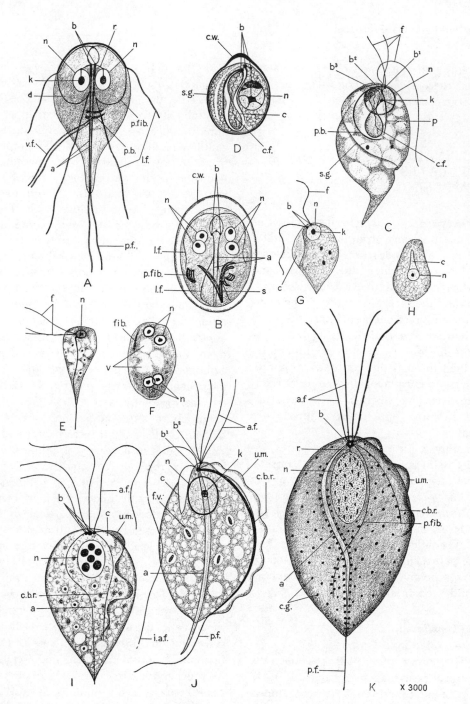

Figure 3-12. The intestinal and atrial flagellates of human beings. A. *Giardia lamblia* trophozoite viewed from dorsal surface. B. *Giardia lamblia* cyst. C. *Chilomastix mesnili* trophozoite, ventral view. D. *Chilomastix mesnili* cyst, ventral view, showing thickening of anterior wall. E. *Enteromonas hominis* trophozoite, showing characteristic caudal protuberance. F. *Enteromonas hominis* quadrinucleated cyst. G. *Retortamonas intestinalis* trophozoite. H. *Retortamonas intestinalis* cyst. I. *Trichomonas tenax* trophozoite. J. *Trichomonas hominis* trophozoite. K. *Trichomonas vaginalis* trophozoite.

a, axostyle; a.f., anterior flagella; b, b¹, b², b³, blepharoplasts; c, cytostome; c.b.r., chromatoid basal rod; c.f., cytotomal flagella; c.g., chromatin granules; c.w., cyst wall; d, sucking disc; f, flagella; f.v., food vacuole; fib., fibril; i.a.f., inferior anterior flagellum; k, karyosome; l.f., lateral flagella; n, nucleus; p, parastyle; p.b., parabasal body; p.f., posterior flagellum; p.fib., parabasal fiber; r, rhizoplast; s, shield; s.g., spiral groove; u.m., undulating membrane; v, vacuole; v.f., ventral flagella.

44

but relatively few trophozoites are passed except in diarrheic stools. When ingested by a new host the cysts pass unharmed through the gastric juices and undergo excystation in the duodenum. In volunteer experiments the ingestion of 100 or more cysts regularly resulted in infections; 10 to 25 cysts infected one-third; but one cyst alone failed to infect. The prepatent period ranged from 6 to 15 days, and infections usually lasted up to 41 days, although several continued for as long as 4 months. Interestingly, no clinical illness could be definitely attributed to experimental *Giardia* infections, although a pattern of increased stools occurred in two-thirds of the infected persons.

Although *G. lamblia* is found in the stools of many children or adults without recent or current symptoms, it is now clear that the parasite can cause diarrheal disease and intestinal malabsorption. Small bowel aspirates and biopsies of symptomatic patients have demonstrated large numbers of trophozoites in the duodenum and proximal jejunum, attachment of the organisms to the intestinal mucosa, with inflammation, and edema of the lamina propria. However, the principal lesion is derangement of normal villous architecture, with shortening of villi and inflammatory foci in the crypts and lamina propria as is seen in other types of malabsorption syndromes. Occasional parasites within mucosal cells or invading below the mucosa have been seen, but mucosal invasion seems to occur rarely and is not necessary to produce disease. Whether the mucosal abnormalities produced by giardia are due to mechanical, toxic, or some other factors is unknown. Functionally, the patient with giardial diarrhea may exhibit steatorrhea, impaired absorption of carotene, folate, and vitamin B_{12}. Disaccharidases and other mucosal enzyme activities can also be greatly reduced. These abnormalities of small bowel function are referred to collectively as *malabsorption syndrome*. Symptomatic manifestations of the syndrome are flatulence, abdominal distention, nausea, and anorexia, passage of foul-smelling and bulky stools, and eventual weight loss. A helpful differential point is that the stool in giardiasis does not contain blood or increase in polymorphonuclear leukocytes as is seen in some of the bacterial dysenteries. The possible role of increased bacterial growth in the small bowel in association with giardiasis is still controversial; it may be a contributing factor in some cases. Both the functional and morphologic abnormalities of the small bowel are reversible after treatment of the giardiasis.

Certain immunodeficiency syndromes are associated to a striking degree with *G. lamblia* infection. These are mainly patients who, for unknown reasons, develop hypogammaglobulinemia, chiefly the IgA and IgM class, in adult life. The predisposition of immunodeficiency patients to giardiasis might be attributable to low or absent secretory IgA in the intestinal tract that normally has a role in immune defense against the infection. However, specific immunologic tests for giardiasis must be developed before immunity in this infection can be evaluated. Since immunodeficient patients may have gastrointestinal disturbances due to other causes, the role of concomitant *Giardia* infection may be difficult to evaluate and require therapeutic response to treatment.

Diagnosis. Diagnosis is usually made by finding cysts in formed stools and trophozoites and cysts in diarrheic feces. The distinctive morphology of *G. lamblia* in saline and iodine mounts and in stained smears distinguishes it from other intestinal protozoa. To find trophozoites, one must examine specimens without delay. Concentration methods increase the chances of detection of cysts. Examination of the duodenal contents for trophozoites gives a somewhat higher percentage of positive findings than that of the feces. A string device* that is swallowed in a weighted gelatin capsule and then retrieved for microscopic examination of adherent intestinal mucus can be used if duodenal aspiration is not possible. Demonstration of organisms in small bowel biopsies has been reported in some patients with negative stools.

---

* Enterotest, HEDECO Company, Palo Alto, California.

Treatment. Quinicrine, uncoated, is given to adults, 100 mg t.i.d. for 5 to 7 days; for children the dosage is 8 mg per kilogram daily for 5 days. The maximum daily dose is 300 mg.

Metronidazole is equally effective but has not been licensed for use in giardiasis. The dosage for adults is 250 mg t.i.d. for 7 days. Children younger than 2 years are given 125 mg daily for 5 days; those from 2 to 4 years old, 250 mg daily for 5 days; those 4 to 8 years old, 375 mg daily for 5 days; those over 9 years old, 500 mg daily for 5 days. See above, pp. 36 and 47 for toxicity to metronidazole. Measures similar to those employed for *E. histolytica* are used in prevention. Drinking water appears to be an important source of some infections.

Trichomonas vaginalis

The genus *Trichomonas* comprises flagellates that have three to five anterior flagella, an undulating membrane, an axostyle, and usually a cytostome. Trichomonads are widely distributed and infect nearly every mammal associated with humans. There are three human species: *T. vaginalis* of the vagina, *T. hominis* of the intestine, and *T. tenax* of the mouth. They may be differentiated by site of origin, morphology (Fig. 3-12), cultural characteristics, and failure to cross infect. *T. vaginalis,* the largest and most robust, is the only pathogen, although it has been suggested that heavy infections with *T. hominis* may cause diarrhea.

Diseases. Trichomonad vaginitis, urethritis, prostatovesiculitis.

T. vaginalis (Fig. 3-12) is a colorless pyriform flagellate, 15 to 18 μ in fresh preparations but smaller when fixed. No cysts have been found. Its habitat is the vagina of the female and the urethra, epididymis, and prostate of the male. Hence, it is frequently found in the urine. It may cause a "nonspecific" urethritis. *T. vaginalis* advances rapidly, rotating through debris by the lashing of the anterior flagella and by the action of the undulating membrane.

In cultures it has been observed to ingest bacteria, starch, and even erythrocytes. Dextrose, maltose, and other carbohydrates stimulate growth. Reproduction takes place by binary longitudinal fission, with mitotic division of the nucleus.

The trophozoite is one of the most resistant of the parasitic protozoa. In cultures it loses its vitality below pH 4.9, hence it cannot live in the normally acid vaginal secretions (pH 3.8 to 4.4) of healthy adults.

Epidemiology. The incidence of infection is about 10 to 25 percent in women. It is higher in groups in which feminine hygiene is deficient. Only about one-seventh of the women with trichomonad infection complain of symptoms, although the vaginal secretions are invariably altered. The detected infection rate in husbands of infected wives is surprisingly low, but this may be due to technical difficulties in securing adequate specimens for diagnosis. Evidently there are several modes of transmission. Sexual intercourse, especially by asymptomatic infected males is probably most important. However, since young virgins are found infected, it appears that direct contact with infected females, contaminated toilet articles, and toilet seats transmits the infection. Infections acquired while passing through the birth canal probably account for some infections in babies.

Pathology and Symptomatology. *T. vaginalis* is the causative agent of a persistent vaginitis. The flagellate is responsible for a low-grade inflammation. Evidence is furnished by its toxic action on cells in tissue cultures and the production of vaginitis in women by bacteria-free cultures. The bacterial flora and the physiologic status of the vagina, including pH, are among the factors that determine infection.

In trichomonad vaginitis the vaginal walls are injected and tender, in some instances showing hyperemia and petechial hemorrhages, and in advanced cases, granular areas. The surface is covered with a frothy, seropurulent, creamy or yellowish discharge, frequently forming a pool in the posterior fornix. Patients present signs of vaginal and cervical inflammation, complain of itching and burning, and have a profuse irritating leukorrheic discharge. Its relationship to cervical cancer is unclear. At times erosion and necrosis are observed. In the male there may be a urethritis and prostatovesiculitis.

Diagnosis. Clinical diagnosis is based on symptoms of burning, a frothy creamy discharge, and punctate lesions and hyperemia of the vagina. The microscopic examination in a drop of saline for motile trichomonads of the fresh vaginal discharge, preferably obtained with a speculum, on a cotton-tipped applicator and dipped in normal saline solution, is the most practical method of diagnosis. Occasionally, cultures will reveal the organism when the microscopic examination is negative. Prostatic secretions following prostatic massage and urine of the male should be examined.

Treatment. The most effective drug for treatment of trichomoniasis in both sexes is metronidazole (Flagyl). Because the drug is carcinogenic and mutagenic under experimental conditions it has been recommended that metronidazole not be used unless other measures have failed or the infection is very severe. Other drugs that have been used with varying success are local therapies to the vaginal mucosa by insufflation or by suppository. These include silver picrate, furazolidone, or iodochlorhydroxyquin. Restoration of the normal acid pH of the vagina will suppress trichomonas since it does poorly below pH 5.0; hence periodic vinegar douches (1 ounce in a quart of water) may control mild infections.

If metronidazole is used, the dose for both males and females is 250 mg t.i.d. for 7 days. Vaginal inserts containing 500 mg of the drug are not effective in therapy. Metronidazole should not be given to pregnant patients. The use of a single large dose of 2 gm of metronidazole has been found to be nearly as effective as a 7- or 10-day course. If prolonged or repeated courses of the drug are given, there may be suppression of the white blood count. Side effects include metallic taste, furry tongue, nausea, and headache. Metronidazole can exert a disulfiramlike effect, so alcohol should be avoided for at least 24 hours after taking the drug.

Prevention. Attention to personal hygiene is the most important preventive measure. The detection and treatment of infected males should help in reducing infections.

COCCIDIA

After more than half a century of uncertain status, *Toxoplasma gondii,* the cause of toxoplasmosis, has been found to be a coccidian. Associated discoveries have also put into a much better perspective the related groups of *Sarcocystis* and *Isospora.* Final classification of all these organisms is not yet settled, partly because complete life cycles for some are still unknown. The coccidia are protozoa belonging to the subphylum Sporozoa, which have a sexual stage in one of their two hosts. The common feature of most coccidia is a sexual cycle in the intestinal mucosa of a carnivorous definitive host (the predator). This results in an oocyst or sporocyst that passes out in the feces to infect an intermediate host (the prey) in which asexual multiplication occurs. However, some species of *Isospora* may have a direct cycle, with both the sexual and asexual stages of multiplication occurring in the intestine of a single host. The most common and important human disease caused by coccidia is toxoplasmosis, but some of the other coccidial infections, although not common in humans are probably often unrecognized. Coccidial infections are very common and economically important in fowl, cattle, cats, and dogs.

Toxoplasma gondii

T. gondii was first found in the African rodent *Ctenodactylus gondii* in 1908. In 1923 Janku described toxoplasmic chorioretinitis, and in 1939 Wolf et al. isolated the parasite and established it as the cause of congenital neonatal disease. Numerous species of *Toxoplasma* have been described, but it appears that there is a single species causing the human infection and capable of infecting a wide variety of hosts.

Morphology. The actively multiplying asexual form in the human host is an obligate, intracellular parasite, pyriform in shape and approximately 3 by 6 μ. This parasite, called a *tachyzoite,* has a cell membrane, nucleus, and various organelles (Fig. 3-13). A collection of tachyzoites can fill up a host cell, develop a parasite membrane around themselves, and become a cyst. The cysts contain 50 to several thousand organisms and measure from 10 to 100 μ in diameter. Within the intestinal epithelial cells of the cat, a variety of morphologic forms has been described, ultimately leading to male and female gametocytes. The fertilized macrogametes develop into nearly spherical oocysts that rupture out of intestinal epithelial cells. When passed in cats' feces, the oocysts measure 10 to 13 μ in diameter. The oocyst wall has 2 layers and contains undifferentiated material, but the contents develop into 2 sporocysts within several days after being passed. Each sporocyst, in turn, contains four sporozoites (Fig. 3-13).

Life Cycle. T. gondii tachyzoites multiply within host cells by a specialized form of division called *endodyogeny,* in which two daughter cells are formed within a mother cell. As the distended host cells fill up with parasites, they rupture, releasing parasites that enter new cells. The infected host cell may swell up, develop a membrane, and become a cyst. The tachyzoites consume oxygen, use dextrose and preformed as well as precursor pyrimidines, and evolve CO_2, but cannot synthesize purines; their respiration is cyanide sensitive. Toxoplasma can grow in any mammalian or avian organs or tissues, developing in the brain, eye, and skeletal muscles. In the natural cycle, mice and rats containing infective cysts are eaten by the cat, which serves as the definitive host for the sexual stage of the parasite. The cyst wall is digested, releasing organisms that penetrate epithelial cells of the small intestine. Several generations of intracellular multiplication occur, finally culminating in development of micro- and macrogametes. Fertilization of the latter results in development of oocysts that are discharged into the intestinal lumen by rupture of infected intestinal epithelial cells. After eating cysts, cats excrete toxoplasma oocysts as early as 4 days later; these increase and then taper off by 14 days. Oocysts require 1 to 5 days, depending upon aeration and temperature, after passage to sporulate. Ingestion of the sporulated oocyst initiates infection by sporozoites in the intermediate host, which can be virtually any animal. The oocyst-induced infection also begins

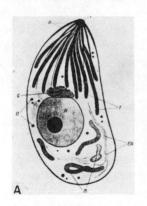

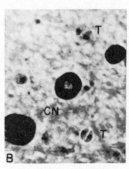

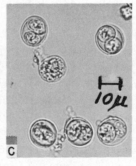

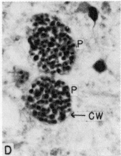

A — SCHEMATIC REPRESENTATION OF MORPHOLOGY SEEN WITH ELECTRON MICROSCOPE.

IN IMPRESSION FILM OF BRAIN
T — TOXOPLASMA
CN — BRAIN CELL NUCLEUS

MICRO-ISOLATED CYST

CYST IN SECTION OF BRAIN
P — PARASITES
CW — CYST WALL

ER — ENDOPLASMIC RETICULUM
G— GOLGI APPARATUS; M— MITOCHONDRIA; N— NUCLEUS; O— OSMIOPHILIC GRANULES
P— POLE RING; R— RADIAL RIBS; T— TOXONEMES

Figure 3-13. *Toxoplasma gondii.* (A and C from Maumenee [ed]: Toxoplasmosis with special reference to uveitis. Williams and Wilkins, 1961. A, courtesy of Ludvik; C, courtesy of R. Lainson; D, courtesy of H. C. Neu.

in the intestinal epithelium, but the tachyzoites multiply and spread to more distant organs to form cysts that are again infective when ingested by a susceptible animal.

Thus, although only the domestic cat or some wild species of *Felidae* can produce the oocyst, a wide variety of animals, including sheep, cattle, and pigs, can become infected by ingestion of the oocyst. These infected animals will, in turn, harbor infective cysts within muscle tissue. Hence, human infections can result (1) from eating raw or partially cooked beef, pork, or mutton containing toxoplasma cysts or (2) by ingestion of material contaminated with infected cat feces.

Epidemiology. Toxoplasmosis is cosmopolitan, and antibody surveys indicate that from 20 to 75 percent of various populations are chronically but asymptomatically infected. In areas where cats are numerous, sanitation is poor, and the climate is humid and mild, the presence of antibodies to *Toxoplasma* is high in children. In urban areas where meat is eaten partially cooked or raw, the rate in adults is high. Raw meat is a gourmet item in France and a "health food" for young children, so it is not surprising that the *Toxoplasma* serology rate in that country is high in both adults and children; cats probably contribute their share also. The senior author, Harold Brown, recalls treating a French child 1 year of age for beef tapeworm; he had been fed raw beef to become a strong Frenchman. Americans eat raw ground beef as steak tartare. On certain Pacific Islands where cats have been absent, antibodies to *Toxoplasma* in humans have been absent as well.

Outbreaks of toxoplasmosis have been recorded, one involving 5 medical students in New York City who patronized a snack bar for their hamburger lunches; presumably, the hamburgers were not well cooked. An interesting recent epidemic at a riding stable could be traced to an indoor riding arena harboring cats that feasted upon the numerous mice. Infection was thought to have occurred via oocysts, ingested directly or by aerosol dispersion. Infection has been traced to white cell or platelet transfusion, probably due to intracellular organisms, but packed red cell transfusions are safe.

Although infection is common, disease is rare. The congenital infection is acquired by transplacental transmission from mothers who develop toxoplasmosis during pregnancy, not from mothers who have already been infected before pregnancy.

Pathology and Symptomatology. Ordinarily, *T. gondii* is a relatively benign, well-adapted parasite, and its disease-producing properties have been attributed to virulent strains, especially susceptible hosts, or the site of the parasite.

CONGENITAL TOXOPLASMOSIS. This occurs in about 1 to 5 per 1000 pregnancies. Unlike that in adults, it is often severe and even fatal, varying in degree of severity with the age of the fetus at infection and the antibody protection from the mother. The child may present the typical syndrome of intracerebral calcification, chorioretinitis, hydrocephaly, microcephaly, psychomotor disturbances, and convulsions. Visceral and muscular lesions are also present. Occasionally the infection is milder, and there may be complete recovery. It is estimated that of the congenital infections, 5 to 15 percent of the babies will die; 8 to 10 percent will have severe brain and eye damage; 10 to 13 percent will have moderate to severe visual handicaps; and 58 to 72 percent will be asymptomatic at birth, with a small proportion developing active retinochoroiditis or mental retardation as children or young adults. Since transplacental transmission takes place during initial exposure to the parasite, second congenital infections rarely, if ever, occur.

There may be spasticity, opisthotonos, retraction of the head, stiff neck, and even paralysis. Anemia and leukocytosis with an absolute increase in monocytes and lymphocytes are present in about half the patients. The spinal fluid shows increased pressure, xanthochromia, round-cell pleocytosis, a high protein content, and, occasionally, the organisms. The cerebral lesions may undergo calcification, appearing in roentgenographs as small round bodies, broad bands, or scattered granules.

Toxoplasmic cysts, which may persist for years without causing tissue reaction, may be present in apparently healthy tissues near the necrotic areas. Occasionally their rupture may give rise to edema, cellular infiltration, and necrosis, possibly an allergic reaction.

The chorioretinal lesions in infants are severe, extensive, and bilateral. There is an intense edema of the retina and various degrees of degeneration and necrotic inflammation, with perivascular and general cellular infiltration. There may be an optic neuritis. Milder forms of the congenital infection are seen as ocular involvement in older children and young adults. This is manifested only as a retinochoroiditis of varying severity, but without other evidence of generalized disease. The exact cause of toxoplasmic retinochoroiditis of this late-onset type is not known; it may be due to localized proliferation of organisms, or an immunologic hypersensitivity reaction.

ACQUIRED OR REACTIVATED TOXOPLASMOSIS. After infection and regional lymph node invasion, the parasite is blood-borne to many organs where intracellular multiplication takes place. Parasitemia persists for several weeks, and with the production of antibody, cysts form in various tissues. The patients are asymptomatic. There are two main clinical types of acquired postnatal toxoplasmosis. (1) The more common, mild lymphatic form, resembling infectious mononucleosis, is characterized by cervical and axillary lymphadenopathy, malaise, muscle pain, and irregular low fever. Slight anemia, low blood pressure, leukopenia, lymphocytosis, and slightly altered liver function may be present. (2) The other type is characterized by acute, fulminating, disseminated infections, often with a skin rash, high fever, chills, and prostration. Meningoencephalitis, hepatitis, pneumonitis, and myocarditis may be present.

Toxoplasmosis has been shown to occur as an opportunistic infection complicating immunosuppression. Fatal outcome due to unsuspected toxoplasmosis has been recognized in recipients of kidney transplants and in patients with neoplastic disease treated with im-

munosuppressive drugs. This probably represents reactivation of previously acquired toxoplasmosis. The ocular involvement that occurs in later life following an inapparent congenital infection is probably a reactivation toxoplasmosis also, although the exact mechanism is unknown. It should be emphasized, however, that there are other causes of retinochoroiditis and uveitis, probably most of it not due to toxoplasma infection.

Diagnosis. Serologic tests are very important in the diagnosis of toxoplasmosis. Because of the common occurrence of antibodies to the parasite in the general population, diagnosis by serologic means requires demonstration of a significant increase in antibody titers. A very high antibody level is not sufficient evidence in itself for a diagnosis of active toxoplasmosis, although it may be a useful clue for further diagnostic measures.

Congenital infections may be difficult to diagnose serologically because maternal IgG crosses the placental barrier and will appear and persist for several months in the circulation of the newborn. But since IgM antibodies do not cross the placenta, demonstration of antitoxoplasma IgM at birth or up to several months of age is presumptive evidence of congenital toxoplasmosis. If tests that measure only IgG are available, it is necessary to show that antibodies persist or increase in titer during the first 6 months or so of life as evidence of congenital infection.

The presence of antitoxoplasma IgM antibodies in suspected acquired toxoplasmosis is also very useful as evidence of active or recent infection. Such antibodies are usually demonstrated by the indirect fluorescent antibody (IFA) test, but they may persist for as long as a year. The IFA test for IgG antibodies, an indirect hemagglutination (IHA) test, and the Sabin–Feldman dye test are the other procedures most commonly used for serodiagnosis of toxoplasmosis.

Although little used, the complement-fixation (CF) test is one of the most helpful in distinguishing recent from old toxoplasma infections. The reason for this is that CF antibodies develop much more slowly than those detected by the dye, IHA, or IFA tests. The CF test also reverts to negative within a few years, in contrast to persisting antibodies demonstrable by the other tests.

A delayed-type skin test has been described in toxoplasmosis, but antigens are not commercially available, and the significance of the test for diagnostic purposes is not clear.

If tissue or fluid suspected of containing parasites is available, a suspension of the material should be inoculated into mice. Laboratory mice are very susceptible to infection, and specimens of biopsied lymph nodes, muscle, spinal fluid, or blood have often been positive, especially in acute cases. A positive result can be shown either by actual isolation of the organism from mice or by their development of antibody. One problem in interpretation of a positive isolation from tissue, especially muscle tissue, is that viable organisms may persist in the encysted state long after the acute phase of an illness.

Treatment. Symptomatic infections should be treated with pyrimethamine (Daraprim); the adult dosage is 25 to 50 mg per day orally for 3 to 4 weeks, plus 2 to 6 gm daily of trisulfapyrimidines orally for the same period. The two drugs act synergistically to inhibit nucleic acid synthesis of microorganisms, the sulfa by preventing incorporation of para-aminobenzoic acid early in the process, and pyrimethamine as a folic acid antagonist at a later stage.

Mild lymphatic toxoplasmosis will often subside without requiring treatment. It is often difficult to decide whether ocular toxoplasmosis, without systemic involvement, should be treated. If the retinochoroiditis is considered to be an active process, most ophthalmologists treat with both corticosteroids and combined sulfapyrimethamine as outlined above.

The usual toxic manifestations of sulfonamides may be encountered; if so, the sulfa drug should be stopped. Large doses of pyrimethamine may cause agranulocytosis, anemia, and thrombocytopenia, which can be prevented or reversed by administration of folinic acid (Leucovorin). Pregnant women should not be treated with pyrimethamine. In this situation, one alternative drug is Spiramycin, which has been used in Europe but is not available in the United States. Another drug that might be used in emergency situations is clindamycin, since it has been effective in experimental infections.

Prevention. Practical measures for prevention of toxoplasmosis are the thorough cooking of all meats and careful attention to cat feces. The oocysts require a few days to sporulate and become infective but then may remain infective up to 18 months in soil.

Pregnant women should follow these suggestions:

1. Handle meat with care, avoid tasting raw meat, and wash hands with soap and water after handling meat.
2. Cook all meats thoroughly, including hamburger and frozen meats.
3. Either get rid of cats or keep them in houses where there are no rodents.
   Feed cats dry or cooked canned cat food.
   Empty litter box *daily,* or delegate this job to other family members. Disinfect litter box with boiling water and wash hands after these activities.
   Children's sandboxes should be covered when not in use to avoid not only toxoplasmosis but also visceral and cutaneous larva migrans from cat and dog feces.

Isospora belli

I. belli is at present the only known coccidial parasite for which humanity is the definitive host; i.e., sexual multiplication takes place in the intestinal mucosa. There was confusion over the fact that oocysts of a smaller size, called *I. hominis,* were also found in human feces. In the light of recent information it is likely that what were called *I. hominis* were actually oocysts of some species of *Sarcocystis,* a related coccidian parasite. *I. belli,* though rare, has a wide distribution. It has been reported from Central and South America, Africa, and

Southeast Asia; the largest concentration is in Chile. Of about 100 cases reported from the United States less than one-fourth have been autochthonus. One similar species, *I. natalensis,* has been described from South Africa.

Morphology. The oocysts, which are the forms found in the stool, are elongated or ovoid and 25 to 33 μ by 12 to 16 μ in size. In fresh feces the granular cytoplasm, contained within a smooth, colorless, two-layered wall, is usually unsegmented, or unsporulated (Fig. 3-14). Division takes place into two sporoblasts that secrete a cystic wall to become sporocysts. Within each sporocyst further division produces four elongated nucleated sporozoites. Since sporulation requires several days, unsporulated oocysts are the forms usually found in feces. In aspirated duodenal contents both sporoblasts and oocysts may be found; the sporocysts are 9 to 14 μ by 7 to 12 μ.

Life Cycle. At present the *Isospora* contain organisms of two biologically and structurally distinct types. One group contains parasites with a direct fecal-oral life cycle without intermediate hosts, in which the infection is confined to intestinal epithelial cells. The other type of *Isospora,* including, for example, *I. felis* and *I. canis,* contains organisms with a two-host life cycle and encysted forms in the tissues of the intermediate host. It is believed that the human parasite, *I. belli,* is of the former group, with a direct, one-host cycle. Thus, humans are probably infected by accidental hand-to-mouth ingestion of the sporulated oocysts or in food or water. Virtually all information about the life cycle is based upon study of intestinal biopsy material from patients. Findings by both light and electron microscopy have shown asexual as well as sexual stages of the parasite in the mucosal epithelium of the upper small intestine. Multiple and indefinite generations of the asexual cycle in the infected individual, or sporulation of oocysts and reinvasion of the bowel could explain the chronic course of some human coccidial infections.

Pathology and Symptomatology. Pathogenicity is variable; excretion of oocysts has been observed in apparently healthy individuals as well as in those with diarrhea. In those with disease, the possible contribution of concomittant bacterial or other parasitic infection has not always been ruled out. Some experimental infections have been associated with fever, malaise, diarrhea, and abdominal pain. Several naturally occurring infections have been studied thoroughly and indicate quite clearly

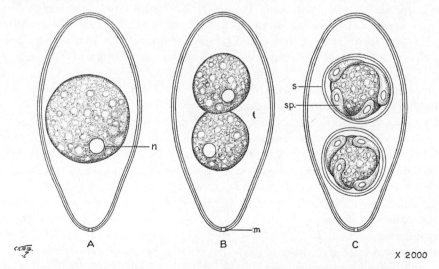

Figure 3-14. *Isopora belli.* A. Unicellular oocyst. B. Oocyst with two sporoblasts. C. Oocyst with two spores, each containing four sporozoites.

m, micropyle; n, nucleus; s, spore; sp., sporozoite. (Modified from Dobell and O'Connor, 1921.)

that serious disease, characterized by malabsorption syndrome, weight loss, and even a fatal outcome, can occur with human coccidial infections. Intestinal biopsies have corroborated the clinical picture of malabsorption, finding mucosal lesions of shortened villi, hypertrophied crypts, and infiltration of the lamina propria, with eosinophils, polys, and round cells. Such biopsies have also disclosed intracellular forms of the parasite in epithelial cells of the involved areas; these are easily overlooked unless the sections are carefully examined under oil immersion.

Diagnosis is made by demonstrating oocysts in the feces, oocysts, and/or sporocysts in duodenal contents and intracellular stages of the parasite in intestinal biopsies. Concentration or floatation techniques of stool examination are helpful in finding the oocysts.

Treatment. For mild or asymptomatic infections, nonspecific measures, such as rest and a bland diet, may be sufficient. Trier *et al.* reported convincing evidence in a well-documented case of a specific response to combined pyrimethamine and sulfadiazine (75 mg and 4 gm daily, respectively). Sulfonamides and furazolidone are used in coccidian infections of poultry and domestic animals.

Prevention. Preventive measures are similar to those for *E. histolytica.*

Genus Sarcocystis

Species of the genus *Sarcocystis* are widely distributed parasites of a variety of mammals and birds. The parasite of humans, designated as *S. lindemanni,* has been found as a cystic stage in striated muscle; but this is usually an incidental finding. Recent work has elucidated the previously unknown life cycle of many species of *Sarcocystis* and has clarified their relationship to the coccidia in general.

Life Cycle. In all *Sarcocystis* species studied there is an obligatory two-host cycle, involving two vertebrate hosts. A schizogonous cycle occurs in the intermediate host, or prey (herbivores and omnivores), and sexual reproduction takes place in the intestine of the predator, or definitive host. The asexual cycle in the intermediate host, however, is more complicated than with most other coccidia, for there is initially a period of intracellular multiplication in vascular endothelial cells of the liver or brain, followed by invasion of muscle cells and development of a characteristic septate cysts containing organisms up to 15 μ in length. When the muscle cysts are eaten by an appropriate definitive host, a sexual stage of multiplication occurs in the intestinal mucosa, resulting in excretion of oocysts and sporocysts, to continue the cycle.

Great surprise and still considerable confusion reigns among protozoologists because organisms comfortably catalogued as isosporan oocysts of various animals have now been found to be stages of *Sarcocystis* instead. Even parasitologists can be wrong!

Pathogenicity. It is the cystic stage of this parasite in striated muscles that has been found in humans, generally as an incidental finding. Local symptoms, such as muscle tenderness, might be associated with the lesion. A recent review concluded that only 16 of the 28 cases reported could be accepted as sarcosporidial infections. Human volunteer experiments in which raw beef or pork containing cysts were eaten also showed that people may be a definitive host for *Sarcocystis,* but naturally occurring disease attributable to this phase of the parasite has not yet been recognized.

Genus Cryptosporidium

Cryptosporidia are protozoan parasites similar to coccidia and capable of causing enterocolitis in a wide variety of vertebrates. They are tiny organisms that form a unique intracellular attachment to the microvillus border of intestinal epithelial cells. Only in the past few years have several instances of human disease been described.

Life Cycle and Diagnosis. The exact cycle of the human parasite is not known, but it can be inferred from what is known of *Cryptosporidia* of other species, especially the guinea pig. Transmission experiments suggest that the parasites are host specific, and different species involve specific areas of the intestinal tract, e.g., stomach or small bowel. Asexual as well as sexual stages have been described for the parasite of guinea pigs, but no oocysts were found and the infective stage has not been described. Yet, a fecal-oral mode of transmission is suspected.

Diagnosis in human cases has been accomplished by biopsy of the small bowel or rectal mucosa and direct demonstration of the characteristic organism attached to the brush border of crypt epithelial cells. The organisms are 2 to 4 μ in diameter. If possible, biopsy tissue should be examined by electron microscopy to demonstrate the attachment zone between the parasite and the cell.

Pathogenicity. The few recognized cases have included a child with a self-limiting enterocolitis and two adults with diarrhea. One of the latter cases may have been related to immunosuppression for underlying disease. Disease caused by this parasite has been recognized in male homosexuals. The portions of the mucosa where parasites were demonstrated showed abnormalities of villi and cellular infiltrate of the lamina propria.

Treatment. There is no known treatment.

REFERENCES

Selected Amebiasis References
Barbour and Juniper: A clinical comparison of amebic and pyogenic abscess of the liver in 66 patients. Am J Med 53: 323-334, 1972.

Juniper, et al: Serologic diagnosis of amebiasis. Am J Trop Med Hyg 21: 157-168, 1972.

Krogstad, et al: Amebiasis: Epidemiologic studies in the United States, 1971-1974. Ann Intern Med 88: 89-97, 1978.

Pittman, et al: Studies of human amebiasis. III. Ameboma: A radiologic manifestation of amebic colitis. Am J Dig Dis 18: 1025-1031, 1973.

Wilmot: Clinical Amoebiasis. Philadelphia, Blackwell Scientific Publications, F. A. Davis Co., 1962.

Diseases Associated with Free-living Amebae
Carter: Primary amebic meningo-encephalitis. An appraisal of present knowledge. Trans R Soc Trop Med Hyg. 66: 193-208, 1972.

Visvesvara, et al: Isolation, identification and biological characterization of *Acanthameba polyphaga* from a human eye. Am J Trop Med Hyg 24: 784-790, 1975.

Balantidiasis
Walzer, et al: Balantidiasis outbreak in Truk. Am J Trop Med Hyg 22: 33-41, 1973.

Giardiasis
Ament and Rubin, Relation of giardiasis to abnormal intestinal structure and function in gastrointestinal immuno-deficiency syndromes. Gastroenterology. 62: 216-226, 1972.

Hoskins, et al: Clinical giardiasis and intestinal malabsorption. Gastroenterology. 53: 265-279, 1967.

Jakubowski and Hoff (editors): Waterborne transmission of giardiasis. Proceedings of a Symposium. Springfield, Va. E.P.A. National Technical Information Service, 1979.

Wolfe: Giardiasis. JAMA 233: 1362-1365, 1975.

Trichomoniasis
Honigberg: Trichomonads of importance in human medicine. In Kreier (ed): Parasitic Protozoa, Vol. II, New York, Academic Press, 1978, pp.275-454.

Coccidiosis, Including Toxoplasmosis
Brandborg, et al: Human coccidiosis—a possible cause of malabsorption. N Engl Med 283; 1306-1313, 1970.

Desmonts, et al: Congenital Toxoplasmosis. N Engl J Med 290: 1110-1116, 1974.

Dubey: Toxoplasma, Hammondia, Besnoita, Sarcocystis and other Tissue Cyst-forming Coccidia of Man and animals. In Kreier (ed): Parasitic Protozoa. Vol. 3, Academic Press, Inc. New York, 1977, pp. 101-237.

Krick and Remington: Toxoplasmosis in the adult. N Engl J Med 298: 550-553, 1978.

Symposium on Toxoplasmosis. Bull NY Acad Med 50: No. 2—Feb., 1974.

Teutsch, et al: Epidemic toxoplasmosis associated with infected cats. N Engl J Med 300: 695-699, 1979.

4

Blood and Tissue Protozoa of Human Beings

PARASITIC TRYPANOSOMES OF HUMAN BEINGS

Trypanosoma (trypomastigote) and *Leishmania* (amastigote) have species pathogenic to man and other mammals. Their transitional forms in insects and cultures resemble species of the genera *Leptomonas* (promastigote) and *Crithidia* (epimastigote), which are found in invertebrates (Table 4-1). The widely distributed members of the genus *Trypanosoma* spend part of the life cycle in vertebrates and, with few exceptions, part in invertebrates. The three species pathogenic to man are *T. gambiense* and *T. rhodesiense* in Africa and *T. cruzi* in America.

Morphology. Trypanosomes are minute, actively motile, fusiform protozoa, flattened from side to side (Fig. 4-1). The long sinuous body has a tapering anterior and a blunt posterior end. Even in the same species the shape varies. The electron microscope reveals surface striations due to spiral bundles of longitudinal contractile fibrils beneath the enveloping pellicle. The flagellum, which consists of five to nine striated parallel fibrils in a cytoplasmic sheath, projects from the anterior end after passing along the margin of the undulating membrane, a wavy fold of the periplast on the convex border of the trypanosome. A large oval nucleus, which has a central karyosome, is situated toward the middle of the body. Near the posterior end there is a kinetoplast, consisting of a spherical or rod-shaped parabasal body of variable size and an anterior connecting basal granule, the blepharoplast. At times, minute refractile volutin granules and vacuoles may be seen in the cytoplasm. Trypanosomes travel with a wavy spiral motion produced by the contractile flagellum and undulating membrane. Reproduction takes place by binary longitudinal fission. Trypanosomes fail to store carbohydrates and thus require as sources of energy the readily available supplies of their hosts. In the blood, dextrose is used by *T. gambiense* and *T. rhodesiense* at a high rate, but by *T. cruzi* at a negligible rate. In cultures *T. cruzi* can use proteins in the absence of available carbohy-

TABLE 4-1
DEVELOPMENTAL FORMS OF TRYPANOSOMIDAE PATHOGENIC FOR MAN

Species	Developmental Forms				Transmission	Insect Vectors	Reservoir Hosts Other Than Man
	Amastigote	Promastigote	Epimastigote	Trypomastigote			
Trypanosoma *T. gambiense*	None	None	1. Salivary glands and gut of insects 2. Culture	1. Blood, lymphatic glands, and spinal fluid of mammals 2. Intestine and salivary glands of insects	Anterior station, bite	Tsetse flies (*Glossina*)	Hog, goat, and cattle
T. rhodesiense	None	None	1. Salivary glands and gut of insects 2. Culture	1. Blood, lymphatic glands, and spinal fluid of mammals 2. Intestine and salivary glands of insects	Anterior station, bite	Tsetse flies (*Glossina*)	Wild game animals and cattle
T. cruzi	1. Intracellular in viscera, particularly myocardium, muscle, and brain, of mammals 2. Tissue culture	Intracellular in mammals but transitional	1. Intracellular in mammals but transitional 2. Intestine of insects 3. Culture	1. Blood and tissues of mammals 2. Intestine and rectum of insects 3. Culture	Posterior station, feces	Reduviid bugs (TRIATOMINAE)	Dog, cat, armadillos, and small wild mammals

T. cruzi	1. Intracellular in viscera, particularly myocardium, muscle, and brain, of mammals 2. Tissue culture	Intracellular in mammals but transitional	1. Intracellular in mammals but transitional 2. Intestine of insects 3. Culture	1. Blood and tissues of mammals 2. Intestine and rectum of insects 3. Culture	Posterior station, feces	Reduviid bugs (TRIATOMINAE)	Dog, cat, armacillos, and small wild mammals
Leishmania *L. donovani*	1. Intracellular in reticuloendothelial system, lymphatic glands, spleen, liver, bone marrow, and phagocytes 2. Tissue culture	1. Midgut and pharynx of insects 2. Culture	None	None	Anterior station, bite	Sandflies (*Phlebotomus*)	Dog
L. tropica and *L. braziliensis*	1. Intracellular in macrophages of skin and mucous membranes of mammals 2. Tissue culture	1. Midgut and pharynx of insects 2. Culture	None	None	Anterior station, bite	Sandflies (*Phlebotomus*)	Wild rodents and dog

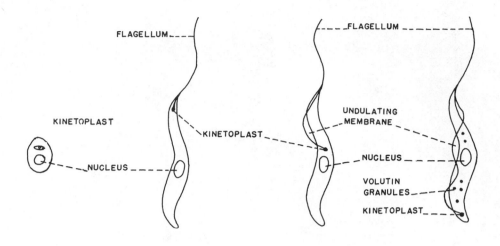

AMASTIGOTE   PROMASTIGOTE   EPIMASTIGOTE   TRYPOMASTIGOTE

Figure 4-1. Developmental forms of Trypanosomidae.

drates. Nourishment is obtained from the blood plasma, lymph, cerebrospinal fluid, and products of cellular disintegration. The original Novy–MacNeal–Nicolle (N.N.N.) medium with its various modifications is still popular for their cultivation.

Life Cycle. The life cycle of mammalian trypanosomes of man involves alternate existence in vertebrate and invertebrate hosts and a cyclic development in a bloodsucking insect before it becomes infective.

Classification. Classifications of trypanosomes have been based on morphology, natural hosts, method of transmission, and pathogenicity. It has been postulated that *T. gambiense* and *T. rhodesiense,* which are common to humans, are varieties or mutants of *T. brucei* of equidae and ruminants because of morphologic similarity and common group antigens. Of the three human species, *T. rhodesiense* morphologically resembles *T. gambiense,* but they differ in various biologic characteristics; *T. cruzi* is distinct.

Pathogenicity. Most species of trypanosomes infecting mammals are not injurious to their natural hosts, but some produce marked pathologic changes. Humans and domesticated animals, apparently more recent hosts, are more susceptible than are wild animals, but as a rule trypanosomes do not produce disease in large domesticated or wild animals.

Trypanosoma gambiense

Diseases. Gambian trypanosomiasis, Mid-African sleeping sickness.

Morphology (Fig. 4-2). In the blood *T. gambiense* is polymorphic, ranging from typical, long, slender trypanosomes to short, blunt forms without free flagella, or even to bizarre degenerate types. In the cerebrospinal fluid all sizes and shapes occur, including multiple and even involuted round or pear-shaped forms. Its length ranges from 15 to 30 μ and its breadth from 1.5 to 3.5 μ.

Life Cycle (Fig. 4-3). The main vertebrate host is humanity. Nonhuman reservoirs are not considered important, but goats, cattle, and pigs may have asymptomatic infections. The principal invertebrate hosts are riverine tsetse flies of the palpalis group, *Glossina palpalis, G. palpalis fuscipes,* and *G. tachinoides,* but other species occasionally may serve as hosts.

Epidemiology. This disease is limited to tropical West and Central Africa, and to the range of its vectors—the palpalis group of tsetse flies. The incidence of Gambian trypanosomiasis is usually less than 3 percent in endemic areas. At times the infection has reached epidemic

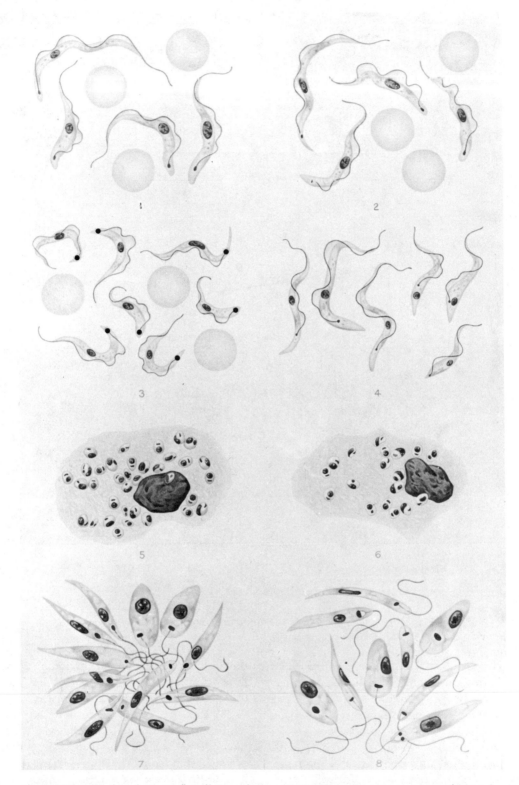

Figure 4-2. Blood and tissue flagellates of man (× 1500). 1. *Trypanosoma gambiense* in blood. 2. *Trypanosoma rhodesiense* in blood. 3. *Trypanosoma cruzi* in blood. 4. *Trypanosoma gambiense,* developmental forms in *Glossina palpalis.* 5. *Leishmania donovani* in endothelial cell. 6. *Leishmania tropica* in large mononuclear cell. 7. *Leishmania donovani,* flagellated forms from culture. 8. *Leishmania tropica,* flagellated forms from culture.

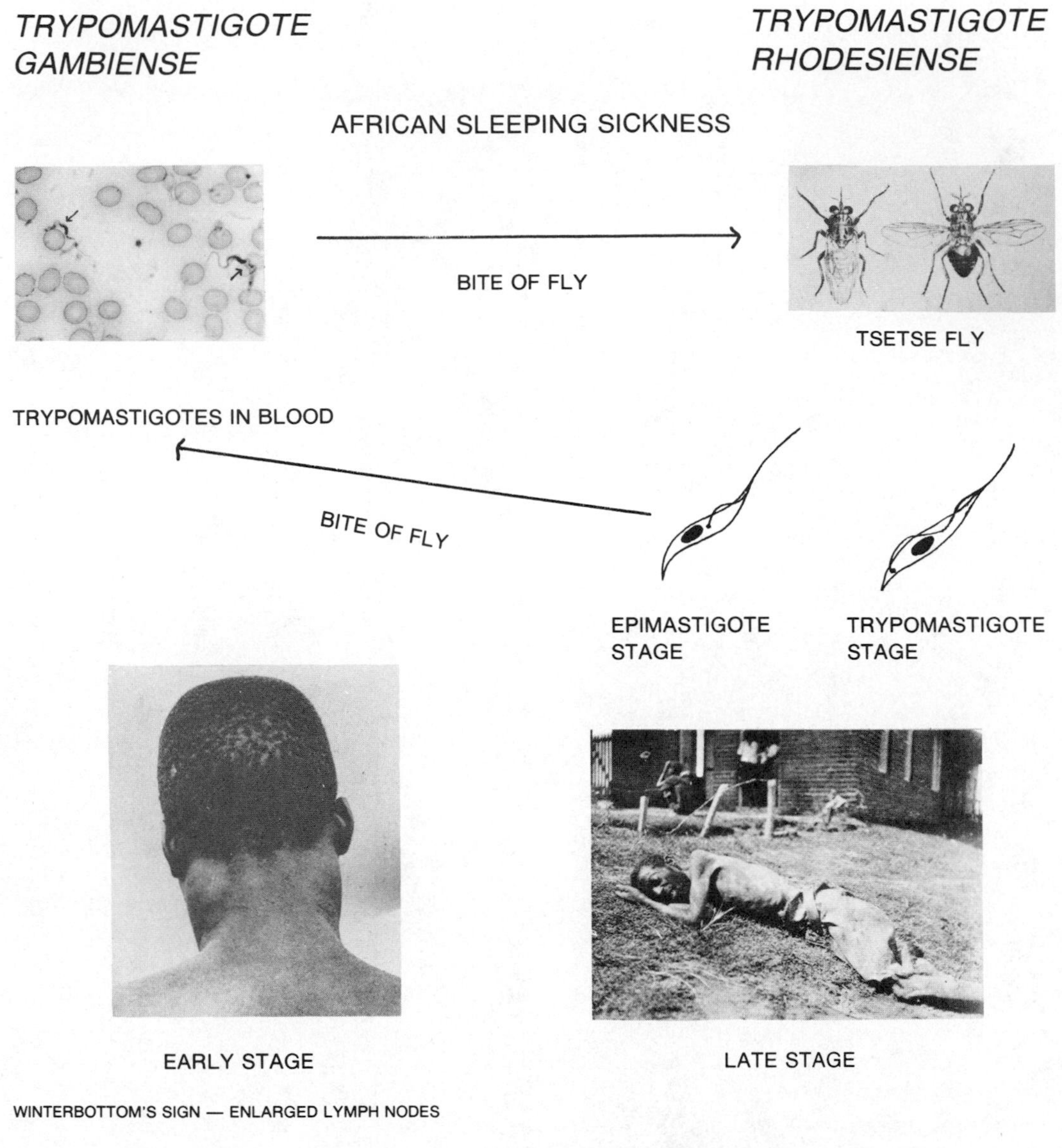

TRYPOMASTIGOTE GAMBIENSE

TRYPOMASTIGOTE RHODESIENSE

AFRICAN SLEEPING SICKNESS

BITE OF FLY

TSETSE FLY

TRYPOMASTIGOTES IN BLOOD

BITE OF FLY

EPIMASTIGOTE STAGE

TRYPOMASTIGOTE STAGE

EARLY STAGE

LATE STAGE

WINTERBOTTOM'S SIGN — ENLARGED LYMPH NODES

Figure 4-3. Life cycle of *Trypanosoma gambiense* and *Trypanosoma rhodesiense.*

proportions, with devastating reductions in population. In recent years the incidence has fallen notably as the result of preventive measures. The disease has disappeared from some old areas and has spread to new ones.

The seasonal incidence is correlated with the distribution and prevalence of the insect vectors. The infection rate is affected by occupation, the proximity of villages, watering places, and trade routes to the habitat of the tsetse flies. Ambulatory carriers in the early stages of the disease provide abundant opportunity for the infection of tsetse flies along trade routes and permanent waterways.

T. gambiense is ordinarily transmitted to humans by the bite of an infected tsetse fly after the cyclic development of the parasite. From a practical standpoint, the disease is spread by a human-fly-human transmission. Infection by mechanical transmission may occur during epidemics when infected individuals and flies are numerous. Occasionally, the disease may be transmitted by coitus and, rarely, congenitally. The percentage of infected flies in endemic areas is only 2 to 4 percent. Their abundance and seasonal incidence are affected by humidity and temperature (optimal 24 to 30 C).

Pathology and Symptomatology. In humans the disease varies in severity from a mild type, with few trypanosomes in the blood (it may be slowly progressive, self-limited, or may revert to serious manifestations) to a severe fulminating type resembling that of *T. rhodesiense.* In the typical case the disease progresses from the acute stage, with trypanosomes multiplying in the blood and lymphatics during the first year, to the chronic sleeping-sickness stage, with invasion of the central nervous system, which starts at the end of the first or the beginning of the second year, and terminates fatally during the second or third year.

At the site of the bite there may be a local inflammatory nodule, or chancre. The incubation period is usually about 14 days but may be delayed for months. The acute disease lasts a year and is characterized by irregular fever, headache, joint and muscle pains, and a rash. There is a slight microcytic anemia, moderate leukocytosis with an increase in the monocytes and lymphocytes, and an increased sedimentation rate. The superficial lymph nodes are enlarged. Winterbottom's sign consists of the enlargement of the postcervical group. The trypanosomes are present in the blood, lymph nodes, and bone marrow. The patient becomes hyperactive.

Gradually the chronic phase of the disease ensues, with the development of characteristic central nervous system changes. There is a perivascular infiltration of endothelial, lymphoid, and plasma cells, leading to ischemic softening of tissues and petechial hemorrhages. A diffuse meningoencephalitis and meningomyelitis develops. The fever and headache now become pronounced. Evidence of nervous impairment becomes prominent with (1) lack of interest and disinclination to work, (2) avoidance of acquaintances, (3) morose and melancholic attitude alternating with exaltation, (4) mental retardation and lethargy, (5)

low and tremulous speech, (6) tremors of tongue and limbs, intention tremors, even choreiform movements, (7) slow and shuffling gait, and (8) altered reflexes. The spinal fluid shows increased protein and cells. The terminal sleeping stage now develops, and gradually the patient becomes more and more difficult to rouse. Death ensues either from the disease or from intercurrent infections, such as malaria, dysentery, and pneumonia, aided by starvation. Prognosis is favorable if treatment is instituted before serious involvement of the nervous system occurs. Untreated infections may progress to a fatal termination or develop into a chronic or latent disease.

Diagnosis. Trypanosomiasis may be suspected when a patient from an endemic area has an acute infection with irregular fever and palpable lymph nodes, particularly in the postcervical triangle, or has developed a chronic disease with somnolence, personality changes, and neurologic symptoms. A definite laboratory diagnosis is made by finding the trypanosomes in the blood, lymph nodes, and bone marrow in the early disease and in the spinal fluid in the late disease, while a presumptive diagnosis is obtained by detecting increases in the cerebrospinal fluid and serum total IgM.

Multiple examinations of thick blood films should be made, since the trypanosomes may be few or present irregularly after the early stages of the disease, and the examination of the centrifuged sediment of 10 to 20 ml of hemolyzed blood is advantageous. The inoculation of laboratory rodents is of limited value. At times trypanosomes may be found in the cerebrospinal fluid.

The protein content and the more sensitive cell count of the spinal fluid, which are indices of the stage of infection, are of therapeutic and prognostic value. For evaluating the results of treatment the disease may be broken down according to the spinal-fluid findings into three stages: (1) early, with normal spinal fluid of under three cells and protein concentration less than 45 mg/100 ml, (2) intermediate, with three to ten cells and protein less than 45 mg/100 ml, and (3) late, with more than 40 cells and protein greater than 45 mg/ 100 ml.

Treatment. The chemotherapy of African sleeping sickness is usually effective when it is begun early in the disease during the blood-lymphatic stage. After the central nervous system becomes involved, therapy is less successful. The available drugs are toxic to humans, and some strains of trypanosomes become resistant to them. Pentamidine isethionate,° 4 mg per kilogram intramuscularly daily for 10 days, or suramin sodium,° 100 to 200 mg test dose intravenously, then 1 gm intravenously on days 1, 3, 7, 14, and 21, is useful during early infection. For late infection with involvement of the central nervous system with either *T. gambiense* or *T. rhodesiense,* melarsoprol° or tryparsamide° is used. Melarsoprol is administered intravenously 2 to 3.6 mg per kilogram daily for 3 doses; after one week, 3.6 mg per kilogram intravenously daily for 3 doses. This may be repeated after 10 and 21 days. Tryparsamide is given as one injection, 30 mg per kilogram intravenously every 5 days to a total of 12 injections, and it can be repeated after one month, in addition to suramin,° one injection intravenously of 10 mg per kilogram every 5 days to a total of 12 injections. It may be repeated after one month.

All these drugs are toxic. Pentamidine can cause hypotension, vomiting, blood dyscrasias, and liver damage. Suramin can cause vomiting, pruritis, urticaria, paresthesia, hyperesthesia of hands and feet, photophobia, peripheral neuropathy, kidney damage (rarely), blood dyscrasia, and shock. Melarsoprol can cause myocardial damage, hypertension, albuminuria, colic, encephalopathy, vomiting, and peripheral neuropathy. Tryparasamide can cause impaired vision, optic atrophy, fever, exfoliative dermatitis, tinnitus, and vomiting. Fortunately, many patients have few or none of these reactions, and without such therapy the disease itself is fatal.

Prevention. Prevention includes pentamidine isethionate° 4 mg per kilogram intramuscularly at 4- to 6-month intervals for Gambian and 2-month intervals for Rhodesian trypanosomiasis, the reduction of sources of infection, the protection of people from infection, and the control of riverine tsetse flies. Chemoprophylaxis and mass treatment have markedly reduced the incidence of Gambian trypanosomiasis in many localities. Successful prophylaxis involves wholesale inoculations, treatment of carriers, persistence of prophylaxis for 4 to 5 years in highly endemic areas, and speedy action to minimize drug resistance.

Exposure to the day-biting riverine species may be lessened by avoidance of streams and waterholes during the warm, dry season, elimination of the flies at watercrossings, restriction of travel in fly-infested regions to nighttime, the use of headnets, leggings, and gloves, and the application of repellents. In some instances, mass removal of local populations from fly-infested areas has proved advantageous, and the spread of the disease may be reduced by border quarantine of infected migrants. The control of the riverine tsetse flies includes the reduction of their habitats and breeding places and their destruction by insecticides and the clearing of stream banks of trees and shrubs.

Trypanosoma rhodesiense

Diseases. Rhodesian trypanosomiasis, East African sleeping sickness.

Life Cycle (Fig. 4-3). Similar to that of *T. gambiense* except in the species of its insect vector. Antelopes and possibly other wild game and domesticated cattle are reservoir hosts. The principal insect vectors are the woodland tsetse flies, *Glossina morsitans, G. pallidipes,* and *G. swynnertoni,* but it is capable of developing in other species. *T. rhodesiense* (Fig. 4-2) is morphologically indistinguishable from *T. gambiense.*

Epidemiology. The incidence of Rhodesian trypanosomiasis is lower and epidemics are less frequent than in the Gambian disease. The disease is endemic among the cattle-raising tribes of East Africa and tends to spread to new territory. It is present in Zimbabwe, Zambia, Malawi, Mozambique, Tanzania, and eastern Uganda. Its endemicity, as well as its geographic distribution, is determined by the woodland habitat of its principal vectors.

The study of reservoir hosts in wild game is complicated by many species' being natural hosts of the pathogenic trypanosomes of domesticated animals. The existence of wildlife reservoirs is indicated by finding infected tsetse flies in areas uninhabited by humans for years and by the acquisition of infection by travelers in areas not traversed by humans for periods exceeding the normal life of this fly. The vector flies feed chiefly upon ungulates and, infrequently, on people.

Pathogenicity. Rhodesian trypanosomiasis runs a more rapid and fatal course than does the Gambian disease, often terminating within a year. The pathologic changes in the acute disease are similar to those of Gambian sleeping sickness, but the febrile paroxysms are more frequent and severe; the glandular enlargement, less pronounced. Edema, myocarditis, weakness, and emaciation are more prominent. Chronic lesions in the central nervous system are less frequently encountered, since death intervenes before marked cerebrospinal changes occur. Thus, while mental disturbances may develop, there are seldom tics, choreic movements, convulsions, or the typical sleeping sickness syndrome. Untreated cases tend to run a fatal course.

Diagnosis. Similar procedures as for *T. gambiense* are called for, except that trypanosomes are more frequently found in the blood and are more readily demonstrated by inoculation into rats or mice.

Treatment. See under Treatment for *T. gambiense.* The Rhodesian disease requires earlier and more intensive treatment than does the Gambian, and suramin is the drug of choice in the early stages of the disease.

Prevention. The prevention of Rhodesian trypanosomiasis involves medical, veterinary, entomologic, agricultural, and social problems arising from the redistribution of populations and the control of vectors. Its control requires constant supervision to detect new cases, to keep track of the old, and to regulate agricul-

ture. The woodland tsetse flies are more difficult to eradicate and control than are the riverine species (see Chap. 15). The detection and treatment of infected persons are the same as for *T. gambiense;* in spite of the scattered foci, the few chronic cases make the task easier. Contact between humans and tsetse flies may be broken by the removal of inhabitants from fly-infested areas to open country in close settlements, by discriminative clearing of bush in essential fly habitats and in the outer fringes of forests, and by spraying insecticides from airplanes. Chemoprophylaxis, repellents, nets, and screens may give some protection to the individual.

Trypanosoma rangeli

T. rangeli is found in Mexico, Central America, and northern South America. Except for the small kinetoplast it may be mistaken for *T. cruzi* in the blood. There is no evidence that it is pathogenic to humans or the many domestic or wild animals it infects. Although *T. rangeli* can circulate in the blood of infected individuals for long periods, unlike *T. cruzi,* it does not invade cells. In fact, where or even whether *T. rangeli* multiplies in the vertebrate host is unknown. This parasite invades the hemolymph and salivary glands of its vector, *Rhodnius prolixus,* or related species, so transmission is through the bite of the bug. In urban areas the reservoir host is humanity's best friend, the dog, and in rural areas monkeys, opossums, and anteaters are common hosts.

Trypanosoma cruzi

Diseases. American trypanosomiasis, Chagas' disease.

Morphology. In the blood the trypanosomes appear either as long, thin flagellates about 20 μ in length or as short, stumpy forms about 15 μ in length, with pointed posterior ends. In stained blood smears they have a U or S shape, a free flagellum about one-third of the body length, a deeply staining central nucleus, and a large kinetoplast (Fig. 4-2). In the tissues the round, intracellular amastigotes are found in small groups of cystlike collections.

Life Cycle. The vertebrate hosts are humans and domesticated and wild animals. At least 28 species of reduviid bugs, of the genera *Panstrongylus, Rhodnius, Eutriatoma,* and *Triatoma,* have been found naturally infected with trypanosomes resembling *T. cruzi,* but the principal vectors are *T. infestans, T. sordida, P. megistus,* and *R. prolixus* (see Chap. 15). Reduviid bugs remain infected as they molt through various stages, probably for life.

After multiplication in the intestine of the reduviid bug as epimastigotes, some parasites transform into infective trypomastigotes that are transmitted to vertebrates by fecal contamination. At night the bugs emerge furtively from cracks in the walls and painlessly extract a blood meal from sleeping people. Since the bugs frequently defecate during or soon after biting, the bite wound is readily contaminated (Fig. 4-4). The sleeping victim may also inadvertently scratch or rub the affected area, thereby transferring parasites from fecal material to ocular and other mucous membranes. Parasites in the blood can be transmitted through blood transfusions. Congenital transmission, another route of infection that does not require the bug as vector, is not unusual.

Epidemiology. Chagas' disease is prevalent throughout South and Central America, where an estimated 10 million persons are infected.

Serologic surveys reveal that as much as 15 to 50 percent of the population is infected in endemic areas. Its prevalence is highest in the rural districts and among the poorer classes living in thatched adobe huts, the walls and ceilings of which offer excellent breeding places for the insect vectors. The acute disease, with parasites in the blood, usually affects children but is often mild and not recognized. Chronic manifestations of the disease are much more common with cardiac and gastrointestinal involvement, occurring in adults later in life. However, chronic Chagas' disease is spotty in its distribution and puzzling in the relative frequency and type of clinical expression. For example, in central and eastern Brazil and northern Argentina, cardiomyopathy is common but mega disease of the esophagus and colon is seen more commonly in Brazil. Chronic Chagasic cardiomyopathy is also present in Chile, Venezuela, and Colombia, but in the latter two countries mega disease seems to be absent. In many of the Latin American countries the real extent of Chagas' disease is unknown. The chronic heart disease also occurs in central America and Mexico, but less commonly and in an older age group than in Brazil.

American trypanosomiasis is clearly a zoonotic infection; i.e., *T. cruzi* is transmitted in nature by sylvatic vectors among a variety of wild rodents and burrowing animals without human participation in the cycle. In those areas where Chagas' disease has become a public health problem, the reason is because certain vectors, such as *T. infestans* and *R. prolixus,* have a great propensity to become adapted to living and breeding in human habitations. Hence, a domiciliary cycle of transmission is established with people as the main reservoir of infection.

T. cruzi has been found in nine species of triatomine bugs and 14 species of mammals in the United States. The distribution covers the southern states from California to Florida and is found as far north as Maryland. Yet only two autochthonous cases of naturally acquired human infection have been recognized, both from Texas. It is possible that some mild infections go unnoticed. Serologic surveys for presence of antibody to the parasite may disclose a few reactors, but such findings are difficult to interpret because false positive reactions occur with about equal frequency. One explanation for the absence of Chagas' disease in the United States is that the vectors are happily sylvatic, living in animal burrows, unwilling or unable to adapt to human dwellings. In addition, whether from politeness or temperament, they tend to be late defecators, depositing their feces well after completing their blood meal, so there is much less chance of contaminative infection.

TRYPOMASTIGOTE CRUZI

CHAGAS' DISEASE

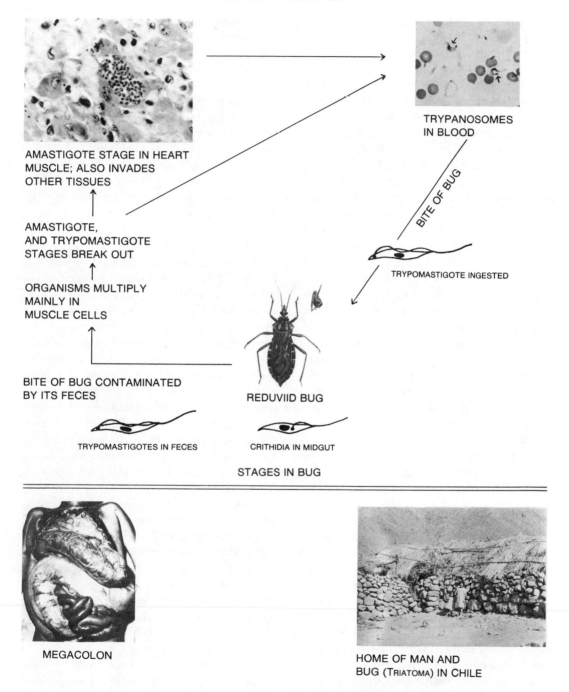

TRYPANOSOMES
IN BLOOD

AMASTIGOTE STAGE IN HEART
MUSCLE; ALSO INVADES
OTHER TISSUES

BITE OF BUG

TRYPOMASTIGOTE INGESTED

AMASTIGOTE,
AND TRYPOMASTIGOTE
STAGES BREAK OUT

ORGANISMS MULTIPLY
MAINLY IN
MUSCLE CELLS

REDUVIID BUG

BITE OF BUG CONTAMINATED
BY ITS FECES

TRYPOMASTIGOTES IN FECES

CRITHIDIA IN MIDGUT

STAGES IN BUG

MEGACOLON

HOME OF MAN AND
BUG (Triatoma) IN CHILE

Figure 4-4. Life cycle of *Trypanosoma cruzi.*

Incidentally, care should be taken in working with *T. cruzi* in the laboratory. There is irony in the fact that more accidental laboratory infections with the parasite have been documented in the United States than naturally acquired cases.

Pathology and Symptomatology. Infective trypanosomes from the bug actively penetrate cells of the mammalian host. After entry into cells they round up and transform into the rounded amastigote forms, undergoing repeated cycles of division until the parasites fill up the cytoplasm of the cell. The amastigotes then transform into flagellate trypanosomes, and after about 5 days the infected cell ruptures, liberating the actively motile trypanosomal forms. Some of these will invade new cells to continue the process of intracellular multiplication, and some find their way to the blood stream, where they circulate. *T. cruzi* can invade and multiply in a variety of cell types, but most strains prefer cardiac, skeletal, and other muscle fibers.

The parasite may initially multiply in cells of the subcutaneous tissue at the site of inoculation, producing a local lesion called the *chagoma*. The individual infected cells remain in good condition until they are finally ruptured by the multiplying parasite. However, after parasites rupture out of the cell there is a prominent inflammatory reaction involving all cell types and local edema. In the early stages of infection, intracellular parasites are readily found in affected tissues, sometimes in large cystlike collections, as well as free trypanosomes in the blood. Glial cells of the central nervous system and meninges can also become infected. As the infection becomes more chronic, intracellular parasites diminish in numbers and trypanosomes can no longer be found in the peripheral blood. Even in those individuals who die with typical manifestations of chronic Chagas' disease, it is usually impossible to demonstrate intracellular organisms in the heart or other tissues, or a few parasites may be found after prolonged search of many serial sections. These chronic cases, however, will generally have a great reduction in numbers of autonomic ganglion cells in the muscle layers of hollow viscera and of the heart. The pathologic changes otherwise in the heart and gut of chronic cases are not very revealing, showing patchy areas of inflammation, fibrosis, and hypertrophy of the organ.

Clinical features of acute Chagas' disease when it does come to medical attention include an incubation period of at least several weeks, fever, and generalized lymphadenopathy. If the portal of entry is the upper face or eye, the unilateral conjunctivitis and orbital edema is called Romaña's sign. Hepatosplenomegaly is common, and there may be a nondescript erythematous rash. Acute disease usually subsides spontaneously, but there can be involvement of the heart with an acute myocarditis, or invasion of the central nervous system with a resultant meningoencephalitis. Either of these manifestations of acute Chagas' disease can be fatal.

But the most common evidence of Chagas' disease are the cardiac and gastrointestinal sequelae that occur many years after initial infection. The factors that determine whether these chronic sequelae will develop in a given infected individual are unknown. An autoimmune mechanism of pathogenesis has been proposed. The heart disease is frequently associated with characteristic conduction disturbances, especially right bundle branch block. Ventricular arrhythmias, demonstrable only by continuous EKG monitoring, are probably responsible for sudden death, which is not unusual in otherwise healthy patients with chronic disease. Other forms of heart involvement are progressive cardiac enlargement, heart failure, and sometimes peripheral emboli from endocardial thrombus formation. Megaesophagus is manifested by substernal discomfort, painful swallowing, progressive dilatation, and hypertrophy of the esophagus with eventual regurgitation of food. The physiologic abnormality responsible for these changes is spasm of the lower esophageal sphincter due to ganglion cell destruction and loss of autonomic function. A similar process, called *megacolon,* can affect the distal alimentary tract, resulting in severe constipation.

Heart and megadisease can occur independently or together. The age at which any form of chronic Chagas' disease develops is variable; in some areas of Brazil victims are frequently in their early twenties, whereas Chagasic cardiomyopathy in Panama is seldom seen before the age of 40.

Diagnosis. The disease may be suspected when general, cardiac, or gastrointestinal symptoms are present in patients who have lived under conditions of economic deprivation in endemic regions. An alert intern in a New York City hospital included Chagas' disease in the differential diagnosis after examining a Colombian male with myocarditis. A serologic test for antibodies to *T. cruzi* was positive by the C.D.C. and radiographs revealed megacolon even though the patient had no gastrointestinal symptoms.

Only in the first month or two of the acute disease can *T. cruzi* be found by direct examination of fresh anticoagulated blood or the centrifuged buffy coat layer or in stained thick blood smears. If parasites are scanty, a better yield can be obtained by culturing the blood or suspected tissue specimen in N.N.N. or other appropriate media. Another method of demonstrating very low concentrations of circulating trypanosomes in the blood is xenodiagnosis. This involves feeding "clean" laboratory-reared reduviid bugs on the patient and examining their intestinal contents later for flagellates. While rather unorthodox, xenodiagnosis is a highly efficient method to demonstrate low-level parasitemia. When a large number of bugs are used, e.g., 30 or 40, xenodiagnosis may be positive in up to 40 percent of patients, even in the chronic stage of Chagas' disease. Unfortunately, this procedure requires a colony of normal bugs. Serologic tests, such as complement-fixation, direct agglutination, and indirect hemagglutination or imunofluorescence, to demonstrate antibodies to *T. cruzi* are required in the diagnosis of Chagas' disease. Such antibodies do not develop until some months after onset of the acute disease, so in this situation they may be absent. However, direct agglutinating antibodies in the IgM fraction would be present even during acute disease. While presence of antibody is needed for diagnosis of chronic Chagas' disease, its presence alone merely indicates that the individual has been infected with the parasite. In addition, diagnosis of chronic Chagas' disease requires exclusion of other known causes of the patient's clinical findings.

Treatment. Treatment is unsatisfactory, since the organisms are within cells in established infections. A nitrofuran derivative, Bayer 2502,° is the best drug currently available, but it is still considered investigational. This drug does have some effect against the intracellular amastigote stages, but it must be used in the acute stage of disease in order to prevent development of chronic disease. When used under these conditions, reversal of serology to negative has been demonstrated. The drug would not be expected to cure established chronic disease. The antimalarial, primaquine, has been recommended by some as being able to destroy bloodstream trypanosomes and, it is hoped, reduce further tissue invasion in the acute stage. It is used in the same dose and duration as for radical cure of relapsing malaria.

Prevention. Preventive measures call for the destruction of the triatomid vectors and the protection of humans from their bites. Since the replacement of unsanitary houses with modern dwellings is economically impractical, the destruction of reduviid bugs in these houses by insecticides seems the best available method of combating the disease. Transfusion-induced infection is a serious hazard in areas of South America where a high proportion of the general population have been infected with *T. cruzi.* Routine addition of gentian violet dye to all blood bottles in a final concentration of .025 percent to kill *T. cruzi* is practiced and is said to be effective.

PARASITIC LEISHMANIA OF HUMAN BEINGS

The genus *Leishmania* includes flagellates that occur as intracellular amastigotes in vertebrate hosts and as flagellate promastigotes in invertebrate hosts and in cultures.

Morphology. The typical leishmanial parasite in the vertebrate host is a small, oval, intracellular organism, 2 to 5 μ by 1 to 3 μ. The organisms are found within phagocytic vacuoles of macrophages and other mononuclear phagocytes. In this form they have no flagellum, and the most conspicuous structure, apart from the nucleus, is a rod-shaped kinetoplast. The kinetoplast is easily recognized by its prominent basophilic staining due to a heavy concentration of DNA. A remarkable feature of the intracellular amastigotes is that they are not only resistant to but apparently thrive in the environment of lysosomal enzymes that are discharged into the macrophage vacuoles they occupy. In cultures or in the invertebrate host, the parasites range in shape from clumps of amastigotes to the more common promastigote flagellates. The latter, equipped with a long, delicate, anterior flagellum, varies from a pyriform to a longer, slender spindle shape, 14 to 20 μ by 1.5 to 4.0 μ (Fig. 4-2).

The motile flagellate has a more active metabolism than the nonmotile amastigote form. Flagellate metabolism is aerobic, can make use of various sugars and requires amino acids and hemin. Reproduction occurs by longitudinal binary division in both the amastigote and the promastigote. *Leishmania* may be cultivated in various noncellular media, such as the diphasic N.N.N. (see Chap. 18) or in completely liquid cultures, where they grow as promastigotes.

Life Cycle. The life cycle involves an alternate existence in a vertebrate and an insect host (Fig. 4-5). The natural reservoir hosts besides humans include the domestic dog and a variety of wild mammals, such as desert or forest rodents and sloths. The invertebrate hosts are sandflies of the genus *Phlebotomus,* which in the Americas has been renamed *Lutzomyia.* There are many species, but only those sandflies that feed on humans are important for human transmission. After parasites within infected cells are ingested with the blood meal they transform into flagellates and multiply in the gut of the insect. In 8 to 20 days the

anterior gut and pharynx are partially blocked by flagellates. When the sandfly attempts a subsequent blood meal, some of the infective promastigotes are dislodged and introduced into the skin. Transmission can also occur by contamination of the bite wound and by contact. Infections have been produced in humans and in experimental animals by injection. When introduced into the tissues the promastigotes gain access to mononuclear phagocytic cells, where they multiply. The rupture of infected cells provides organisms to be phagocytosed by other cells that may spread the infection to other organs or more distant sites, depending upon the infecting species or the immune status of the host.

Temperature is one important factor that may determine localization of leishmanial lesions. The strains of parasites causing cutaneous leishmaniasis cannot grow at core body temperature whereas strains that cause visceral leishmaniasis can do so.

At least four major species of parasites, similar in morphology but differing in cultural characteristics, clinical manifestations, geographic distribution, and sandfly vectors cause disease in humans: (1) *L. donovani,* the etiologic agent of visceral leishmaniasis, or kala-azar, (2) *L. tropica* of Old World cutaneous leishmaniasis, or oriental sore, (3) the *L. braziliensis* complex of cutaneous and mucocutaneous disease in the Americas, and (4) the *L. mexicana* complex associated mainly with cutaneous lesions in the Americas. Within each major group are strains and possibly subspecies with their own distinctive characteristics. A new approach to classification that appears promising is based upon isoenzyme patterns and buoyant density of nuclear and kinetoplast DNA, as well as the serotype of certain antigens. Whatever taxonomic schemes are used for the leishmania, however, a considerable range of clinical involvement in humans may result from infection with a strain of any species depending upon such factors as nutritional state, race, integrity of lymphatic drainage, and, most importantly, host immune response.

Immunity. Malnutrition and debility predispose to visceral leishmaniasis. Recovery from

LEISHMANIA DONOVANI

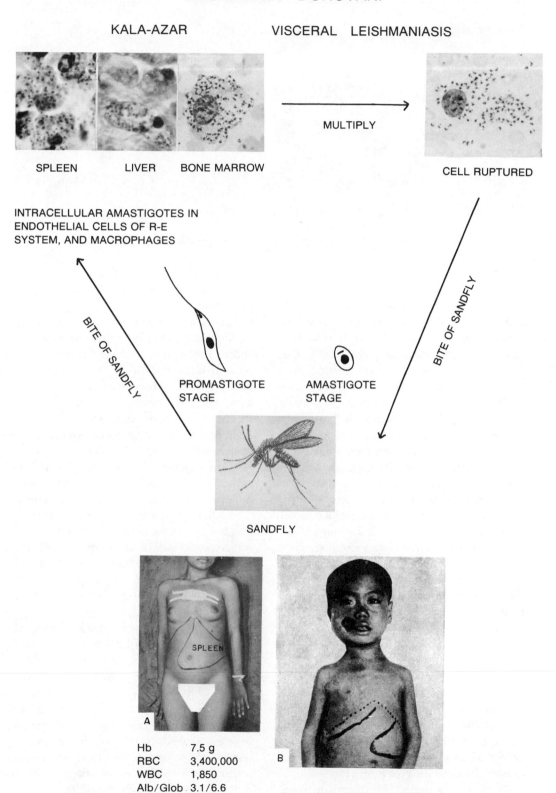

KALA-AZAR   **VISCERAL LEISHMANIASIS**

SPLEEN   LIVER   BONE MARROW

MULTIPLY

CELL RUPTURED

INTRACELLULAR AMASTIGOTES IN
ENDOTHELIAL CELLS OF R-E
SYSTEM, AND MACROPHAGES

BITE OF SANDFLY

BITE OF SANDFLY

PROMASTIGOTE
STAGE

AMASTIGOTE
STAGE

SANDFLY

SPLEEN

A

Hb   7.5 g
RBC   3,400,000
WBC   1,850
Alb/Glob 3.1/6.6

B

Figure 4-5. Life cycle of *Leishmania donovani*. A. Diagnosed by sternal puncture. B.
Cancrum oris and enlargement of liver and spleen. (Photograph from China.)

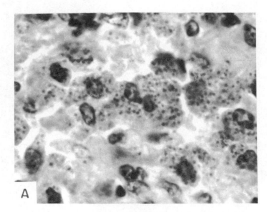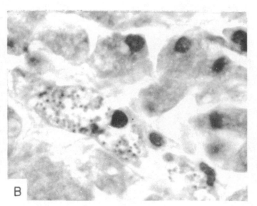

Figure 4-6. *Leishmania donovani.* A. Spleen (× 900). B. Liver (× 950).

kala-azar and oriental sore gives lasting immunity to the homologous disease, but probably no cross protection. Deliberate scarification of extremities with material from human lesions was once practiced in the Middle East to prevent scarring that might result from a later natural infection of the face. The presence of delayed-type skin reactivity to promastigote antigens in a patient with leishmanial infection is generally indicative of a normal immune response. Such skin tests are negative during active visceral leishmaniasis but become positive with recovery. Most patients with cutaneous disease have positive skin tests of the delayed type. Humoral antibodies can usually be demonstrated in the serums of patients with leishmaniasis with various serologic tests. Yet, from clinical observations and from an increasing body of experimental studies it appears that cell-mediated immune reactions are of primary importance in recovery from disease.

Leishmania donovani

Diseases. Kala-azar, or black disease; visceral leishmaniasis; dumdum fever.

In mammalian tissues *L. donovani* is a small, intracellular, nonflagellated oval body of uniform size—4.2 by 2.8 μ (Figs. 4-2 and 4-6). In the gut of infected sandflies or in cultures, it assumes the promastigote form (Fig. 4-2).

Life Cycle (Fig. 4-5). The important insect vectors are sandflies, *Phlebotomus* or *Lutzomyia.*

In addition to humans, the dog is the most important host.

Epidemiology. There are three main epidemiologic pattens: (1) the classic kala-azar of India, which affects chiefly adults, does not occur in dogs, and has no nonhuman reservoir host; (2) the Mediterranean or infantile kala-azar, which is sporadic in children throughout the Mediterranean countries, China, Middle Asia, and Central and South America, occurs frequently in dogs, and has wild reservoir hosts in jackals and possibly foxes in Middle Asia and wild dogs in South America; and (3) Sudanese kala-azar, which affects adults, is somewhat resistant to antimony treatment, and has rats as the reservoir. In Kenya ground squirrels and gerbils are reservoirs. All strains causing visceral leishmaniasis produce a similar disease in hamsters, and appear to belong to a common group on the basis of the new biochemical taxonomy.

Age, sex, and general resistance apparently affect susceptibility. In Mediterranean Europe the infection is chiefly confined to children; in Middle Asia it is rare in those over 10 years of age; in China about one-third of the infections are in children under 10 years; and in Brazil about half of the cases occur in children under 6 years. Males acquire the disease more frequently than females. Its incidence is highest in rural areas and in surroundings where conditions are favorable for sandflies.

Humans and domestic dogs are the chief

sources of infection. The disease is transmitted from human to human or from dog to dog to human by various species of *Phlebotomus*. A well-documented infection in a female who had never been out of England showed that transmission by venereal contact is possible. Her husband had been infected in 1941 when serving in Africa and was inadequately treated. They married in 1953, and in 1955 the wife developed a vaginal lesion which, after much confusion, was eventually found to contain leishmania and was correctly diagnosed. A positive lymph-node biopsy in the husband was then found with a culture of the organisms. A post–kala-azar skin lesion in the husband was undoubtedly the source of infection.

Pathology and Symptomatology. A primary lesion at the site of infection is rarely observed, but minute papules have been described in infants, and in Africa dermal lesions of the legs can occur (leishmaniomas). The phagocytosed parasites are present only in small numbers in the blood, but they are numerous in the reticuloendothelial cells of the spleen, liver, lymph nodes, bone marrow, intestinal mucosa, and other organs (Fig. 4-6), and there is marked hyperplasia of the reticular cells.

The incubation period is usually 1 to 4 months, but it can be much longer. The initial fever, which lasts from 2 to 4 weeks, is usually intermittent, with a daily rise to 102 to 104 F (39 to 40 C). Sometimes there is a pathognomonic double daily rise. Chills and sweating may be present, and the patient may present a septic picture similar to tuberculosis, endocarditis, or brucellosis. Diarrhea and dysentery are not uncommon and are related to heavy intestinal infection. Despite these symptoms, the patient has a good appetite, and toxemia is absent. Later there is considerable weight loss and emaciation. The spleen gradually enlarges, owing to the enormous increase of reticuloendothelial cells, many of which are heavily parasitized. This may be the first evidence of the disease (Fig. 4-6A). Likewise, the liver may be enlarged, owing to proliferation of the Küpffer cells, which contain parasites. Serum glutamic oxalacetic transaminase is in-

creased. Amyloid degeneration of renal glomeruli is found at autopsy.

A marked leukopenia with a relative monocytosis and lymphocytosis, anemia, and thrombocytopenia develop. The anemia is due to a reduced red cell life span and a mild degree of ineffective erythropoiesis. The plasma proteins undergo marked changes, with a reversal of the albumin to globulin ratio due largely to the elevation in the gamma globulins of a polyclonal nature.

Skin changes develop as the disease continues and may consist of darkly pigmented erythematous, granulomatous areas with numerous parasites, or hypopigmented areas with few parasites. Sometimes visceral disease may be arrested spontaneously or by treatment, with development of nodular skin lesions containing many organisms, a condition called *post–kala-azar dermal leishmaniasis*.

General debility and leukopenia render the patient especially susceptible to secondary infection, e.g., cancrum oris, noma, pulmonary infections, and gastrointestinal complications. The untreated disease usually progresses to a fatal termination within 2 years, although fulminating infections may cause death within a few weeks, and, alternatively, chronic infections may persist for years. The clinical manifestations of the disease have been regarded as an expression of the breakdown in the parasite-host relationship due to failure of an adequate immune response.

Diagnosis. In endemic areas, kala-azar may be suspected in a patient who has a persistent, irregular, or remittent fever, often with a double daily peak, leukopenia, and splenomegaly. Absolute diagnosis is made by finding the parasite in material from blood and tissues by smear, culture, or inoculation of animals. In untreated patients the blood is usually examined first by smear or, preferably, by culture. If the result is negative, sternal, splenic, hepatic, or lymph-node punctures are performed. Splenic puncture reveals the highest percentage of positive findings and is the method of choice in skilled hands, but sternal and hepatic puncture, although less certain, are safer procedures. When the parasites are relatively few, multiple cultures in N.N.N. medium of splenic or hepatic material give the most reliable results.

Fluorescent antibody and other serologic tests are used but are not in themselves diagnostic. The presence of elevated serum globulin levels can be a helpful clue to kala-azar; these were formerly detected by formol-gel and other nonspecific floccidation tests.

Treatment. Patients require bedrest during the acute disease, as well as a well-balanced high-protein and high-vitamin diet, good nursing care, and auxillary treatment with appropriate antibiotics for secondary bacterial infections, such as bronchopneumonia, diarrhea, and cancrum oris. Preliminary blood transfusions should be given to patients with severe anemia, edema, or bleeding from the mucous membranes. Systemic chemotherapy includes the antimonials or aromatic diamidines. The pentavalent antimonials are the standard chemotherapeutic agents. Sodium antimony gluconate° (stibogluconate),° 600 mg intramuscularly or intravenously daily for 6 to 10 days, may be repeated in resistant cases. Pentamidine isethionate,° 2 to 4 mg per kilogram intramuscularly daily for up to 15 doses, should be used for failures with antimony.

Prevention. The treatment of infected persons and the elimination of diseased dogs will reduce the sources of infection. Sandflies may be controlled by the destruction of their breeding grounds near human habitations and by the use of insecticides, particularly the residual spraying of houses with DDT (see Chap. 15). Human beings can be protected by compactly built houses with fine mesh screening and by repellents.

Leishmania tropica

Diseases. Oriental sore, Delhi ulcer, Aleppo, Delhi or Baghdad boil, cutaneous leishmaniasis.

The amastigote (Fig. 4-5) and the promastigote (Fig. 4-5) parasites are indistinguishable from those of *L. donovani.* In smears from the cutaneous lesions, amastigotes may be observed intracellularly in mononuclear phagocytic cells, or extracellularly when released by the rupture of these cells.

There are two clinico-epidemiologic types of oriental sore due to different strains: (1) the dry or urban type, which runs a chronic course with late ulceration, and (2) the moist or rural type, which has an acute course with early ulceration and exudation.

Life Cycle. The reservoir hosts for the moist type are gerbils and other wild rodents. Experimental infections have been produced in mice, hamsters, rats, dogs, and monkeys, but results vary from strain to strain and according to the genetic background of animals. The insect vectors are species of *Phlebotomus.*

Epidemiology. Oriental sore is endemic in Asia Minor and in Middle and Southwest Asia; it is prevalent to a lesser extent in North and West Africa and Mediterranean Europe. The incidence of oriental sore is high in some endemic regions, such as the Dead Sea area of Jordan, Iraq, and Iran, and the southern part of the Soviet Union bordering Asia Minor. At times the disease may even assume an epidemic form. Experimentally, infections have been transmitted cyclically by *P. papatasii* after feeding on cultures or lesions, and mechanically by the bite of the stable fly, *Stomoxys calcitrans,* and by the contamination of wounds with infective material from insects or lesions. The moist type is transmitted from gerbil to human being and from person to person by sandflies in rural areas. The infection rate, which remains constant during the year in gerbils because of the optimal conditions in their burrows, explains the high incidence in humans in isolated settlements during the seasons when sandflies attack humans. Dogs and foxes also harbor the infection.

Pathology and Symptomatology. In humans the disease is limited to the cutaneous tissues and occasionally to the mucous membranes. The difference between the moist and dry types is quantitative rather than qualitative. In the infected area there is hypertrophy of the corium and cellular infiltration of the dermal layers with epithelioid and lymphoid elements. The parasites are found intracellularly in macrophages and histiocytes. The infiltrative stage is followed by a papular or nodular stage with dilated and anastomosing capillaries and a prominent infiltrate of mononuclear cells. Ulceration of the epithelium finally results secondarily to anoxia from the infiltrate or perhaps from an immunopathologic reaction. The neighboring satellite lesions, which have a tuberculoid structure with few or no parasites, may be a hypersensitivity reaction.

The usual incubation period varies from at least 1 or 2 weeks to several months, but periods as long as 3 years have been recorded in experimental infections. The small initial papule continues to enlarge, acquires a glazed purplish appearance, and becomes covered with brown scales. After a period of weeks it becomes an indurated, crusted ulcer that discharges a thin, offensive pus. Single or multiple lesions may occur at the site of sandfly biting, but additional metastatic lesions may form, as well as one or more subcutaneous nodules proximal to an ulcer, as with sporotrichosis. Secondary bacterial infection of lesions is possible, but generally systemic signs and symptoms are absent in cutaneous leishmaniasis. Uncomplicated sores heal in 2 to 10 months but leave depigmented retracted scars, which are often disfiguring (Fig. 4-7). A disseminated disease with multiple nodular lesions containing abundant parasites in vacuolated macrophages has been described in Ethiopia. This is due to anergy to leishmanial antigens rather than infection with a different parasite.

Diagnosis. The type of lesion, with elevated and indurated margin of the ulcer, is a helpful feature. Amastigotes with the characteristic kinetoplast may be seen in impression smears of biopsied tissues or scrapings of the lesion edges. But culture of the organisms from lesions is preferable for diagnosis. A delayed intradermal reaction to an *L. tropica* antigen becomes positive within several months after appearance of the lesion and remains positive for years. Generally, 90 percent or more of cases show tests with induration and erythema of 5 mm or more in diameter.

Treatment. Healing without chemotherapy can occur, but it requires many months. Nonspecific measures, such as local heat and cleanliness to prevent secondary infection, contribute to spontaneous healing. Treatment of choice, however, is pentavalent antimony, sodium stibogluconate, 10 mg per kilogram per day (maximum 600 mg) intramuscularly for 6 to 10 days. Pentavalent antimonials are much less toxic than trivalent, so a second or even a third course of treatment can be given

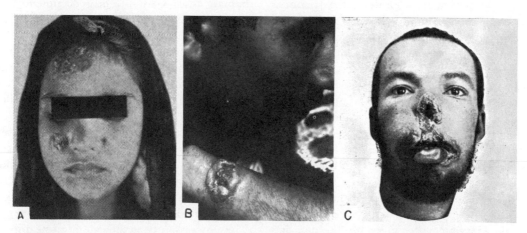

Figure 4-7. Dermal and mucocutaneous leishmaniasis. A. Lesions on forehead, right and left cheek. (Courtesy of Dr. H. K. Giffen, American Mission Hospital, Assiut, Egypt.) B. Lesion on arm. (Courtesy of Army Medical Museum.) C. Mucocutaneous form. (From Strong: Stitt's Diagnosis, Prevention and Treatment of Tropical Diseases, 7th ed., 1944. Courtesy of The Blakiston Co.)

over 6 to 8 weeks if healing is not progressive. Depending upon the site and size of the lesion, local infiltration, instead of systemic therapy, may be tried. Poor response to usual treatment has been noted in some localities, e.g., in Iraq; recourse to drugs used in American leishmaniasis may be required.

Leishmania mexicana *and* Leishmania braziliensis *complexes*

Diseases. American leishmaniasis, mucocutaneous leishmaniasis, espundia, uta and chiclero ulcer. (Fig. 4-7C)

Cutaneous leishmaniasis in the Americas separates into two nosologic varieties, each represented by a group or complex of parasites with common biologic and biochemical properties. They are (1) the *L. mexicana* complex, parasites that cause mainly cutaneous lesions in humans, tend to grow well in culture, but produce prominent metastatic lesions when inoculated into hamsters, and (2) the *L. braziliensis* complex, parasites that are also capable of causing mucocutaneous lesions in humans, grow relatively poorly in culture, and have low virulence for hamsters. Isolates representative of these two complexes can also be distinguished on the basis of buoyant density of their kinetoplast DNA and isoenzyme patterns. The issue of classification is confusing because some authorities use a trinomial system of nomenclature. Therefore, within the *L. braziliensis* complex strains may be referred to as *L. braziliensis braziliensis, L. b. panamensis,* etc. While these characteristics, especially those of growth in culture, of the two broad groups of leishmania causing cutaneous disease are generally consistent, some discrepancies are observed. *L. braziliensis* from Panama, for example, can be cultivated reasonably well; further variables may result from lack of standardized culture media.

Life Cycle. The vectors for all human leishmania in the New World are sandflies of the genus *Lutzomyia.* After ingestion, the parasites transform to promastigotes and multiply in the gut of the fly. The level of the gut, i.e., anterior, mid, or hind, at which most promastigotes multiply may be of significance. No special morphologic features have been found to distinguish those forms that are infective for the vertebrate host. Certain features of the parasite-vector relationship, such as large numbers of promastigotes at various levels in the gut, but no particular concentration in mouth parts, have made it difficult to be certain about the way the parasite is transferred to the vertebrate host. Experts believe that parasites are regurgitated into the bite wound rather than injected; others think that infected flies may be swatted and squashed so that the parasites are rubbed into bite sites secondarily to pain and the irritation of biting flies. In contrast to *Phlebotomus* vectors for Old World leishmanial strains, there seems to be no specificity of New World parasites for American sandflies; they can develop in various species of *Lutzomyia.* Animal reservoir hosts are mainly various species of forest rodents, marsupials, and, only occasionally, the domestic dog. The skin of reservoir hosts from which parasites are readily cultured, such as the nose, ear, or base of the tail, is often normal in appearance or only slightly altered.

Epidemiology. Organisms of the *L. mexicana* and *L. braziliensis* complexes are distributed mainly from the Yucatan peninsula of Mexico into Central and South America, except for Chile and Argentina. Several autochthonous human cases were recently documented in south-central Texas, and an unusual new focus has been found in the Dominican Republic. The Caribbean is otherwise free of leishmaniasis. The disease is a zoonosis, with jungle or forest animal reservoir hosts. Only in the Peruvian Andes, where the disease is called *uta,* is the domestic dog known to be a reservoir. Activities in clearing land and agricultural, recreational, or industrial pursuits bring humans into contact with infected sandflies. Leishmaniasis was common in workers building the trans-Amazon highway and in soldiers taking jungle military training in Panama. The proportion of sandflies that are captured and found infected with flagellates presumed to be leishmania varies from a fraction of 1 up to 10 percent; usually the rate is around 1 percent. It should be remembered, however, that some of these flagellates in the gut of sandflies may be animal trypanosomes or leishmania of lizards that are not necessarily pathogenic for humans.

Pathology and Symptomatology. The clinical appearance and histopathology of American cutaneous leishmaniasis are identical to that of oriental sore, except that it may produce later mucous membrane involvement. The initial lesion at the bite site is a papule that later develops into an indolent ulcer with elevated indurated edges. The location of lesions may be distinctive, e.g., the chiclero ulcer that erodes the pinna of the ear in forest workers who gather chicle gum. That organisms can metastasize is evidenced by the development of nearby satellite lesions or subcutaneous nodules in a linear drainage pattern. Regional adenopathy is common.

A variable proportion of patients, fortunately a minority, of those with cutaneous lesions later develop mucous membrane involvement. Rarely, the mucosal lesion may be the initial one. The mucocutaneous form is much more likely with infections caused by the *L. braziliensis* complex of organisms, occurring in jungle areas of Brazil, Venezuela, Bolivia, and Ecuador. The mucosal lesions are painful and can cause great deformity, with erosion of the nasal septum, palate, or larynx. Edema, tissue destruction, and secondary bacterial infection can combine to produce considerable mutilation of the face. The form of disease with mucosal features is called *espundia.* In Mexico and in most of Central America the causative strains belong to the *L. mexicana* complex and seem less likely to cause mucous membrane lesions.

Disseminated cutaneous leishmaniasis, or the diffuse type, is an unusual form of the disease characterized clinically by multiple nodular lesions, resistance to chemotherapy, and anergy to leishmanin skin-test antigen. The diffuse disease has been reported as isolated cases from a number of Latin American countries, but it has been best described in Venezuela. It also has been reported from Ethiopia and, more recently, from the Dominican Republic of the Caribbean. The non-ulcerating chronic skin lesions resemble those of lepromatous leprosy. The organism causing the diffuse form of leishmaniasis was initially thought to represent a unique variety of parasite, but it is now felt that the disease can be caused by any cutaneous strain of parasite. The basic abnormality for disseminated cutaneous leishmaniasis is failure of immune response, manifested by a negative delayed hypersensitivity skin test.

Diagnosis. In clinical appearance leishmaniasis must be differentiated from other chronic skin diseases, such as nonspecific or bacterial tropical ulcers, sporotrichosis, atypical mycobacterioses, yaws, and syphilis. South American blastomycosis may resemble mucocutaneous leishmaniasis. Every attempt should be made to establish a specific diagnosis by demonstration of organisms in lesions, by smear or, preferably, by culture. For smears or cultures material can be aspirated or scraped from the edge of lesions. However, the likelihood of demonstrating organisms from a fragment of biopsied tissue is best. If a biopsy is done, a portion of tissue should be fixed and submitted for histologic examination. Organisms can often be demonstrated in tissue sections also. Parasites are more numerous in early than in late lesions. A positive intradermal Montenegro test using antigen from cultured promastigotes may be helpful as confirmatory evidence of cutaneous leishmaniasis. But since the delayed-type skin test remains positive indefinitely, the reaction can indicate a past infection.

Treatment. Pentavalent antimony as sodium antimony gluconate,° 600 mg intramuscularly daily for 10 days, is the recommended treatment. Two, and sometimes even three, courses of antimony may be needed. In the most resistant cases Amphotericin B is used, 0.25 to 1 mg per kilogram intravenously, daily or every other day, for a total dosage of 1.0 to 2.5 gm for adults. Amphotericin is toxic; cortisone is often given concurrently with each dose to control fever, and hemoglobin and renal function must be monitored. Although not available in the United States, cycloguanil pamoate, a repository injectable drug is reasonably effective for situations in which frequent visits to a clinic are impractical.

Prevention. Preventive measures include protection against sandflies (see Chap. 15) and avoidance of contact infection. Infected persons should be treated, and the lesions should be protected from sandflies. Protection of forest workers is a difficult problem. Immunization with a killed promastigote vaccine has been tried in Israel, but results are inconclusive.

PNEUMOCYSTIS: A PATHOGENIC TISSUE PARASITE

Pneumocystis carinii

P. carinii, an extracellular organism that causes an interstitial plasma cell pneumonia, is presently classed as a protozoan, although its taxonomic status is uncertain.

Morphology and Life Cycle. Because the organism can only be cultured for short periods in vitro, classification of *Pneumocystis* is based mainly on morphology of the parasite from involved tissues. Several morphologic forms have been described. One is a unicellular, pleomorphic form usually 1 to 2 μ in diameter, but ranging up to 5 μ, that some refer to as a *trophozoite.* More characteristic, however, is a spherical or crescentic, thick-walled structure, 6 to 8 μ in diameter, called a *cyst.* Small intracystic bodies, 1 to 2 μ in size and termed *sporozoites,* may sometimes be seen within the cysts. From observations during short-term culture of *Pneumocystis* in chick lung epithelial cells, attachment to but not invasion of host cells by the parasite was prominent. The exact type of multiplication of the organism is unknown. A similar or identical organism to that found in humans can be recovered from the lungs of rats given cortisone or from nude mice inoculated with material from infected humans or rats. Organisms are abundant in the pulmonary exudate; hence, transmission is probably by droplet to close contacts. Such contact transmission has been shown with rat *Pneumocystis.*

Epidemiology. Pneumocystis infection is cosmopolitan in humans, rodents, and dogs and several other domestic animals. In humans clinical infections are more common in infants than in adults. Institutional epidemics of fatal pneumonia have been described in premature and malnourished infants. When found clinically in older children and adults, this infection is usually associated with hypogammaglobulinemia, debilitating diseases such as leukemia, Hodgkin's disease, or other malignancies, or administration of immunosuppressive drugs. Its relationship to use of corticosteroids, especially in large doses, is particularly striking, suggesting that *Pneumocystis* is an opportunist, smouldering in the body asymptomatically. Even allowing for age and type of patient populations served, the frequency of this disease can vary considerably.

Pathology and Symptomatology. The lungs are firm and the cut surfaces are gray and airless. Microscopically, the most striking change is the thickened alveolar septa, infiltrated with plasma cells—hence the name, "interstitial plasma cell pneumonia." The alveolar epithelium is partly desquamated, and the alveoli are filled with fat-laden cells, parasites and foamy, vacuolated material. The presence of *Pneumocystis* within the alveoli may be suspected but can be identified with certainty only with the use of special stains. With appropriate treatment the alveolar exudate (Fig. 4-8) can be completely resorbed. The organisms are found only in the lungs.

With the infantile disease associated with malnutrition, onset is insidious over weeks with poor feeding; there is failure to thrive, leading finally to a rapid respiratory rate of up to 100 respirations per minute, and cyanosis. The disease in immunosuppressed children and adults has a rapid onset over a few days, associated with fever, rapid respirations, nonproductive cough, and cyanosis. In both types, rales are not heard in the chest and radiographs show a diffuse infiltrate that is usually bilateral and often has a "ground-glass" appearance. The arterial oxygen tension (PO_2) is low, and the carbon dioxide tension (Pco_2) is normal or low. Death is due to asphyxia.

Diagnosis. In outbreaks or epidemics the ep-

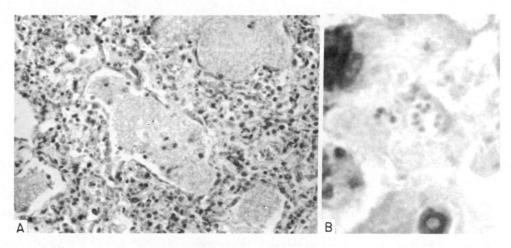

Figure 4-8. *Pneumocystis carinii* in lungs. A. Note "ground-glass" appearance of exudate and interstitial plasma cells (× 250). B. Organism showing 8 daughter cells (× 2000).

idemiologic circumstances associated with radiographic appearance of interstitial pneumonia suggests pneumocystosis. More commonly, *P. carinii* pneumonia occurs sporadically. So the diagnosis should be suspected when an immunosuppressed person or one on large doses of steroids develops fever and characteristic pneumonitis that cannot otherwise be explained. For specific diagnosis, *P. carinii* must be demonstrated in affected lung tissue or pulmonary secretions. This is most reliably done with a specimen obtained by surgical open-lung biopsy for tissue imprints and tissue sections. Bronchoscopy to obtain specimens by brush-biopsy and lung puncture by needle aspiration have been used; tracheal aspirates have been used as well. The success of the latter techniques varies with the skill and experience of the operator, but the methods are generally not as dependable as is open-lung biopsy. Toluidine blue or methenamine-silver stains are needed to identify the thick-walled cysts. Serologic tests for antibody to *P. carinii*, and even demonstration of antigen in the serum, are not yet sufficiently specific and reliable to diagnose active disease.

Treatment. Two different chemotherapeutic agents are effective, although mortality is still considerable. The treatment of choice is the fixed combination of trimethoprim-sulfamethoxazole (Bactrim),° 120 mg per kilogram per day, every 6 hours for 14 days for both adults and children. An equally effective but much more toxic drug is pentamidine isethionate,° which must be given intramuscularly for 12 to 14 days. Supportive measures are important, e.g., oxygen and antibiotics, if indicated. In certain groups of patients and in some institutions where the risk of *P. carinii* pneumonia is high, prophylaxis has been successful with trimethoprim and sulfamethoxazole, 150 and 750 mg per square meter per day, respectively, divided into two equal doses at 12-hour intervals. This chemoprophylaxis has been continued in some patients for up to 2 years.

Genus Babesia

The *Babesia* are sporozoan parasites of the red blood cell that have only recently been found to cause human infections. *B. microti* is a species in New England that has caused both sporadic and epidemic cases in humans of a febrile illness associated with hemolysis. There are multiple species of *Babesia*, such as *B. bigemina*, which was shown by Smith and Kilborne to be the cause of Texas cattle fever in 1893. This discovery was one of the first examples of microbial transmission by an arthropod vector (see Chap. 16).

Morphology and Life Cycle. B. microti appear as small rings within the red cell, very much like *P. falciparum*, with a darkly staining nucleus and very little cytoplasm. In contrast to malaria parasites, *Babesia* have no associated pigment in the red cell. The morphology of different species is variable, some may be pear-shaped, with pointed ends in contact, or in fours like a Maltese cross. Asexual multiplication by binary fission occurs in the red cell, with production of merozoites to invade new cells; there are no known sexual stages. When taken up by the tick, there is a complex cycle of multiplication, resulting ultimately in the presence of the parasite in salivary glands. The parasite is transmitted transovarially and from stage to stage in the tick.

Epidemiology. People are accidental hosts when activity brings them into the usual animal-tick cycle and when an infected tick finds the person an acceptable host. Even with appropriate exposure to infected ticks, humans are not susceptible to some species of *Babesia* unless the spleen is absent. Four fatal cases of babesiosis, due to several different species, have been reported in humans who had been splenectomized for various reasons. During the summer of 1975 the genteel vacation atmosphere of affluent Nantucket Island was shattered by an outbreak of babesiosis among five of its inhabitants. A few sporadic cases had occurred earlier and there were some later cases on Martha's Vineyard and nearby coastal islands, including Long Island. The species of parasite in New England is *B. microti,* which has been commonly found in voles and field mice. The vector is the tick *Ixodes dammini,* normally feeding on wild deer in the adult stage. In contrast to other species, *B. microti* is able to cause disease in individuals with intact spleens. The New England cases have virtually all been in people over 40 years of age. Serologic studies suggest that some infections may be inapparent or unrecognized, and hence they may be transmitted by transfusion to others.

Pathology and Symptomatology. Babesiosis is basically a hemolytic anemia, associated with fever, weakness, jaundice, and hepatosplenomegaly. In patients with intact spleens up to 25 percent of the red cells can be parasitized, and in those without spleens the parasitemia is higher. The hemolytic process probably involves other mechanisms besides simple rupture of red cells by parasites. The incubation period is often difficult to determine and can probably be prolonged, but in those instances where exposure could be established, it was about 7 to 16 days.

Diagnosis and Treatment. A history of exposure to ticks and residence in endemic areas are helpful in suggesting the possibility of babesiosis. Diagnosis of active infection can only be made by demonstrating the parasites in the blood, by stained smears, or by inoculation of 1 to 2 ml of blood into a hamster. Unless babesiosis is suspected, parasites in the blood smear are likely to be called malaria. The IFA test may be helpful in identifying recent past infections when parasitemia is no longer present. The duration that IFA antibodies remain elevated is not known.

Because the parasite invades the red cell and resembles malaria, chloroquine has been given to treat babesiosis. However, a critical examination of the literature discloses no evidence of its effectiveness. Persistence of parasitemia has been documented in several patients with *B. microti* infection after a week or more of chloroquine treatment, and the drug is without effect in experimental infections of the hamster. Berenil and pentamidine show some effect in experimental *B. microti* infections, and several cases have responded to pentamidine in a dose of 4 mg per kilogram daily for 10 days. But these drugs are toxic and their possible benefit must be carefully weighed against risk. Individuals do recover spontaneously, so supportive treatment may be all that is needed in most cases. In patients desperately ill with very high parasitemia, exchange transfusion may be lifesaving.

MALARIA PARASITES OF HUMAN BEINGS

Genus Plasmodium. The malarial parasites of humans are species of the genus *Plasmodium* of the class SPOROZOA in which the asexual cycle (schizogony) takes place in the red blood cells of vertebrates and the sexual cycle (sporogony) in mosquitoes. The members of this genus, which cause malaria in mammals and birds, have closely similar morphology and life cycles.

Diseases. Malaria, paludism, intermittent fever, chills and fever, Roman fever, Chagres fever, marsh fever, tropical fever, coastal fever, and ague. The term *malaria* is derived from two Italian words, *mal* (bad) and *aria* (air). Hippocrates divided miasmic fevers into continuous, quotidian, tertian, and quartan types, the last three being attributed to malaria. Legend, or possibly history, suggests that in 1638 the Countess d'El Chinchon, wife of the Viceroy of Peru, was cured of malaria by the bark of certain trees, later called cinchona, from which the material quinine was found to be extractable.

Species. P. *malariae* was described in 1880 by Laveran; P. *vivax* was named in 1890 by Grassi and Feletti; P. *falciparum* in 1897 by Welch; and P. *ovale* in 1922 by Stephens. In 1898 Ross published a description of the sporogony of the avian species P. *relictum* in culicine mosquitoes. About the same time Grassi *et al.* reported a similar sexual cycle in P. *falciparum* in anopheline mosquitoes. Yet it was not until 1948 that Shortt *et al.* demonstrated the exoerythrocytic cycle of human malaria. Monkeys are naturally infected with various species of malaria parasites, some of which are capable of infecting humans. Asian species of simian malaria are probably the ancestors of human malaria, while European explorers in the Americas were the likely source of the malaria found in New World monkeys.

Morphology. The diagnostic morphology of the human plasmodia as seen in blood smears stained by Giemsa or Wrights is shown in the color plates found between p. 84 and p. 85. Some general characteristics are common to all malaria parasites, but differential features make it possible to identify species. The earliest form after invasion of the red cell is a ring of bluish cytoplasm with a dotlike nucleus of red chromatin. As this early stage, the *trophozoite,* grows the erythrocyte hemoglobin is metabolized to produce a darkly staining malarial pigment, hemozoin. Depending upon the species of parasite, the cytoplasm may become irregular in shape, and the red cell may show pink granules. When the growing parasite divides, it is called a *schizont,* showing multiple masses of nuclear chromatin. Some of the trophozoites develop into *gametocytes,* or sexual stages, which are differentiated by compact cytoplasm and the absence of nuclear division. In endemic areas, mixed infections with two or more species are encountered, depending upon the local prevalence of infecting species. The most common combination is P. *vivax* and P. *falciparum;* infection with three species is very rare.

The number of parasites observed in the peripheral blood, or parasite density, varies with the species. P. *falciparum* gives the highest parasitemia, at times infecting 10 to 40 percent of the red blood cells. The different species of malaria parasites have a predilection for red blood cells of certain ages. P. *vivax* and P. *ovale* prefer to invade young red cells, P. *malariae* has an affinity for mature or older red cells, while P. *falciparum* infects cells of all ages. Further morphologic features of the different malaria species are summarized below, while differential characteristics of clinical significance are outlined in Table 4-2.

PLASMODIUM VIVAX (see color plate). The infected red cell is enlarged, but this may be partly explained by affinity of the parasite for the larger reticulocytes. As the signet-ring–appearing trophozoite grows, it becomes irregular in shape, with ameboid extensions of the cytoplasm. At about this point Schüffner's dots make their appearance in properly stained smears of P. *vivax*-infected cells; these are fine, round, pink or reddish granules, distributed uniformly over the red cell. Increasing amounts of pigment accumulate in the parasite cytoplasm. After 36 hours the parasite fills over half the enlarged red cell, and the nucleus divides, becoming a shizont. By 48 hours the schizont has segmented into 16 distinct cells, the merozoites, 1.5 to 2.0 μ in diameter, each with a red nucleus and blue cytoplasm condensed about it, and rupture of the erythrocyte takes place. The gametocytes re-

TABLE 4-2
CLINICAL DIFFERENTIATION OF THE MALARIAS

	P. vivax	*P. malariae*	*P. falciparum*	*P. ovale*
Other names	Benign tertian	Quartan	Malignant tertian aestivo-autumnal	Benign tertian or ovale
Incubation period (days)	14 (8–27) [sometimes 7–10 mo]	15–30	12 (8–25)	15 (9–17)
Erythrocytic cycle (hr)	48	72	48	48
Persistent EE stages	Yes	No	No	Yes
Parasitemia (mm³)				
Average	20,000	6,000	50,000–500,000	9,000
Maximum	50,000	20,000	Up to 2,500,000	30,000
Duration of untreated infection (yr)	1.5–4.0	1–30	0.5–2.0	Probably 1.5–4.0

PLASMODIUM FALCIPARUM

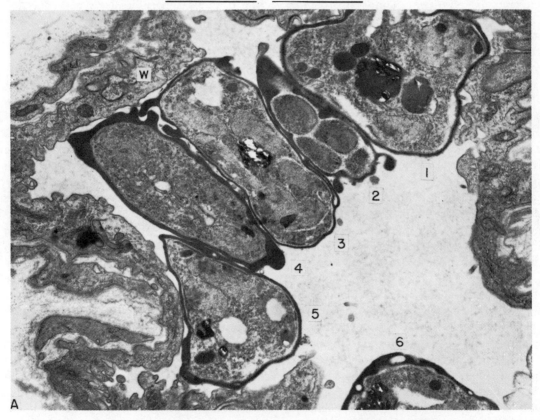

Figure 4-9. A. *Plasmodium Falciparum.* Electron micrograph of schizonts in red blood cells in a capillary. Note distortion of red blood cells that are closely adhering to wall of the capillary. 1-6, infected red cells; W, wall of vein. (Courtesy of S. Luse and L. H. Miller.)

semble a late trophozoite prior to segmentation. They are oval, nearly filling the red cell—the microgametocyte with less deeply staining nucleus and cytoplasm, the macrogametocyte with darker blue cytoplasm and more compact nucleus.

PLASMODIUM MALARIAE (see color plate). The early ring form of *P. malariae* resembles that of *P. vivax,* but the parasite is smaller, less irregular, and more compact, and the cytoplasm is a deeper blue. The growing trophozoite acquires coarse granules of dark brown or black pigment and may assume a band shape across the cell. Infected red cells are normal or even smaller than most in size since old cells are preferentially infected. In contrast to other species, a period of 72 hours is required for the development of the mature schizont, which

resembles a daisy or rosette with only eight to ten oval merozoites. A compact mass of greenish black pigment is often located centrally, surrounded by the merozoites. The gametocytes are similar to those of *P. vivax* but are smaller.

PLASMODIUM FALCIPARUM (see color plate). This differs from other plasmodia of humans in that, except in infections with very high parasitemia, only the ring forms of early trophozoites and the gametocytes are ordinarily seen in the peripheral blood. Schizogony takes place in capillaries of the muscles and viscera, and very few schizonts are found in the peripheral blood (Fig. 4-9). The infected red blood cells are of normal size. The presence of more than one ring form in a cell is relatively common. Double chromatin dots (nuclei) are

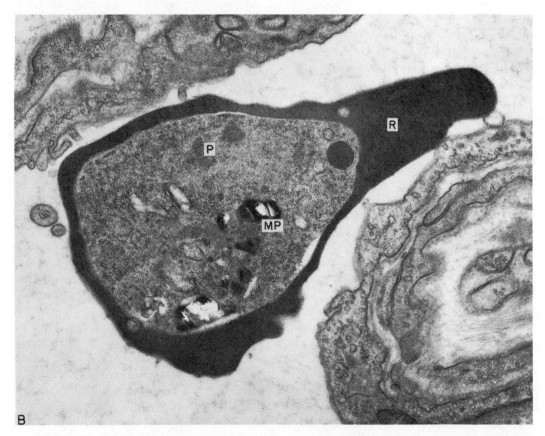

Figure 4-9. B. Electron micrograph of schizont in red blood cell in a capillary. Note distortion of red cell.

R, red cell; P, parasite; MP, malarial pigment. (Courtesy of S. Luse and L. H. Miller.)

frequently found in *P. falciparum* ring forms, and only occasionally in the rings of other species. The schizonts, seldom found in the blood, resemble those of *P. vivax* but have smaller and a few more merozoites when mature and ready to rupture. The immature gametocytes gradually acquire an elliptical shape, stretching but remaining within the red cell. When fully developed, they have a characteristic banana shape, the so-called crescent. In cells infected with *P. falciparum* there are sometimes cytoplasmic precipitates known as Maurer's dots that appear as irregularly distributed red spots or clefts.

PLASMODIUM OVALE. Commonly found in West Africa, but infrequently encountered elsewhere, is similar to *P. vivax* and *P. malariae* in several characteristics. The infected red blood cells are slightly enlarged, can be of oval shape, and show Schüffner's dots. An important diagnostic feature is the irregular or fimbriated appearance of the edges of the infected red cell. Schizonts have centrally massed pigment and only about eight merozoites when mature.

Physiology. A procedure for in vitro maintenance of malaria-infected blood that permitted development to the schizont stage was described as early as 1912. Research efforts during World War II resulted in better but still inefficient methods for short-term culture, and not until 1976 was a practical system for continuous culture of asexual stages of *P. falciparum* finally achieved. Critical conditions for successful culture include a reduced O_2 tension and the presence of CO_2. However, considerable difficulty has been encountered thus far in obtaining substantial numbers of gametocytes by in vitro culture that are infective for mosquitoes. Glucose is necessary and avidly consumed by malaria parasites, leading to an acid medium. Methionine and isoleucine are required amino acids. Purines must be supplied in the medium, but the parasites are capable of pyrimidine biosynthesis. This observation is consistent with the well-known sensitivity of plasmodia to inhibitors of folate metabolism. The earliest step in folic acid synthesis, namely the incorporation of p-amino-

benzoic acid (PABA), is also vital for malaria parasites. Deficiency of PABA has been noted to suppress the infection in vitro in experimental animals and even in human populations. Malaria parasites are capable of lipid biosynthesis from glucose, but plasma or serum appears to be a necessary constituent of culture media.

After entry into the red cell, the malaria parasite pinches off, in a pinocytotic process, host cell contents through openings called *cytostomes*. The resulting food vacuoles coalesce and malarial pigment in the form of hemazoin crystals, which are breakdown products of hemoglobin, accumulate in the vacuoles. Another ultrastructural feature of red cells infected with certain species of malaria is the development of knoblike protrusions on the cell surface as the parasite matures. Properties of these knobs are believed responsible for adherence of infected cells to vascular endothelium and to each other, resulting in partial obstruction of visceral capillaries in falciparum malaria.

Life Cycle. The life of the plasmodia is passed in two hosts, a vertebrate and a mosquito (Fig. 4-10). The asexual cycle in the vertebrate host is known as *schizogony*, and the sporulating sexual cycle in the mosquito as *sporogony*.

SCHIZOGONY. The infectious sporozoite from the salivary glands of an infected female *Anopheles* mosquito is injected during biting into the human blood stream. Within 30 minutes this slender motile organism enters a liver parenchymal cell, initiating what is called the *exoerythrocytic* (EE) portion of the life cycle, because the red blood cells have not yet been invaded. Within the liver cell the parasite begins an extensive multiplication and is called a *schizont,* producing thousands of merozoites within the liver cell after 8 to 15 days, depending upon the species of malaria. The parasitized liver cell then ruptures, freeing merozoites to initiate the erythrocytic cycle. It is still not known whether late relapses of *P. vivax* and *P. ovale* are due to multiple cycles within the liver or are simply a dormant state of some of the originally formed hepatic schizonts that

EXOERYTHROCYTIC CYCLE IN HEPATIC CELLS

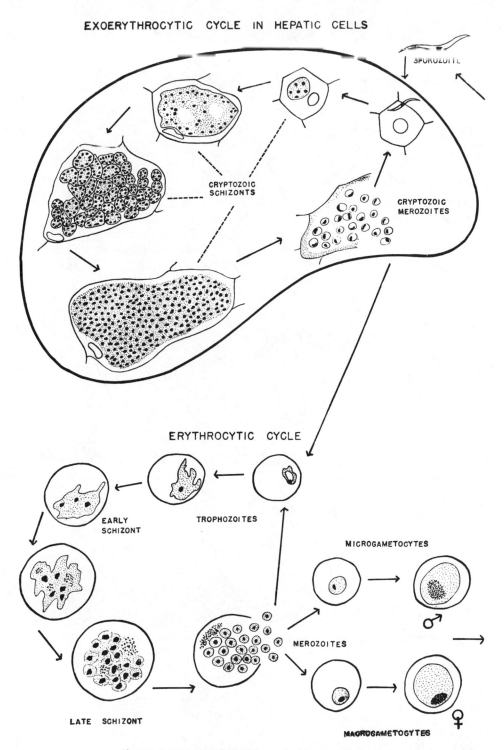

SPOROZOITE

CRYPTOZOIC
SCHIZONTS

CRYPTOZOIC
MEROZOITES

ERYTHROCYTIC CYCLE

EARLY
SCHIZONT

TROPHOZOITES

MICROGAMETOCYTES

MEROZOITES

LATE SCHIZONT

MACROGAMETOCYTES

Figure 4-10. A. Malaria life cycle in man; asexual.

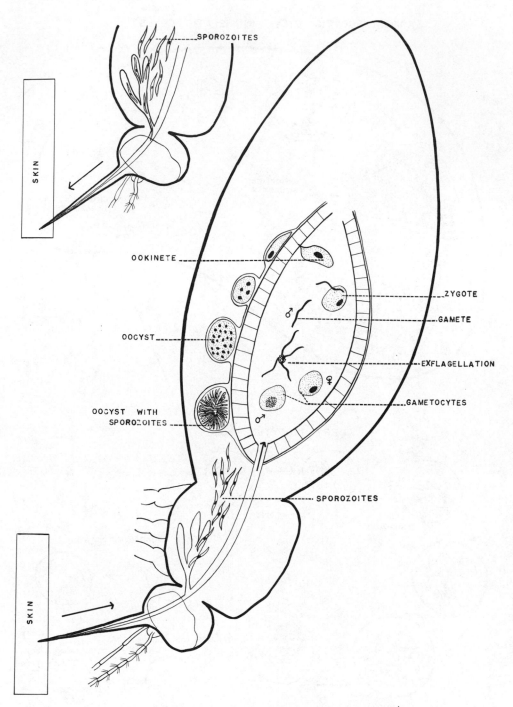

Figure 4-10. B. Malaria life cycle in mosquito; sexual.

Trophozoites; ring forms, basophilic stippling.

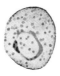
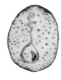
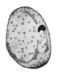
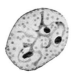

Ameboid trophozoites; enlarged red cells; Schüffner's granules.

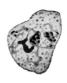

Older trophozoites; note pigment and double infection.

Late trophozoites and 1 early schizont.

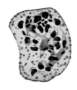
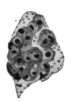

Schizonts; young to mature.

Developing gametocytes; mature macrogametocyte.

Plasmodium vivax.

Trophozoites; ring **forms.**

 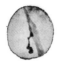

Young trophozoites; red cells not enlarged.

Older trophozoites; 1 band form.

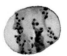

Mature trophozoites and early s**chizonts.**

Schizonts; young to mature rosette form.

Immature gametocytes; micro- and macrogametocytes.

Plasmodium malariae.

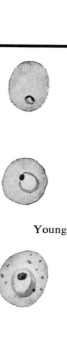

Trophozoites; ring forms; 1 applique form.

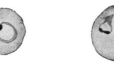

Young trophozoites; double chromatin dot; multiple infection.

Maturing trophozoites; note Maurer's dots.

Young to mature trophozoites. Early schizont.

Schizonts; rarely found in peripheral blood.

Developing gametocytes.

Immature, mature macrogametocytes; immature, mature microgametocytes.

INEZ DEMONET

Plasmodium falciparum.

will later release their merozoites. A morphologic form persisting in liver cells, appropriately termed a *hypnozoite* and presumably responsible for late relapses, has been described for a vivax-like malaria of monkeys. In any event, with *P. falciparum* and *P. malariae,* in which true relapse does not occur, the hepatic schizonts apparently survive only a short time.

A relapse signifies that parasitemia develops from EE stages in the liver; a recrudescence means an increase in parasites that has persisted at low levels in the blood. Inadequately treatd *P. malariae* infections may persist at low levels in the peripheral blood for as long as 25 or 30 years. Even with a variable number of relapses, *P. vivax* infections die out within 3 or 4 years. *P. ovale* may initiate relapses up to 4 or 5 years after primary infection from persistent EE stages. Certain strains of *P. vivax* exhibit what must be an evolutionary adaptation to survival in temperate climates or in tropical areas that have a long dry season. Strains that existed in northern Europe and Korea, for example, could have a prolonged incubation period of up to 7 to 10 months, and some central American strains have an interval of 5 to 7 months between the primary attack and subsequent relapses. Such a long interval is likely to span the winter or a dry season, increasing the chance of vector availability for transmission.

The erythrocytic cycle consists of the invasion of red cells by merozoites, their development through trophozoites, then schizonts, the rupturing of the cell, and the reinvasion of new cells. The process of invasion involves recognition by the merozoite of a specific receptor site on the red cell membrane and proper orientation of the anterior end of the merozoite, exposing special organelles to the red cell surface. Then, after a few seconds, the red cell becomes deformed and the merozoite enters through an invagination of the red cell membrane (Fig. 4-10). The receptor site on the red cell for *P. vivax* malaria has been found to be associated with the Duffy blood-group antigen. The Duffy blood-group status is determined by three alleles, Fy^a, Fy^b and Fy. Absence of the a and b antigens indicates a Duffy negative genotype, $FyFy$. Black Africans, most of whom lack the Duffy antigen, are resistant to both experimental and natural infection with *P. vivax*. However, those individuals whose red cells contain either the Fy^a or Fy^b determinant are susceptible to infection. This explains the absence of *P. vivax* in West Africa, where the frequency of $FyFy$ is greater than 90 percent, and the resistance of many American blacks to this species of malaria, since about 60 percent are Duffy negative. As repeated cycles of asexual multiplication occur, some parasites that invade red cells do not undergo division as schizonts but, instead, transform into male and female gametocytes.

SPOROGONY. Sporogony, the sexual cycle, takes place in the mosquito. The gametocytes ingested with the blood meal, unlike the schizonts, are not digested. In the male microgametocyte the chromatin dot divides into 6 to 8 nuclei that migrate to the periphery of the parasite (Fig. 4-11). There, several whiplike, actively motile filaments, the uninuclear microgametes, are thrust out and detached from the parent cell, a process known as *exflagellation.* In the meantime, the female macrogametocyte has matured into a macrogamete. Fertilization is achieved by the entry of the microgamete, forming a zygote. MacCallum, the noted pathologist, was the first to observe this phenomenon as a second-year medical student. He reported his findings at a scientific meeting of his august elders and, because of his youth, had great difficulty in convincing them. Yet this was the key that opened to Ronald Ross the riddle of the life cycle of malaria in the insect vector, for which he received a Nobel Prize.

In 12 to 24 hours after the mosquito's blood meal, the zygote changes into a wormlike form, the ookinete, which penetrates the wall of the mosquito's gut and develops into a spherical oocyst between the epithelium and the basement membrane. Here it increases to many times its original size (Fig. 4-11), with thousands of sporozoites developing inside. With rupture of the oocyst, sporozoites are liberated into the body cavity and migrate to the salivary glands. When the mosquito feeds

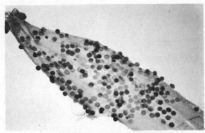
OOCYSTS ON STOMACH
OF MOSQUITO

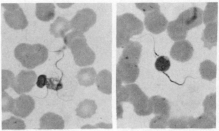
EXFLAGELLATION OF
MICROGAMETOCYTE

Figure 4-11. Stages of sexual life cycle of malaria in mosquito.

on humans, the sporozoites gain access to the blood and tissues and enter upon their exoerythrocytic cycle. The sporogonic cycle in the mosquito takes from 10 to 17 days.

Transmission of malaria occurs by other mechanisms, such as blood transfusion, contaminated syringes, or across the placenta. Malaria may be accidentally transfused from an infected but asymptomatic donor to a recipient. Most transfusion malaria in temperate climates has been due to *P. malariae*. Transfusion-induced *P. falciparum* has increased in recent years, probably because it has become increasingly resistant to drugs. Malaria outbreaks have resulted from multiple use of a syringe among "mainlining" drug addicts. Transfusion malaria initiates only the erythrocytic cycle and therefore is usually easily eradicated, since there is no exoerythrocytic cycle. A rare type of nonmosquito transmission is congenital infection. When it does occur it indicates some placental defect, and it can involve any species of parasite.

Pathology. The pathologic changes associated with all types of malaria have certain features in common, but the best known are those for *P. falciparum* malaria, the cause of virtually all fatalities. The reticuloendothelial system is activated by the rupture of infected red cells and intravascular release of parasites, malarial pigment, and cellular debris. The liver and spleen bear the brunt of disposing of this particulate material by hyperplasia of Küpffer cells and macrophages, resulting in

enlargement of the liver and spleen. In acute infections the soft, enlarged spleen is susceptible to spontaneous or traumatic rupture. Fixed macrophages of the spleen and liver exhibit phagocytosis of infected and even some normal erythrocytes, as well as the presence of ingested malarial pigment. With the increased red cell destruction there is increased turnover of iron and blood pigments, and excess iron not immediately used to form new hemoglobin is deposited as hemosiderin in parenchymatous cells. In chronic or repeated infections the liver and spleen especially, but also other organs, become slate-gray or black in color from the deposition of malarial pigment. Continued activity of malaria leads to a firm, fibrotic spleen that shrinks back to normal size. Hepatic dysfunction is minimal, showing only slight elevation of bilirubin and liver enzyme levels. There is little or no reaction to the exoerythrocytic stages in liver cells.

If the malarial infection continues, anemia develops, and often the anemia is of greater degree than can be explained by direct destruction of red cells by the parasite. This suggests the operation of some additional hemolytic process, possibly autoimmune, although the Coombs test is usually negative. The complement system is activated, with consumption of complement components via the classical pathway. Immune complexes are formed and may be deposited in the kidneys.

With *P. falciparum* infections there is an additional and much more serious component to the pathologic picture, which is primarily due to vascular obstruction. The main reasons for this are (1) the tendency for red cells infected with this parasite to stick to the endothelium of vessels and to each other and (2) the ability of *P. falciparum* to infect red cells of all ages and thus produce a high parasitemia. Adherence of infected cells to capillary walls appears related to the development of electron-dense, knoblike structures on the red cell membrane as the parasite matures. Thus, schizonts tend to sequester in visceral capillaries and not circulate in the periphery. Infected red cells are more rigid than normal erythrocytes. All these factors contribute to congestion and reduced blood flow. The result is functional, if not actual mechanical, obstruction of small blood vessels with anoxia of affected organs. Pathologic changes of *P. falciparum* infections, therefore, are basically vascular in nature and may affect any organ, including the brain, kidney, heart, lungs, or gastrointestinal tract.

In fatal *P. falciparum* infections the brain is edematous and markedly congested. Macroscopically, the cortex is dusky gray or brown, and petechial hemorrhages may be visible in the perivascular tissues. Cerebral capillaries are dilated and packed with infected red cells and pigment (Fig. 4-12). Interstitial pneumonitis may occur in acute falciparum infections, and the heart may show petechial hemorrhages, partially blocked myocardial capillaries, edema of cardiac muscles, and foci of degeneration. Other findings include adrenal hemorrhage, retinal hemorrhages, and a concentration of plasmodia in the placenta, resulting in spontaneous abortion.

Several types of kidney involvement are seen in malaria. During or soon after the acute stage, and especially with *P. falciparum* infections, transient abnormalities of the urinary sediment compatible with glomerulonephritis are not unusual. If the infection is associated with severe hemolysis and hypotension, acute tubular necrosis, with all its related findings, can complicate an already serious disease. *Blackwater fever* is a term given to the clinical syndrome of acute and massive hemolysis during malaria. It was more common in the past when quinine was the main antimalarial, and

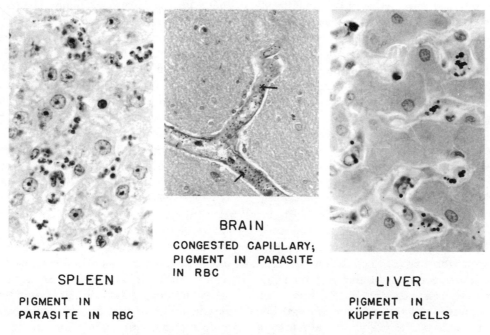

SPLEEN

PIGMENT IN
PARASITE IN RBC

BRAIN

CONGESTED CAPILLARY;
PIGMENT IN PARASITE
IN RBC

LIVER

PIGMENT IN
KÜPFFER CELLS

Figure 4-12. Malaria parasites and pigment in organs.

the syndrome is probably etiologically related to the administration of quinine. Another form of kidney disease in malaria is an immune-complex nephrosis, seen mainly with chronic *P. malariae* infections.

A number of physiologic and metabolic abnormalities, especially in *P. falciparum* infections, can lead to serious complications. One of these is disseminated intravascular coagulation, which is manifested by thrombocytopenia, increased levels of fibrin split products, and abnormalities in blood clotting. Reduced blood sodium may be caused by both salt depletion and water retention. In acute malaria the blood volume is often increased; this, plus increased capillary permeability, may lead to problems when parenteral administration of fluids is needed. Pulmonary edema associated with hyaline membrane formation has been described.

Symptomatology. The incubation period, which generally varies from 9 to 30 days, may be prolonged for months. Strains of *P. vivax* from certain geographic regions can have an incubation period of as long as 10 months. Another reason is that clinical *P. vivax* and *P. ovale* infections may develop many months after cessation of suppressive chemotherapy. Small numbers of parasites are actually present in the circulation a day or two before symptoms begin. Then, as numbers of parasites increase, the infected individual begins to experience various general symptoms, such as headache, lassitude, vague pains in the bones and joints, chilly sensations, and fever. In non-endemic areas, such symptoms are often diagnosed as influenza or some other viral infection. Within a few more days regular episodes of chills and fever become prominent, but other systemic symptoms, especially headache, muscle aches, and pains, persist.

The malarial paroxysm occurs at the end of the schizogonic cycle, when the merozoites of the mature schizonts, together with their pigments and residual erythrocyte debris, erupt from infected red cells and are released into the circulation. The relationship of schizogonic cycle to the fever curve is shown in Figure 4-13. It can be seen that the intervals between

febrile paroxysms represent the periods required for development of asexual forms from entry of the merozoite into the red cell to rupture of the schizont. These intervals are 48 hours for *P. vivax, P. ovale,* and *P. falciparum,* and 72 hours for *P. malariae.* Different vivax strains actually require slightly less than 48 hours, varying from 43.6 to 45. Confusion results from the common names given to different types of malaria based upon febrile interval. Thus, vivax malaria is called *benign tertian,* falciparum is *malignant tertian,* and malariae is referred to as *quartan.* The ancients counted the first paroxysm as day one, rather than day zero, so the next fever came on the third day for *P. vivax* and the fourth day for *P. malariae;* hence the terms *tertian* and *quartan.*

The malarial paroxysm is one of the most dramatic and frightening events in clinical medicine. It begins with a cold stage of up to an hour, with chilly sensations that progress to a teeth-chattering, frankly shaking chill. Peripheral blood vessels are constricted and the lips and nails are cyanotic. At the end of the cold stage the body temperature begins to mount rapidly, ushering in the hot stage, which lasts from 6 to 12 hours. Nausea and even vomiting, headache, and a rapid pulse occur; the circulation opens up, and the temperature peaks at 103 to 106 F (39 to 41 C), with the skin hot and the face flushed. The patient may become euphoric; the high fever may produce convulsions in children. Then the patient perspires profusely; the temperature falls and the headache disappears. In a few hours the patient is exhausted but symptomless. The next day the patient can feel quite well before the next paroxysm occurs.

When malarial paroxysms are discrete and occur at regular intervals, they are said to be synchronized. Synchrony depends upon all the parasites reaching maturity at the same time, like the climax of a well-rehearsed symphony. However, at the start of a primary attack, infection may be initiated from several hepatic schizonts that did not develop at exactly the same rate. Therefore, in the early stages of malaria there may be multiple broods of parasites. However, with the passage

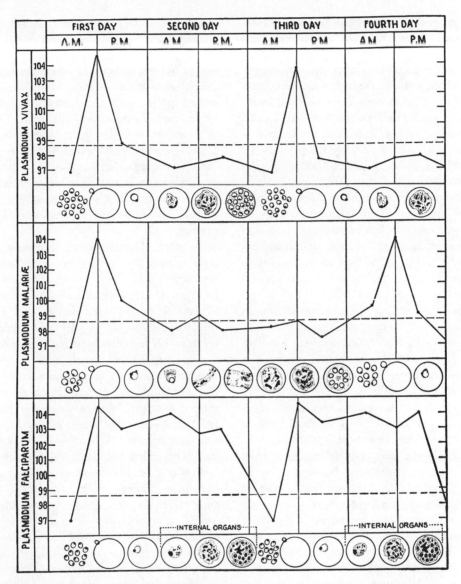

Figure 4-13. Temperature curves in malaria showing relation to growth and schizogony of malarial parasites.

of time the broods tend to become synchronous in their development. This explains why the fever pattern usually does not have a regular periodicity during the first week of the primary attack. This is particularly true of *P. falciparum* infections, which in the primary attack may have a very irregular, daily, or even continuous fever. The exact mechanism causing the febrile paroxysm is still unknown, although it very much resembles the pyrogen effect of endotoxin. A tolerance phenomenon appears to operate in the sense that higher degrees of parasitemia later in the infection produce no greater degree of fever than in the early stages, and partially immune individuals often have parasitemia without fever.

The primary attack of acute malaria comprises a series of paroxysms over a period of at least 2 weeks or more. The spleen becomes enlarged and can be palpated in most patients within a week or two of the primary attack. Stretching of the splenic capsule often results in left upper quadrant pain, and the spleen may rupture secondary to trauma or coughing. Although fluctuations in total leukocytes occur during paroxysms, the white cell count generally remains within normal limits. Thrombocytopenia is common. Anemia is usually only moderate during the primary attack, unless some drug-induced hemolytic process, such as blackwater fever, supervenes. Anemia can be more severe with chronic malaria. Kidney function is not disturbed in patients with uncomplicated malaria, although evidence of transient glomerulonephritis occurs in a small proportion of patients with acute malaria. Herpes labialis is not uncommon.

Without treatment, all species of human malaria may ultimately result in spontaneous self-cure, but with *P. falciparum* there is a likelihood of progressively increasing parasitemia and fatal outcome. The phenomenon of capillary sequestration of infected cells can result in a great variety of symptoms and involvement of any organ system. The cerebral type is characterized by headache, delirium, psychotic behavior, and convulsions, or it may feature apathy and stupor before leading to coma. Cerebral malaria has been found at autopsy in individuals who have died in jail after being mistakenly picked up in the street for drunkenness. Sometimes gastrointestinal symptoms may be prominent, e.g., vomiting, abdominal pain, diarrhea, and even intestinal hemorrhage. Weakness, hypotension, and circulatory collapse are sometimes seen, as are pulmonary edema, cyanosis, and impaired oxygenation of the blood.

Two complications of chronic malaria, nephrotic syndrome and tropical splenomegaly, are immune complex disorders. Renal biopsies in patients with malarial nephrosis show variable histologic patterns and the presence of glomerular deposits of antibody, complement, and antigen. The nephrotic syndrome of quartan malaria is a chronic process, does not respond to antimalarial treatment, and usually does not respond to steroid treatment. The other entity, tropical splenomegaly, is seen where malaria is endemic, but it is not related to one particular species of parasite. In addition to hypersplenism, the disease is characterized by rather striking elevation of serum IgM values, presence of circulating immune complexes, and lymphocytic infiltration of hepatic sinusoids as seen by liver biopsy. In many patients with tropical splenomegaly syndrome the abnormalities will regress if antimalarial prophylaxis is initiated and continued for at least 6 months. Epidemiologic studies suggest that there may be a genetic or familial predisposition.

Diagnosis. The definitive diagnosis of malaria is made by microscopic identification of the parasites in blood smears. Specimens can be taken at any time, since infections are usually not so highly synchronized that a few of the later asexual stages will not be present in the blood, even after schizont rupture. A few laggard organisms, out of step, "listening to another drummer," are usually found in the blood throughout the cycle. If a high degree of synchrony exists, it may be easier to detect later developmental stages of the parasite in repeated smears taken at 4- to 6-hour intervals. This is less helpful in *P. falciparum* infections, since the late stages sequester in visceral capillaries and only ring forms are in the peripheral blood. However, taking additional smears at intervals for several days is recommended if parasites are not found initially and malaria is suspected on clinical grounds. Gametocytes of all species may be present in the blood continuously, but those of *P. falciparum* do not appear until 10 days after symptoms begin. A thin blood film (see p. 322) should be examined for at least 15 minutes, whereas a 5-minute search of a thick film (p. 322) should reveal parasites if present. The thick film is the most efficient method of detecting malarial parasites, but interpretation requires an experienced worker. Available serologic tests cannot differentiate current from past infections and are therefore helpful only in epidemiologic studies. Serologic tests can also be useful in identifying an infected individual among multiple donors responsible for transfusion

TABLE 4-3
CHEMOTHERAPY OF MALARIA

Chemotherapeutic Agent		Drug Acts Against				
			RBC Phase			
Type	Drug	EE Phase	Asexual Forms	Sexual Forms	Mosquito Phase	Main Toxicity
Cinchona alka-loid	Quinine	−	+	−	−	Cinchonism
9-amino-acridine	Quinicrine	−	+	−	−	Dermatitis, G-I, and CNS
4-amino-quinoline	Chloroquine	−	+	−	−	Dermatitis, ocu-lar with chronic dosage
	Amodiaquine	−	+	−	−	
8-amino-quinoline	Primaquine	+	−	+	−	G-6-PD deficient hemolysis
Dihydro-folate reductase inhibitors	Chloroguanide	−	+*	−	+	Minimal in recommended doses
	Pyrimethamine	−	+*	−	+	Minimal in recommended doses

Action too slow for treatment of acute attack.

malaria in a setting where malaria is uncommon. If no facilities are available for laboratory diagnosis, or even if blood smears are reported as negative, treatment is justified when malaria is suspected clinically in a severely ill patient.

Treatment. The treatment of malaria involves general and supportive measures and chemotherapy (Table 4-3). During the acute attack the patient should have bedrest, cold sponging for the relief of fever, aspirin or sedatives for headache and general discomfort, and regulation of fluid intake and salt balance. If fluid replacement or blood transfusion is necessary, it must be administered with care because of hypervolemia, increased capillary permeability, and hyponatremia, which often accompany acute malaria.

The chemotherapeutic agents may be classed as (1) suppressive, for preventing the development of clinical symptoms, (2) therapeutic, for the treatment of the acute attack by destroying the asexual erythrocytic parasites, (3) radical cure, for the destruction of the late exoerythrocytic forms, and (4) gametocytic and gametostatic.

The treatment of all uncomplicated attacks (all plasmodia except resistant *P. falciparum*) consists of chloroquine phosphate, orally, 1 gm (600-mg base), then 0.5 gm in 6 hours and 0.5 gm daily for 2 days. Amodiaquine dihydrochloride, orally, is an alternative drug, 760 mg (600-mg base) the first day and 520 mg (400-mg base) daily for the next 2 days. In *P. falciparum* malaria, if the patient has not shown a prompt response to the usual doses of chloroquine, parasite resistance to this drug must be considered (see below).

The treatment of severe illness (all plasmodia except resistant *P. falciparum*) consists of chloroquine hydrochloride 250 mg (200-mg base) intramuscularly every 6 hours; the maximum dosage is 1 gm daily until oral therapy with chloroquine phosphate is possible or until a total of 3 gm has been given.

The prevention of relapses—a radical cure,

after the clinical cure (not needed for *P. falciparum* and *P. malariae*)—requires primaquine phosphate, 26.3 mg (15-mg base) orally daily for 14 days. Exoerythrocytic stages of some strains of *P. vivax* are not always eradicated by primaquine—but such failure is unusual.

Infections of *P. falciparum* resistant to chloroquine are treated by combined therapy, with quinine sulfate orally, 650 mg t.i.d. for 3 to 10 days; pyrimethamine, 25 mg b.i.d. for 3 days; and sulfadiazine, 500 mg q.i.d. for 5 days. Another possible combination of drugs for the treatment of chloroquine-resistant *P. falciparum* malaria is quinine for 3 days, accompanied by either tetracycline or clindamycin for 7 days. The dosages of these drugs for adults are as indicated above for quinine, and for tetracycline and clindamycin the dosage is 500 mg t.i.d. These antibiotics are slow in their action against *P. falciparum,* so the quinine is essential for its rapid action against asexual forms. Mefloquine, a new drug that should become commercially available, is effective against *P. falciparum* that is resistant to all known drugs, including quinine.

Severe resistant *P. falciparum* infections in coma or vomiting are treated by intravenous quinine dihydrochloride, 600 mg in 300 ml saline or 5 percent glucose over at least 45 minutes. This is repeated in 6 to 8 hours until oral quinine therapy is possible. Intravenous administration of quinine can be hazardous but is preferred in seriously ill patients. Pulse and blood pressure should be monitored for arrhythmias or hypotension. The use of steroids in large doses, which has been advocated for cerebral malaria, is without value. It might reduce cerebral edema in some instances, but specific antimalarial treatment is the most important.

P. falciparum strains resistant to chloroquine are found principally in southeast Asia, including New Guinea, Indonesia, the Philippines, and eastern India, and in northern South America, with extension into Panama. While strains of *P. falciparum* on the African continent vary in susceptibility to chloroquine, the great majority are still responsive to the drug. Recently, the presence of chloroquine-resistant strains has been documented in East Africa (Tanzania, Kenya and Madagascar).

The suppression of malaria while in endemic areas and after departure is achieved by chloroquine phosphate, if resistance to this drug is absent or uncommon. It is taken orally, 500 mg (300-mg base) once weekly, a week before entering the area and for 6 weeks after last exposure. The dosage for children is appropriately reduced in amount but is of the same duration (Table 4-4). Since infection with *P. vivax* and *P. ovale* can be acquired while on chloroquine suppression, additional treatment is needed to prevent later relapse with these species of malaria. A 14-day course of primaquine phosphate, 26.3 mg (15-mg base) daily, is given for this purpose, after the last exposure. Primaquine is the only drug effective against persisting exoerythrocytic

TABLE 4-4
ORAL DOSAGE OF CHLOROQUINE (BASE) FOR SUPPRESSION AND TREATMENT OF MALARIA

Age (yr)	Suppressive Dose per Week,* Usual Range (mg)	Dose for Treatment† Usual Range (mg)	
		Initial	6 Hours later and Daily, next 2 days
1	37.5–50	75–100	37.5–50
1–3	50–75	100–150	50–75
4–6	75–100	150–200	75–100
7–10	120–160	250–325	120–160
11–15	175–275	350–550	175–275
Adults	300	600	300

* 5 mg (base) per kilogram of body weight.
† 10 mg (base) per kilogram initially, then half this dose for next three doses.

liver stages of *P. vivax* and *P. ovale*. Since primaquine can cause hemolysis, the routine use of primaquine for all who have been potentially exposed to malaria is questionable and depends upon the intensity of exposure, the relapse potential of parasite strains in the area of exposure, and the availability of future health care.

The above recommendations for suppressive therapy must be modified for areas of the world where resistance of *P. falciparum* to chloroquine is widespread. In this situation, weekly administration of a combination of a sulfonamide drug, such as sulfadoxine (500 mg), with pyrimethamine (25 mg), either separately or in a fixed dose (Fansidar) is suggested.

Toxicity of Antimalarials. Some toxic manifestations are very common in people receiving 2 gm of quinine per day, and in about 5 percent the side effects are severe enough to require discontinuation of treatment. Symptoms of cinchonism include tinnitus, visual disturbances, dizziness, headache, and nausea. More severe reactions, such as skin rashes, asthma, and hemolytic anemia, probably represent idiosyncratic or hypersensitivity reactions to quinine.

Chloroquine is remarkably free of toxic side effects in the doses used for the treatment of malaria, and even for long periods of chemoprophylaxis. Pruritus and mild visual disturbances are the most common complaints. Exfoliative dermatitis exacerbated by exposure to sunlight sometimes results from chloroquine, especially in individuals with psoriasis. When used for treatment of other diseases, chloroquine in doses of 250 to 750 mg daily for months or years can deposit in the eye and produce a progressive retinopathy. The margin between toxic and therapeutic levels of chloroquine for children is much narrower than for adults, so overdosage must be carefully avoided.

Primaquine, an 8-aminoquinoline, causes hemolysis of red cells deficient in glucose-6 phosphate dehydrogenase (G-6-PD). The degree of hemolysis produced is dependent upon the severity of G-6-PD deficiency, which is common but usually mild in blacks. Tests for presence and severity of enzyme deficiency can be done before primaquine is used. Abdominal cramps and leukopenia can be produced by primaquine.

The frequency and range of toxic effects of sulfadoxine, the long-acting sulfonamide most commonly used in combination with pyrimethamine for treatment of malaria, has not been established. The incidence of untoward effects with other long-acting sulfonamides is about 5 percent and includes various types of skin eruptions, fever, hepatitis, and hematologic abnormalities. Some of these reactions can be serious if the drug is not withdrawn. The toxicity of pyrimethamine and other dihydrofolate reductase inhibitors is mainly bone-marrow depression, but this rarely, if ever, occurs when the dose is no greater than 25 mg weekly.

Drug Resistance and the Development of New Drugs. The problem of drug-resistant malaria involves mainly chloroquine and strains of *P. falciparum*. Such strains are often resistant to other antimalarial drugs as well. Asexual parasites of sensitive strains are generally cleared from the blood by 3 days after the initiation of treatment and definitely by 6 or 7 days. Resistance of a parasite to drugs is graded according to patterns of asexual parasitemia after initiation of treatment. R I, the mildest form, is characterized by initial clearance of parasites but recrudescence within a month after start of treatment. R II refers to a reduction in parasitemia after treatment but failure to clear and subsequent increase. With R III, the most severe form of resistance, parasitemia shows no significant change with treatment or even an increase. Resistance of human malaria to pyrimethamine and chloroguanide can develop in communities where there is widespread use of these drugs as chemoprophylaxis for long periods of time.

These problems of drug resistance have stimulated efforts to develop and evaluate better antimalarial drugs. The Walter Reed Army Institute of Research has supported the testing of several hundred thousand compounds over the past 20 years. Several drugs that are active against chloroquine-resistant *P. falciparum* have emerged from this program. Although not yet in general use at the time of this writing, the new drugs include a quinoline methanol, mefloquine, and a series of amino-alcohols.

Epidemiology. Human malaria was acquired from our simian ancestors. Cross infections between modern human and simian tertian and quartan plasmodia have been produced in the laboratory and have occurred naturally in the field. People, however, are the only important reservoir of human malaria. One of the most important parasitic diseases of humanity, it has a worldwide distribution in the tropics and subtropics and also in areas in the temperate zone. It is not present in Hawaii, many southeastern Pacific Islands, or New Zealand, since anopheline mosquitoes are absent from these areas. More than a billion people live in malarious areas; it is estimated that millions are infected and that many die of it each year (Fig. 4-14). Surveys designed to determine the prevalence and intensity of the disease and the factors governing its local spread include (1) the collection of statistics of past and present morbidity and mortality, (2) spleen index, (3) parasite index, (4) mosquito density and infection rate, and (5) environmental features affecting transmission.

Splenic enlargement is a useful index of the prevalence of malaria. The largest spleens are found in *P. vivax* and the smallest in *P. malariae* infections; the highest incidence is in the younger age groups. The spleen index represents the percentage of children of 2 to 9 years of age with enlarged spleens. Since the spleen decreases rapidly in size after the cessation of an attack, the index should be taken at the height of the malarial season. With repeated exposure to malaria, the spleen becomes fibrotic and shrinks to near normal size. So in areas with heavy transmission, the spleen index in adults may be normal.

The parasite index of a community is the percentage of children from 2 to 9 years of age with detectable plasmodia in a single thick blood smear. Children, especially the very young in hyperendemic areas, show a higher parasite index than do adults. Age-specific parasite rates will reflect the degree of malaria transmission, with a lower frequency of parasitemia in the older age groups, whose members have developed immunity.

The presence and intensity of infection in female *Anopheles* mosquitoes may be determined by the dissection of the stomach for oocysts and of the salivary glands for sporozoites. The blood-sucking habits in relation to humans (anthropophilic) and animals (zoophilic) may be determined by precipitin tests on their blood meals. The percentage of infected mosquitoes, usually 0 to 10 percent in endemic areas, varies with the species and strain of the parasite, the susceptibility of the mosquito species, and its proximity and attraction to humans.

The epidemiology of malaria is determined by the climatic and ecologic requirements of the mosquito vector, coupled with the habits of the human population. Temperatures between 16 and 34 C and a relative humidity greater than 60 percent are suitable for the transmission of malaria by favoring the breeding of mosquitoes and the development of sporogonic stages of the parasite. Breeding habitats for anopheline vectors can vary tremendously, depending upon the species. Some can breed in tiny collections of water in depressions of animal footprints; others require large ponds. Many anophelines prefer to enter houses or shelters to bite (endophilic), but some will bite outside (exophilic). Agricultural practices, such as water use or wastage that provides breeding sites, or the use of agricultural insecticides, are often closely linked to malarial epidemiology. A variety of nonspecific factors, including improved economic conditions (to buy antimalarials), better housing (screens) and industrial development (eliminates breeding sites) can contribute greatly to the reduction of malaria.

Beginning in the 1950s, a global malaria-eradication program, based largely upon twice-yearly spraying of houses with residual insecticides, was sponsored by the World Health Organization (WHO) (Fig. 4-15). The eradication of malaria was accomplished in

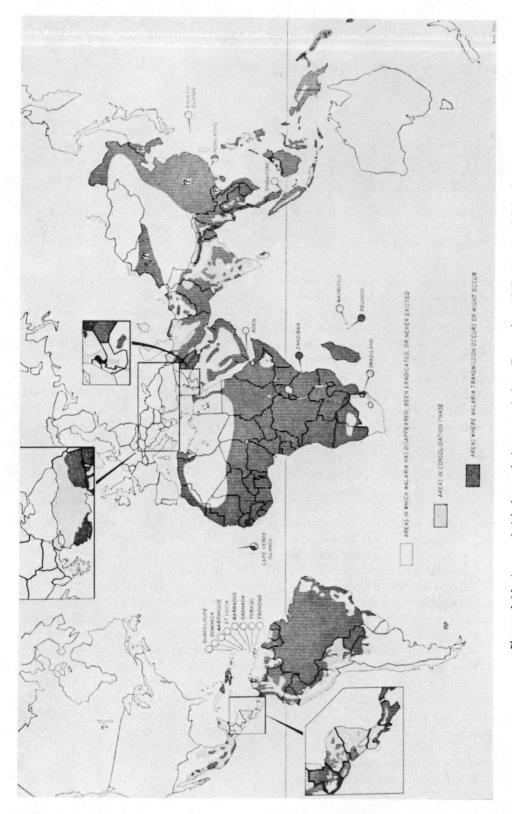

Figure 4-14. Areas of risk for malaria transmission, December 1978. (Map published in WHO Weekly Epidemiologic Record, No. 31, 1980.)

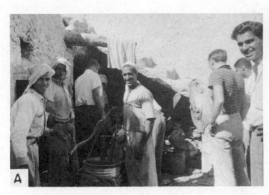 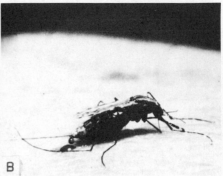

Figure 4-15. Malaria control. A. DDT spray team in a village in Saudi Arabia. B. Greedy *Anopheles* female overeating. She will fly, we hope, to a DDT'd wall in the house. (Courtesy of Dr. J. B. Poole.)

many countries, and there was reasonable control of the disease in others, but a variety of factors led to a resurgence of malaria so that the WHO global eradication approach was abandoned in the early 1970s. The main reasons for the recent increase in malaria include the widespread development of anopheline resistance to insecticides, often accelerated by the profligate use of insecticides in agriculture, and the development of chloroquine resistance by *P. falciparum*. Another factor was the lack of trained personnel and the expense involved for poor countries to set up and maintain health organizations required for an eradication program.

Currently, most countries in the temperate zone are free of malaria, but transmission continues in virtually all of tropical Africa. The most serious area for drug resistance is Southeast Asia. Between 400 and 800 cases of malaria were reported to occur annually in the United States in the years 1975–79, but practically all of these cases were acquired elsewhere. A large increase in cases for 1980 was the result of the influx of refugees from Southeast Asia. In the United States a small focus of indigenous mosquito transmission occasionally occurs, and a few cases of transfusion or congenital malaria are reported. More recent details on the status of malaria risk in different countries, advice on chemoprophylaxis, and regions with chloroquine-resistant malaria can

be found in annual summaries of malaria surveillance from the CDC.

Immunity. An important distinction must be made between conditions that confer resistance to malaria and acquired immunity, which develops after infection or after immunization. One example of innate resistance is the long-known, but only recently understood, insusceptibility of most blacks to *P. vivax* malaria because of the absence of the merozoite receptor associated with the Duffy factor on red cells. The presence of the sickle hemoglobin trait confers another form of resistance to *P. falciparum*, which does not prevent infection but limits high degrees of parasitemia that might be fatal. In some parts of the world G-6-PD deficiency of red cells also appears to limit parasitemia.

Much knowledge of acquired immunity to malaria has come from observations on the course of infections induced in syphilitic patients for fever therapy and in volunteers. These findings have shown that response to infection can be quite variable, with intermittent parasitemia lasting anywhere from 1 to many weeks or even months if treatment was not given. Immunity to one species of parasite does not protect against other species, and it also could be strain-specific within the species. Generally, repeated infections have been required for immunity.

The epidemiology of malaria in hyperendemic areas where transmission is intense provides another good source of information on natural immunity. Infants do not become infected during the first 3 to 4 months of age because of transplacental immunity from their mothers and also because of the reduced ability of fetal hemoglobin to support development of the parasite. P-aminobenzoic acid deficiency from a milk diet due to nursing may also contribute to lack of infection in infants. Thereafter, over the first few years of life, children suffer repeated infections. Without treatment, many die if *P. falciparum* is present; those who survive become immune by late childhood. The age at which immunity develops will depend upon the intensity of transmission. Malaria surveys in endemic areas will therefore disclose many individuals with parasites in the blood but with no or few clinical symptoms of malaria.

Although the operation of various mechanisms contributing to acquired immunity in malaria is known, their relative importance at different stages of infection is still not clear. For example, a role for serum antibody was demonstrated by the clearance of parasites from the peripheral circulation in semiimmune children given repeated doses of immune globulin. But parasitemia recurred after the immune serum was discontinued. An inhibiting effect of serum antibody can be shown on in vitro asexual multiplication, but this may be largely due to agglutination of merozoites released from schizonts, rather than to specific inhibition of the merozoite invasion of red cells. The fixed macrophage system is required to dispose of parasitized red cells and perhaps merozoites as well. The presence of the spleen is important, but it seems to function as much as a mechanical filter for infected erythrocytes as an immunologic organ. Removal of the spleen before or during infection results in a much higher parasitemia or, if done later, in exacerbation of latent infection. Yet in some chronic malarial infections the continued presence of the spleen inhibits the eradication of parasites and hence a cure. Enhanced reactivity of T lymphocytes to malar-

ial antigens can be demonstrated in infected individuals. Polyclonal B cell activation, which is common in malaria, may be due to nonspecific stimulation of helper cells. It is also clear, however, that suppression of various immune functions frequently occurs during malarial infection. This is much more conspicuous in experimental animals, but it also occurs in human malaria. Decreased antibody responses to tetanus toxoid and to certain bacterial vaccines, for example, has been shown in populations with malaria, but there is no clear evidence that the immunosuppression is clinically important. However, the clinical consequences of malarial immunosuppression are likely to be indirect and reflect the results of immunoregulatory effects. Thus, one theory explains the frequency of Burkitt's lymphoma in malarious Africa as due to suppression of normal immunologic surveillance. On a more practical level, the slow and relatively inefficient development of immunity to natural malarial infection may be a manifestation of immunosuppression.

Specific antibodies demonstrable by various tests (IFA, IHA, ELISA, and CF) are found in the serum after infection, but their presence does not signify protective immunity. Circulating malarial antigens can be present in the blood of endemic populations, but they have not been well characterized. Complement activation is a feature of malaria during early stages, and sharp reductions in components of the classical pathway of complement occur with the malarial paroxysm during schizont rupture later in the infection.

Prevention. The prevention of malaria includes (1) the reduction of gametocyte carriers, the source of infection, (2) mosquito control, and (3) the protection of susceptible people against mosquitoes. There is ample evidence that districts and even countries can be made malaria-free by mosquito control measures, although the cost may be beyond the resources of some countries. Intensive efforts have recently been directed to a fourth method of prevention, namely, the use of vaccines. These efforts are being stimulated by the same factors that led to abandonment of a global malaria-eradication strategy. One approach uses immunization by irradiated sporozoites to block the invasion of liver cells. This procedure has been shown to be effective in rodents, monkeys, and even a few human volunteers, but protection lasts only up to 6 months' duration. Another approach uses antigens from asexual parasites, but adjuvants are needed for immunization. Immunization against sexual stages is a third method in which serum antibody acts upon ingested gametocytes in the mosquito gut to block fertilization.

REFERENCES

African Trypanosomiasis

Brun, et al: In-vitro cultivation of bloodstream forms of *Trypanosoma brucei, T. Rhodesiense,* and *T. gambiense.* J Protozool. 28: 470-479, 1981.

Cross: Identification, purification, and properties of clone-specific glycoprotein antigens constituting the surface coat of *T. brucei.* Parasitolology 71: 393-417, 1975.

Gray: Variable agglutinogenic antigens of *T. gambiense* and their distribution among isolates of the trypanosome collected in different places in Nigeria. Trans R Soc Trop Med Hyg 66: 263-284, 1972.

Mulligan and Potts (eds): The African Trypanosomiases. London, Allen and Unwin, 1970.

Spencer, et al: Imported African trypanosomiasis in the United States. Ann Intern Med 82: 633-638, 1975.

Malaria

Boyd (ed): Malariology: A comprehensive survey of all aspects of this group of diseases from a global standpoint (by 65 contributors)—2 vols. Philadelphia, Saunders, 1949.

Krogstad and Pfaller: Prophylaxis and treatment of malaria. In: Remington and Swartz (ed): Current Clinical Topics in Infectious Diseases. Vol. 3. New York McGraw-Hill, 1982, pp. 56-73.

Miller, et al: The resistance factor to *Plasmodium vivax* in blacks—the Duffy-blood group genotype, Fy Fy. N Engl J Med 295: 302-304, 1976.

Neva, et al: Malaria: Host-defense mechanisms and complications. Ann Intern Med 73: 295-306, 1970.

Trager and Jensen: Human malaria parasites in continuous culture. Science 193: 673-674, 1976.

American Trypanosomiasis

Cerisola: Chemotherapy of Chagas' infection in man, in Publication No. 347 of Pan Am. Health Organization. A symposium on Chagas' Disease. Wash., D.C. Pan Am. Health Organization. 1977.

Koberle: Pathogenesis of Chagas' disease. Chapt. in Ciba Foundation Symposium 20 (new series). New York, Associated Scientific Publishers, 1974.

Marsden: South American trypanosomiasis (Chagas' disease). Int Rev Trop Med 4: 97-121, 1971.

Puigbo, et al: Clinical and epidemiological study of chronic heart involvement in Chagas' disease. Bull WHO 34: 655-669, 1966.

Raizman, et al: A clinical trial with pre- and post-treatment manometry comparing pneumatic dilation with bouginage for treatment of Chagas' megaesophagus. Am J Gastroenterol 74: 405-409, 1980.

Leishmaniasis

Hoogstraal and Heyneman: Leishmaniasis in the Sudan Republic. 30. Final epidemiological report. Am J Trop Med Hyg 18: 1091-1210. 1969 (Part 2—Supplement to Nov. issue)

Neva: Diagnosis and Treatment of cutaneous leishmaniasis. In Remington and Swartz (eds): Current Clinical Topics in Infectious Diseases. Vol. 3, New York, McGraw-Hill, 1982.

Petersen, et al: Specific inhibition of lymphocyte-proliferation responses by adherent suppressor cells in diffuse cutaneous leishmaniasis. N Engl J Med 306: 387-392, 1982.

Pneumocystis and Babesia

Dammin: Babesiosis, In Weinstein and Fields (eds): Seminars in Infectious Diseases, New York, Stratton Intercont. Medical Book Corp., 1978, pp. 169-199

Ruebush: Human babesiosis in North America. Trans R Soc Trop Med Hyg 74: 149-152, 1980.

Walzer, et al: *Pneumocystis carinii* pneumonia in the United States: epidemiologic, diagnostic, and clinical features. Ann Intern Med 80: 83-93, 1974.

Winston, et al: Trimethoprim-sulfamethoxazole for the treatment of *Pneumocystis carinii* pneumonia. Ann Intern Med 92: 762-769, 1980.

THE NEMATHELMINTHES, OR ROUNDWORMS

5

Nematodes

HELMINTHS

The term *vermes* designates wormlike animals of three phyla:

Annelida, (segmented worms)
Nemathelminthes (roundworms)
  Nematoda
Platyhelminthes (flatworms)
  Cestoda (tapeworms)
  Trematoda (flukes)

Annelida

The ectoparasitic leeches comprise the parasitic members of the phylum. The species of medical importance are either aquatic or terrestrial. They have variously sized, muscular, often pigmented, oval bodies with a tough cuticle, suckers at both ends, hard jaws, and a muscular pharynx.

The aquatic leeches, usually species of *Limnatis,* are injurious to humans. The larger suck the blood of bathers. The smaller, taken in drinking water, infest the upper respiratory or digestive passages. At times they invade the vagina, urethra, and eyes of bathers.

The terrestrial leeches, especially species of *Haemadipsa* found in the Far East, live in damp tropical forests, where they attach themselves to travelers, even crawling inside clothing and boots. The painless and often unnoticed wound caused by the bite bleeds readily because of an anticoagulative secretion, hirudin, and heals slowly. Leeches may be removed, after loosening their hold, by applying a local anesthetic, a strong salt solution, or a lighted match. Travelers may be protected by impregnating their clothing with a repellent, such as dimethyl phthalate.

Nemathelminthes—Nematoda

The nematoda include numerous free-living and parasitic species. The free-living forms are widely distributed in water and soil. The parasitic species live in plants, mollusks, annelids, arthropods, and vertebrates. It is estimated that more than 80,000 species are parasites of vertebrates. The species parasitic in humans range in length from 2 mm *(Stronglyoides sterco-ralis)* to more than a meter *(Dracunculus medinensis)*. The sexes are usually separate. The male, which is smaller than the female, commonly has a curved posterior end and, in some species, copulatory spicules and a bursa.

Morphology and Physiology (Fig. 5-1). The adult nematode is an elongate cylindrical worm, primarily bilaterally symmetrical. The anterior end may be equipped with hooks, teeth, plates, setae, and papillae for purposes of abrasion, attachment, and sensory response. The supporting body wall consists of (1) an outer, hyaline, noncellular cuticle, which the electron microscope has demonstrated to be rather complex, (2) a subcuticular epithelium, and (3) a layer of muscle cells. The cuticle has various surface markings and spines, bosses, or sensory papillae. The thin, syncytial, subcuticular layer is thickened into four longitudinal cords—dorsal, ventral, and two lateral—that project into the body cavity and separate the somatic muscle cells into four groups. These cords carry longitudinal nerves and often lateral excretory canals. The body wall surrounds a cavity, within which lie the digestive, reproductive, and parts of the nervous and excretory systems. This cavity is lined by delicate connective tissue and a single layer of muscle cells.

The alimentary tract is a simple tube extending from the mouth to the anus, which opens on the ventral surface a short distance from the posterior extremity (Fig. 5-1). The mouth is usually surrounded by lips or papillae and, in some species, is equipped with teeth or plates. It leads into a tubular or funnel-shaped buccal cavity, which in some species is expanded for sucking purposes. The esophagus, lined with an extension of the buccal cuticle, has a striated muscular wall, a triradiate lumen, and associated esophageal glands. It usually terminates in a bulbar extension equipped with strong valves. Its size and shape are useful for species identification. The intestine or midgut is a flattened tube with a wide lumen that follows a straight course from the esophagus to the rectum. Its wall consists of a single layer of columnar cells.

In the female the intestine leads into a short rectum lined with cuticle. In the male it joins with the genital duct to form the common cloaca, which opens through the anus. Around the anal orifice are papillae, the number and pattern of which aid in the identification of species.

There is no circulatory system. The fluid of the body cavity contains hemoglobin, glucose, proteins, salts, and vitamins and fulfills the functions of blood. The nervous system consists of a ring or commissure of connected ganglia surrounding the esophagus (Fig. 5-1). From this commissure six nerve trunks pass forward to the head and circumoral region, and six nerve trunks connected by commissures extend posteriorly. Sensory organs are situated in the labial, cervical, anal, and genital regions.

The male reproductive organs are situated in the posterior third of the body as a single coiled or convoluted tube, the various parts of which are differentiated as testis, vas deferens, seminal vesicle, and ejaculatory duct (Fig. 5-1). The ameboid spermatozoa traverse the vas deferens to the dilated seminal vesicle and pass through the muscular ejaculatory duct into the cloaca. The accessory copulatory apparatus consists of one or two ensheathed spicules and, at times, a gubernaculum. In some species winglike appendages or a copulatory bursa serve to attach the male to the female.

The female reproductive system (Fig. 5-1) may be either a single or a bifurcated tube, differentiated into ovary, oviduct, seminal receptacle, uterus, ovejector, and vagina. The ovum passes from the ovary into the oviduct, where it is fertilized. The true shell, a secretory product of the egg, begins to form immediately after sperm penetration, the vitelline membrane separating from the inner layer of the shell. In the uterus the protein coat is added as a secretion of the uterine wall. There is considerable variation in relative thickness of these layers. The daily output of a gravid female ranges from 20 to 200,000 eggs.

The excretory system consists of two lateral canals that lie in the lateral longitudinal cords. Near the anterior end of the body the

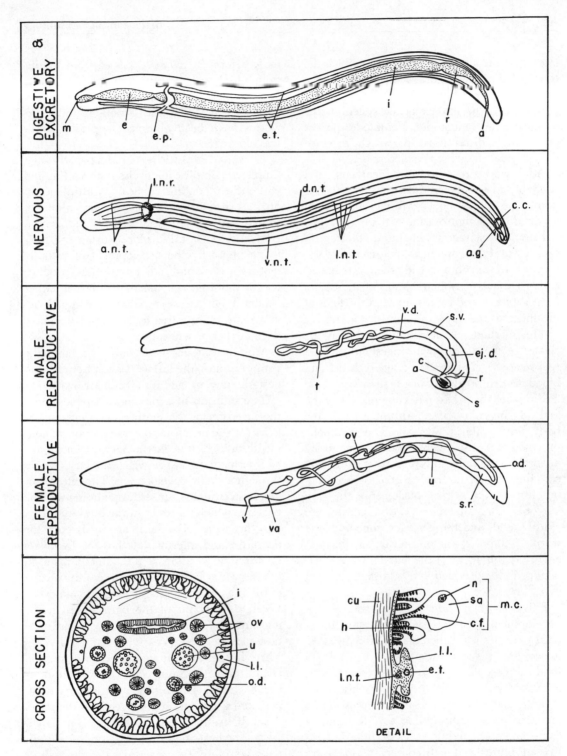

Figure 5-1. Morphology of a nematode, based on *Ascaris*.
  a, anus; a.g., anal ganglion; a.n.t., anterior nerve trunks; c, cloaca; cu, cuticle; c.c., circumcloacal commissure (male); c.f., contractile fibers; d.n.t., dorsal nerve trunk; e, esophagus; e.p., excretory pore; e.t., excretory tubules; ej.d., ejaculatory duct; h, hypodermis; i, intestine; l.l., lateral line; l.n.r., circumesophageal ring; l.n.t., lateral nerve trunks; m, mouth; m.c., muscle cells; n, nucleus; ov, ovary; o.d., oviduct; r, rectum; s, spicules; sa., sarcoplasm; s.r., seminal receptacle; s.v., seminal vesicle; t, testis; u, uterus; v, vulva; va, vagina; v.d., vas deferens; v.n.t., ventral nerve trunk.

101

lateral canals join in a bridge from which the terminal duct leads to a ventral pore in the region of the esophagus. Variations from this pattern, even to absence of the system, occur in some adult nematodes. Nematodes possess only longitudinal muscles, which produce their typical sinuous movements.

Adult worms react to touch, heat, cold, and probably to chemical stimulus. The penetration of the skin by hookworm larvae has been ascribed to thigmotropism.

Intestinal nematodes maintain their positions by oral attachment to the mucosa *(Ancylostoma)*, by anchorage with their attenuated ends *(Trichuris)*, by penetration of the tissues *(Strongyloides)*, and by retention in the folds of the mucosa and pressure against it *(Ascaris)*.

The methods of obtaining food may be classed as (1) sucking with ingestion of blood *(Ancylostoma)*, (2) ingestion of lysed tissues and blood by embedded worms *(Trichuris)*, (3) feeding on the intestinal contents *(Ascaris)*, and (4) ingestion of nourishment from the body fluids (filarial worms). The metabolic processes of parasitic nematodes are essentially anaerobic, since the intestinal tract ordinarily contains little or no free oxygen. Aerobic metabolism may also take place, since they are not obligatory anaerobes. Carbohydrates are readily used, and the glycogen content of the worms is high. A major portion of the total energy requirement of the female worm is expended in the production of a large number of ova.

Existence within the host necessitates the development of protective mechanisms. Intestinal parasites resist the action of the digestive juices, and tissue invaders that of the body fluids. Protection against digestive action is afforded by the cuticle and by the elaboration of antienzymes. The free-living larval forms are capable of withstanding a wide range of environmental conditions. Desiccation, excessive moisture, and extremes of temperature retard growth and may even kill the larvae. The growth of both the larval and adult worms follows the typical logistic curve of animal growth.

The life span of nematodes varies: The female *Trichinella spiralis* is passed from the intestine in 4 to 16 weeks; *Enterobius vermicularis* has a life span of 1 to 2 months; *Ascaris lumbricoides* may live for about 12 months; and hookworms have been observed to persist for at least 14 years.

Life Cycle. Parasitic nematodes pass through simple or complex life cycles both within and without the definitive host. Multiplication during the larval stages, so prevalent in trematodes, rarely occurs. In some genera *(Strongyloides)* it takes place during the free-living phase by the development of sexually mature free-living individuals that produce one or more generations. These larvae either resume their parasitic existence or again develop into mature free-living worms that produce further generations.

Most nematodes have only one host (the definitive one), the larvae passing from host to host directly or after a free-living existence.

Transmission to a new host depends upon the ingestion of the mature infectious egg or larva, or the penetration of the skin or mucous membranes by the larva. Some species have an intermediate host in which the larva passes through a cyclic development. The intermediate host, usually an arthropod, ingests the parasite, which passes from the intestinal tract into the tissues. The same animal is both the definitive and intermediate host of *Trichinella spiralis*. The location of the adult parasite in the host, to a large extent, governs the escape of the eggs and the character of the life cycle. When the habitat of the parasites is in the intestinal tract, the eggs or larvae leave the host via the feces. When its habitat is elsewhere in the body, there are other avenues of escape: urine, sputum, skin, blood, lymph, or tissue fluids. During larval development, nematodes pass through several molts or ecdyses, both inside and outside the host. Invasion of the host takes place through the intestinal tract or by the penetration of the skin or mucous membranes. In many instances the infective larvae within the egg shells are ingested in food. Nematodes, with few exceptions, do not multiply in humans, thus differing from many other pathogenic organisms.

Pathogenicity. The effect of parasitic nematodes upon the host depends upon the species and location of the parasite. Since nematodes can only rarely multiply in humans, the number of parasites present, or the intensity of infection, is a critical factor in determining the amount of damage to the host. The local reactions to adult worms in the intestine are generally minimal; there may be some local irritation, some degree of invasion of the intestinal wall, or mucosal damage from blood sucking. A single adult *Ascaris* worm may penetrate the bowel or obstruct the bile duct; in large numbers they can cause intestinal obstruction. The larvae of certain species may produce local and general reactions during their invasion, migration, and development in the host. Under some conditions the circuitous routes of migration of the larvae result in damage to organs not affected by the adult parasite. In unnatural hosts the larvae may remain viable and continue to migrate, causing injury to the host, but never become established as adult parasites.

The infected individual can become sensitized to either adult or larval nematodes so that the immune response results in tissue damage. This is seen, for example, in onchocerciasis with pathologic reactions to microfilariae in the skin and eye, or in the intense myositis that occurs around *Trichinella* larvae in the muscles. Tissue reactions to nematode parasites can involve both immediate hypersensitivity, or allergic reactions, as well as delayed-type cell-mediated reactions with granuloma and giant cell formation.

Resistance and Immunity. Inability of a nematode parasite to infect a host may be due to some innate, preexisting incompatibility that renders the host resistant or to immunity acquired from previous exposure to the parasite. While the factors that determine host specificity of a nematode usually cannot be defined, they undoubtedly involve certain biochemical requirements that render the environment suitable for the parasite. But host specificity is not always absolute. *Ascaris lumbricoides* develops to the adult stage almost exclusively only in humans, although its larval development

may take place in other animals. The *Ascaris* of the pig similarly will undergo at least partial development in humans. Embryonated eggs of the dog *Ascaris* hatch when ingested by humans, and the larvae stay alive for months, migrating in the tissues, but development to the adult stage does not occur. There may be racial differences in susceptibility to infection; blacks, for instance, seem to be less susceptible than whites to pinworm infection.

Specific immunologic responses and acquired immunity because of previous exposure can also be demonstrated. These involve the development of specific immunoglobulins as well as different types of cell-mediated responses. Some of the first experiments on immunology of parasites demonstrated precipitates at the oral and anal regions of nematode larvae when incubated in immune serum. Protective immunity to otherwise lethal challenge as a result of previous smaller infections has been shown with experimental hookworm and trichinella infections in animals. Nematodes that do not invade the tissues or secrete absorbable products produce slight if any immunity; human pinworms provide an example. Little success has attended attempts in the past to immunize animals against nematodes by the injection of worm antigens. A recent exception is the demonstration that antigens prepared from secretory granules of an organ called the stichosome are unusually active in protecting against trichinella and trichuris infections of animals. On the other hand, larvae attenuated by irradiation generally stimulate a much better immunity; veterinary vaccines of this type have been used.

Immune response to experimental nematode infections has been analyzed in great detail. One such phenomenon involves expulsion of adult worms from the small intestine, with evidence for the operation of both humoral and cell-mediated events. A variety of immunologic reactions have been shown to take place at the surface membrane of nematodes, such as complement activation, neutrophil interaction to generate chemotactic factors for eosinophils, and direct attack of larval nematodes by eosinophils. Production of reaginic antibodies of the immunoglobulin class IgE, which fix to mast cells and mediate immediate hypersensitivity reactions, is a prominent feature of many nematode infections.

The various immunologic mechanisms that can be demonstrated so elegantly in experimental animals are often not so clear-cut and may even be irrelevant when the same type of parasite is in the human patient. Whether acquired protective immunity exists and, if so, the exact mechanisms by which it operates in human nematode infections are more difficult to answer. The lower frequency of infection with common intestinal worms that is seen in adults as compared to children may be largely attributable to less exposure rather than to acquired immunity. Epidemiologic and clinical observations suggest that in humans trichinosis results to some extent in immunity against subsequent infections. Very little is known of the extent and possible mechanisms of protective immunity to the human filarial infections.

The immune response to nematode infections can be deleterious as well as beneficial. Immunopathology can be manifested by allergic reactions, such as urticarial skin eruptions during acute trichinosis or visceral larva migrans, or the bronchospasm and cough of tropical pulmonary eosinophilia of filariasis. Immunopathologic tissue damage to the skin and eye, which may be both immediate and delayed, is a prominent feature of onchocerciasis.

REFERENCES

Nematodes
Levine: Nematode parasites of domestic animals and man. Minneapolis, Burgess Publishing Co., 1968.
Lee and Atkinson: Physiology of nematodes. 2nd Ed. New York, Columbia University Press, 1977.

6

Intestinal Nematodes of Human Beings

Trichinella spiralis

Diseases. Trichinosis, trichiniasis, trichinelliasis.

Morphology (Fig. 6-1). The infrequently seen adult is a small worm, the male measuring 1.50 mm by 0.04 mm, the female 3.50 mm by 0.06 mm. It is characterized by (1) a slender anterior end with a small, orbicular, nonpapillated mouth, (2) a posterior end bluntly rounded in the female and ventrally curved with two lobular caudal appendages in the male, (3) a single ovary with vulva in the anterior fifth of the female, and (4) a long, narrow digestive tract. The larva has a spearlike burrowing tip at its tapering anterior end. It measures 80 to 120 μ by 5.6 μ at birth and grows but little until it has entered a muscle fiber, where it attains a size of 900 to 1300 μ by 35 to 40 μ. The mature encysted larva has a digestive tract similar to that of the adult, and although the reproductive organs are not fully developed, it is often possible to differentiate the sexes.

Life Cycle. The same animal acts as final and intermediate host, harboring the adult parasite temporarily and the larva for a longer period. In order to complete the life cycle, flesh containing the encysted larvae must be ingested by another host (Fig. 6-2). The larval parasite is found chiefly in humans, hogs, rats, bears, foxes, walruses, dogs, and cats, but any carnivorous or omnivorous animal may be infected. Adult birds may temporarily harbor the adult parasite, but the larvae do not encyst in the muscles. Poikilothermal animals do not harbor the parasite.

When infective larvae are ingested by humans, usually in pork, they pass to the upper small intestine, where the capsules are digested and the larvae released in a few hours. The liberated larvae immediately invade the intestinal mucosa. The sexes may be differentiated in 18 to 24 hours. After fertilization the males are dislodged from the mucosa and carried out of the intestine, although they sometimes remain for several days. The female increases in size and, in about 48 hours, burrows deeply into the mucosa of the intestinal villi, from the duodenum to the cecum and even in the large intestine in heavy infections. At

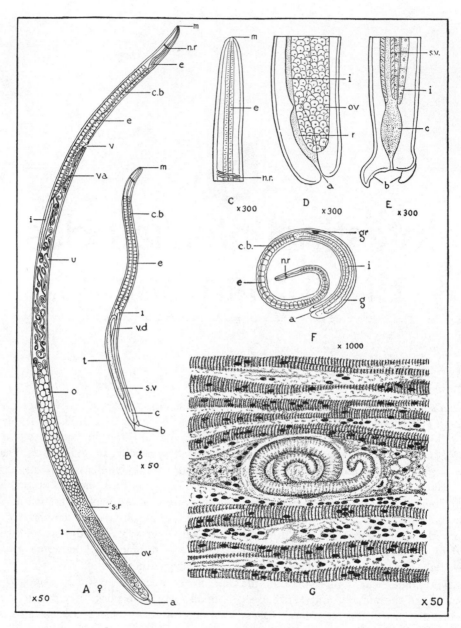

Figure 6-1. Schematic representation of *Trichinella spiralis.* A. Adult female. B. Adult male.
C. Anterior end of worm. D. Posterior end of female. E. Posterior end of male. F. Young
larval worm. G. Early encysted larva in muscle. (C adapted from Leuckart, 1868.)
   a, anus; b, bursa; c, cloaca; c.b, cell bodies; e, esophagus; g, gonads (anlage); gr,
granules; i, intestine; m, mouth; n.r., nerve ring; o, ova; ov., ovary; r, rectum; s.r, seminal
receptacle; s.v., seminal vesicle; t, testis; u, uterus containing larvae; v, vulva; va, vagina;
v.d, vas deferens.

TRICHINELLA SPIRALIS

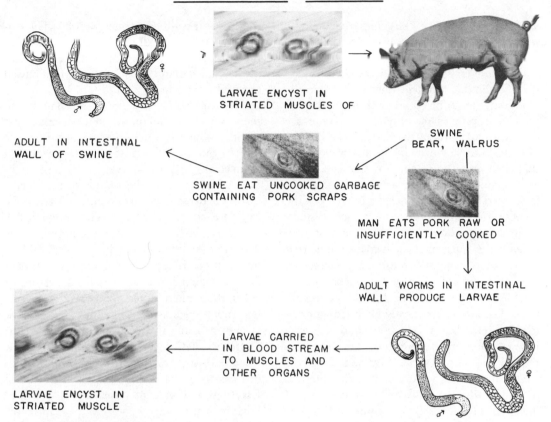

LARVAE ENCYST IN
STRIATED MUSCLES OF

SWINE
BEAR, WALRUS

ADULT IN INTESTINAL
WALL OF SWINE

SWINE EAT UNCOOKED GARBAGE
CONTAINING PORK SCRAPS

MAN EATS PORK RAW OR
INSUFFICIENTLY COOKED

ADULT WORMS IN INTESTINAL
WALL PRODUCE LARVAE

LARVAE CARRIED
IN BLOOD STREAM
TO MUSCLES AND
OTHER ORGANS

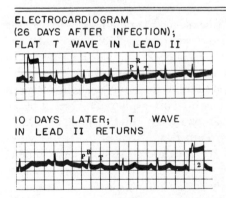

LARVAE ENCYST IN
STRIATED MUSCLE

ELECTROCARDIOGRAM
(26 DAYS AFTER INFECTION);
FLAT T WAVE IN LEAD II

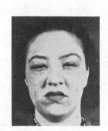

10 DAYS LATER; T WAVE
IN LEAD II RETURNS

PERIORBITAL EDEMA

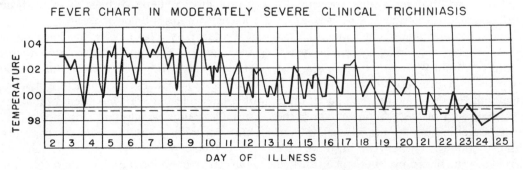

FEVER CHART IN MODERATELY SEVERE CLINICAL TRICHINIASIS

Figure 6-2. Life cycle of *Trichinella spiralis*.

about the fifth day the viviparous female worm begins to deposit larvae into the mucosa and, sometimes, directly into the lymphatics and the mesenteric lymph nodes, from which they reach the thoracic duct and enter the blood stream. After passing through the hepatic and pulmonary filters, the larvae are carried to all parts of the body. They burrow into the muscle fibers by means of a spear-shaped apparatus at the anterior end. They are capable of encysting and developing only in striated muscle. In other tissues, such as the myocardium and brain, they soon disintegrate, cause inflammation, and are absorbed. Among the muscles most heavily parasitized are the diaphragmatic, masseteric, intercostal, laryngeal, lingual, extraocular, nuchal, pectoral, deltoid, gluteus, biceps, and gastrocnemius. The larvae are mostly liberated within 4 to 16 weeks, but production continues with lessened intensity as long as the female worms remain in the intestine. Live female adults containing larvae were found in the intestine of a man who died on the fifty-fourth day of infection. His diaphragm contained 2677 larvae per gram of muscle. A female worm produces approximately 1500 larvae. Occasionally, larvae may be liberated into the intestinal lumen.

The larva grows rapidly in the long axis of the muscle, begins to coil on the seventeenth day, and attains its maximal size about the twentieth day. Encapsulation begins about the twenty-first day. The larva is enclosed in a blunt, ellipsoidal, lemon-shaped capsule of muscle fiber origin, 0.40 by 0.25 mm, which is composed of an inner mantle of basophilic degenerative muscle plus epithelioid cells and fibroblasts and an outer hyaline covering derived from the sarcolemma. The permanent capsule is completed in about 3 months.

Calcification, which may begin as early as 6 months or within 2 years, ordinarily starts at the poles and proceeds toward the center. Usually the capsule calcifies first, but at times there may be a primary impregnation of the larva. Calcification is usually completed within 18 months. The newly formed cysts are invisible to the naked eye, but when calcified they appear as fine opaque granules. The calcified cysts are seldom if ever revealed by radiograph. The adult female dies after passing her larvae and then is digested or passed out of the intestine.

Epidemiology. In 1947 Stoll estimated that there were 27.8 million infected persons in the world, of which three-quarters were in the United States. This number has been greatly reduced in the past 30 years. It is cosmopolitan, except in Asia, the islands of the Pacific (though present in wild pigs in Hawaii), Puerto Rico, and Australia. The prevalence of trichinosis in humans may be determined by detecting encysted larvae in cadavers and by intracutaneous tests. Recent autopsy surveys have revealed a prevalence of 2.2 percent or less in the United States, compared to 15 or 25 percent 40 years ago. The number of new, largely subclinical, infections annually in the United States is unknown, but only a few hundred are reported, including several deaths. In garbage-fed hogs the incidence is less than 0.5 percent, whereas in grain-fed hogs it is 0.1 percent or less. In nature the enzootic disease is maintained by cannibalistic rats.

The prevalence of trichinosis is less in the tropics and subtropics, chiefly owing to low consumption of pork products. Poor people in many countries cannot afford meat; an occasional bit of fish is their only protein. Religious bans on eating pork explain the absence of the disease among some Hindus, Jews, and Moslems. Seventh-Day Adventists and other vegetarians are not exposed to infection. Chinese, who consume large quantities of pork, are protected by their culinary custom of cooking it thoroughly, and the garbage of these thrifty people contains little or no meat.

People may also acquire the infection by the ingestion of ground beef, as hamburger or steak tartar, which is diluted with its cheaper competitor, pork. Beef, ground in a machine in which infected pork has been ground is a possible source of infection. Instances of human infection from bear and walrus meat have been reported. As bears leave their sylvan retreats and join humanity in picnic areas and suburbia, banqueting on our raw or poorly cooked pork garbage, they will become an even greater threat to the nimrod. The prevalence of *Trichinella* in New England bears is 1.3 percent.

Pathology. Except for the early intestinal lesions caused by the adult worms, the pathology of trichinosis is concerned with the presence of the larvae in the striated muscles and vital organs and with the reaction of the host to their activities, metabolic products, and, possibly, toxic secretions. The characteristic pathologic picture is found in the striated muscles that contain the encysted larvae. The muscle fibers, in 3 to 4 days after the invasion of the larva, increase in size, become edematous, develop a spindle shape, lose their cross-striations, and undergo basophilic degeneration. The nuclei increase in number and size, stain intensely, and migrate toward the interior of the muscle cell. There is an acute interstitial inflammation about the parasitized muscle fiber, which reaches its peak in 5 to 6 weeks, with edematous swelling and cellular infiltration of polymorphonuclear neutrophils, eosinophils, lymphocytes, and, at times, foreign body giant cells. The adjacent muscle fibers undergo hydropic degeneration and hyaline necrosis.

Symptomatology (Table 6-1). Because of the involvement of many organs, the protean symptoms of trichinosis resemble those of many other diseases. The variability and severity of the clinical symptoms depend upon

TABLE 6-1
TRICHINOSIS SYMPTOMATOLOGY AND CLINICAL DIFFERENTIAL DIAGNOSIS

Site of Parasites	Signs and Symptoms	Simulating Disease
Young adults migrating into mucosa of small intestine 24–72 hours	Nausea Vomiting Diarrhea Headache Abdominal pain	Food poisoning Intestinal influenza Appendicitis
Larvae in bloodstream and striated muscles 10–21 days	Edema, periorbital* Conjunctivitis* Photophobia* Fever, chills, sweating* Muscle pain and spasm* Headache Eosinophilia* Dyspnea Sore throat Skin eruptions Pleurisy Hypostatic pneumonia Diarrhea or constipation	Conjunctivitis Measles Rheumatism Arthritis Intercostal neuritis Periarteritis nodosa Dermatomyositis Laryngitis Influenza Pleurisy Pneumonia
Larvae in myocardium 10–21 days	Precordial pain Tachycardia Hypotension EKG changes Edema of extremities	Myocarditis Endocarditis
Larvae in brain and meninges 14–28 days	Headache, supraorbital Mental apathy Delirium, stupor, coma Reflexes absent	Frontal sinusitis Meningitis Encephalitis

* *Very common.*

the number of worms, the size and age of the patient, the tissues invaded, and the general resistance of the patient. A distinction should be made between zoologic and clinical infection. Only a small percentage of infected persons has sufficient parasites to produce clinical trichinosis. As early as 24 hours after ingestion of the infected pork, the migration of the young worms into the intestinal wall may produce a diarrhea, especially in one previously infected, and the gastroenteritis may persist for a week. This may be mild in light infections but very severe in heavy infections. From digests of muscle biopsies in patients, a rough correlation has been made between clinical severity of illness and larvae per gram of muscle tissue. Infections with one to ten larvae tend to be mild or moderate; those with 10 to 100 can vary from moderate to severe, while infections with 100 or more larvae per gram are likely to be very severe or even fatal.

The predominating symptoms depend upon the organs affected. In typical cases the findings in order of frequency are eosinophilia; edema, chiefly orbital; muscular pain and tenderness; headache, fever; shallow and painful breathing; and general weakness. There can be evidence of myocardial and central nervous system involvement. Trichinosis is one of the few helminthic infections that often run a consistent fever during its course that may persist for several weeks. Increasing eosinophilia associated with fever, facial edema, myalgia, and gastrointestinal disturbance provide strong presumptive evidence of trichinosis, especially if there is a history of eating pork.

The disease is commonly divided into three clinical phases corresponding to the periods of (1) intestinal invasion by adult worms, (2) migration of the larvae, and (3) encystment and repair. In the first there may be diarrhea; in the second and third, muscle pain and discomfort; in the third, weakness and cachexia. If the patient survives the acute illness, he or she usually will recover slowly and show no residual ill effects, although muscle pain may persist for months. In overwhelming infections death may take place in 2 to 3 weeks, but more often it occurs in 4 to 8 weeks from exhaustion, pneumonia, pulmonary embolism,

cerebral involvement, or cardiac failure. Weakness, stiffness, rheumatic pain, and loss of dexterity can persist for up to a year or more after an acute attack, but permanent sequelae are very rare.

Trichinella infection results in the development of serum antibodies, including IgE, and cell-mediated immune responses. In experimental animals, resistance to reinfection can be demonstrated by an allergic IgE-mediated inflammatory response that expels adult worms from the intestine. Another immune mechanism is the destruction of newborn larvae by eosinophils, which requires the presence of specific serum antibody. The role of the eosinophil in immunity to trichinosis appears to be specific and functionally important because increased numbers of larvae can be recovered from infected animals in which eosinophils have been depleted. Suppression of the IgE antibody response also reduced resistance to infection by *T. spiralis*.

Diagnosis. The definitive diagnosis often depends upon several laboratory tests. None of them is 100 percent accurate, and, even if negative, they do not rule out a diagnosis based upon sound clinical judgment. Early in the infection, the skin test and serologic tests are usually negative. Therefore, an initial negative test, followed by a positive test or increase in antibody level is of great diagnostic significance.

The intradermal test, using an antigen prepared from *Trichinella* larvae, gives an immediate reaction (within 30 minutes) in a high proportion of infected individuals. A positive test is characterized by a blanched wheal of 5 mm or more diameter surrounded by an area of erythema. The skin test usually becomes positive 2 to 3 weeks after infection and may remain positive for several years. In recent years there have been problems with the activity of commercial skin-test antigens.

The bentonite flocculation and latex agglutination tests are the most common of a variety of serologic tests that can be used for diagnosis of trichinosis. They have the advantage of not remaining positive for more than a year or so. A strongly positive test, therefore, is indicative of recent infection.

Eosinophilia is a useful diagnostic aid in trichinosis, especially when it can be shown to rise as the illness progresses. Eosinophilia of 40 to 80 percent is not unusual, and an accompanying leukocytosis is common. Secondary bacterial infection or an overwhelmingly severe *Trichinella* infection can cause a decrease or even disappearance of eosinophilia. The time course of the eosinophilia begins in the second week, reaches a maximum during the third or fourth week of infection, and then gradually declines. But up to 6 months may elapse before eosinophil levels return to normal.

Interestingly, the erythrocyte sedimentation rate may remain within normal limits.

Although serum IgE levels are elevated, this in itself would not be diagnostic unless specific IgE for *T. spiralis* were measured.

Muscle Biopsy. Demonstration of living larvae in a fragment of biopsied skeletal muscle is the most definitive diagnostic procedure. The invading larvae do not begin to coil up and encyst until the seventeenth day of infection, making their detection easier. Since most patients do not relish the idea of multiple biopsies, the third or fourth week of infection is the best time to do one. The biopsy is taken from one of the larger muscles, such as the gastrocnemius or deltoid, preferably near the tendinous attachments. Some of the tissue can be compressed between two microscope slides and/or digested in pepsin-hydrochloric acid for examination under low power or a dissecting microscope for living larvae. Some of the muscle should also be fixed for histopathologic examination. The presence of old calcified cysts or larvae, with no surrounding inflammatory response, must be carefully evaluated, since they probably represent a previous and not a recent infection.

Treatment. Patients with symptomatic trichinosis should be confined to bed and given general supportive treatment. Salicylates are usually enough to relieve headache and muscle pain, although the latter may require codeine or even stronger analgesics. Barbiturates may be useful for sedation. Fluid and electrolyte balance should be watched since impaired capillary permeability can lead to general edema and later mobilization of fluid. This may be especially important if there is acute myocarditis and congestive heart failure.

Steroids give symptomatic relief in trichinosis but are generally not indicated unless acute myocarditis or central nervous system involvement are complications. EKG conduction defects, for example, due to myocardial inflammation might be reversed or improved by corticosteroids. Oral prednisone in a dose of 20 to 40 mg daily, with reduction and tapering after 3 to 5 days, is recommended for this purpose. Corticosteroid therapy, however, will increase the total number of larvae that invade the muscles by inhibiting the inflammation reaction. In experimental animals thiabendazole can be a very effective drug, but its usefulness in human infections has been difficult to evaluate. Some case reports indicate that the drug damages larvae in the tissues, and it could also give symptomatic relief by inhibiting inflammatory responses. If used, the dosage of thiabendazole is 25 mg per kilogram of body weight, twice daily for 5 to 7 days.

Prevention. The ultimate eradication of trichinosis in humans is dependent upon its elimination in hogs. Its prevalence in these animals can be greatly reduced by sterilizing garbage containing raw meat scraps. Laws to this effect are in force in every state. Federal inspection, which covers about 70 percent of the pork products in the United States, is macroscopic and therefore unreliable. The microscopic examination of pork, once used for exported pork in the United States from 1891 to 1906, was abandoned because of its unreliability under American conditions of abattoir automation.

The general public should be continuously informed, through educational campaigns, of the danger of trichinosis, its method of transmission, and the necessity of thoroughly cooking pork until its attractive pink color turns to a drab gray.

Trichuris trichiura

Diseases. Trichuriasis, trichocephaliasis, whipworm infection.

Life Cycle. People are the principal hosts of *T. trichiura,* but it has also been reported in monkeys and hogs. Closely allied species are found in sheep, cattle, dogs, cats, rabbits, rats, and mice.

The morphologic characteristics of *T. trichiura* (Fig. 6-3) are (1) an attenuated whiplike anterior, three-fifths traversed by a narrow esophagus resembling a string of beads, (2) a more robust posterior, two-fifths containing the intestine and a single set of reproductive organs, (3) similarity in length of male (30 to 45 mm) and female (35 to 50 mm) and (4) the bluntly rounded posterior end of the female and the coiled posterior extremity of the male with its single spicule and retractile sheath. The number of eggs produced per day by a female has been variously estimated at 3000 to 10,000. The eggs, 50 to 54 μ by 23 μ, are lemon-shaped with pluglike translucent polar prominences. They have a yellowish outer and a transparent inner shell. The fertilized eggs are unsegmented at oviposition. Embryonic development takes place outside the host. An unhatched, infective, first-stage larva is produced in 3 weeks in a favorable environment, i.e., warm, moist, shaded soil. The eggs are less resistant to desiccation, heat, and cold than are those of *Ascaris lumbricoides.*

When the embryonated egg is ingested by humans, the activated larva escapes from the weakened egg shell in the upper small intestine and penetrates an intestinal villus, where it remains 3 to 10 days near the crypts of Lieberkühn. Upon reaching adolescence, it gradually passes downward to the cecum. A spearlike projection at its anterior extremity enables the worm to penetrate into and embed its whiplike anterior portion in the intestinal mucosa of the host, whence it derives its nourishment. Its secretions possibly may liquefy the adjacent mucosal cells. The developmental period from the ingested egg to ovipositing adult covers about 30 to 90 days. Its life span is usually given as 4 to 6 years—the senior author's light infection persisted for 8 years.

Epidemiology. The prevalence of whipworm infection is high, but its intensity is usually light. Hundreds of millions of people throughout the world are infected, the prevalence ranging as high as 80 percent in certain tropical countries. In the United States whipworm

infection is found in the warm, moist South. Its distribution is coextensive with that of *A. lumbricoides.* The highest incidence is found in the regions of heavy rainfall, subtropical climate, and highly polluted soil.

Children are more frequently infected than adults. The heaviest infections are in young children, who live largely at ground level, habitually contaminate the soil, and pick up infection from polluted dooryards. Infection results from the ingestion of embryonated eggs via hands, food, or drink that have been contaminated directly by infested soil or indirectly by playthings, domestic animals, or dust.

Pathology and Symptomatology. *Trichuris* lives primarily in the human cecum, but it is also found in the appendix and lower ileum. In heavily parasitized individuals, the worms are distributed throughout the colon and rectum, and they may be seen on the edematous, prolapsed rectal mucosa that results from straining at the frequent stools (Figs. 6-4 and 6-5).

Light infections usually do not give rise to recognizable clinical manifestations, and the presence of the parasite is discovered only on routine stool examination.

Patients with very heavy chronic *Trichuris* infections present a characteristic clinical picture consisting of (1) frequent small blood-streaked diarrheal stools, (2) abdominal pain and tenderness, (3) nausea and vomiting, (4) anemia, (5) weight loss, and (6) occasional rectal prolapse, with worms embedded in the mucosa. Headache and slight fever may occur. Extreme cachexia is sometimes seen with a fatal termination. Getz reported four infections with fatal terminations in malnourished Panamanian children who harbored from 400 to 4100 worms.

The anemia that accompanies *Trichuris* infections may sometimes be marked, and hemoglobin levels as low as 3 gm per 100 ml have been reported. The worms apparently suck some blood of their host, but the hemorrhage that may occur at their attachment sites is probably a greater source of blood loss. Approximately 0.005 ml of blood is lost per day per each *Trichuris.* We removed 1500

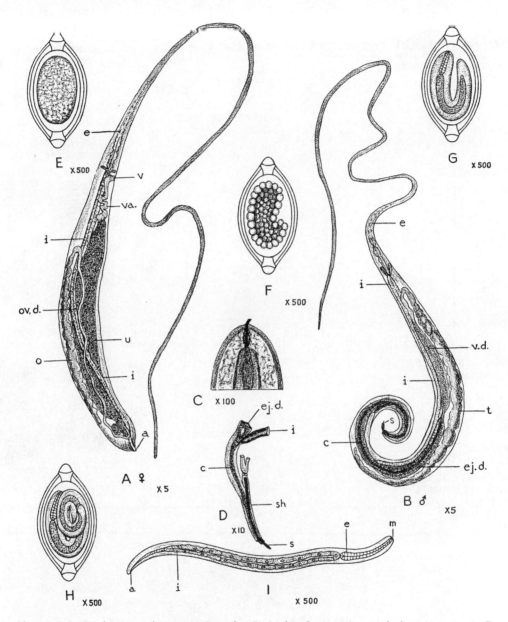

Figure 6-3. *Trichuris trichiura*. A. Female. B. Male. C. Anterior end showing spear. D. Cloaca and copulatory organs of male. E. Unicellular stage of egg. F. Multicellular stage of egg. G. Early larva in egg shell. H. Mature larva in egg shell. I. Newly hatched larva. (A,B,D-I adapted from Leuckart, 1876. C drawn from photograph by Li, 1933.)

a, anus; c, cloaca; e, esophagus; ej.d., ejaculatory duct; i, intestine; m, mouth; o, ovary; ov.d., oviduct; s, spicule; sh, sheath of spicule; t, testis; u, uterus; v, vulva; va., vagina; v.d., vas deferens.

TRICHURIS TRICHIURA

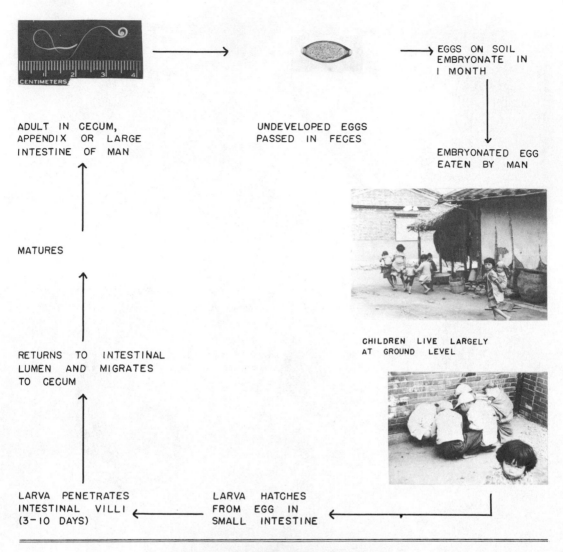

ADULT IN CECUM, APPENDIX OR LARGE INTESTINE OF MAN

UNDEVELOPED EGGS PASSED IN FECES

EGGS ON SOIL EMBRYONATE IN 1 MONTH

EMBRYONATED EGG EATEN BY MAN

MATURES

CHILDREN LIVE LARGELY AT GROUND LEVEL

RETURNS TO INTESTINAL LUMEN AND MIGRATES TO CECUM

LARVA PENETRATES INTESTINAL VILLI (3-10 DAYS)

LARVA HATCHES FROM EGG IN SMALL INTESTINE

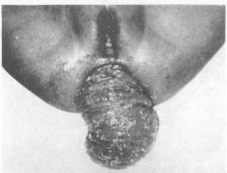

VERY HEAVY TRICHURIS INFECTION WITH WORMS ON PROLAPSED RECTUM

Figure 6-4. Life cycle of *Trichuris trichiura*.

114

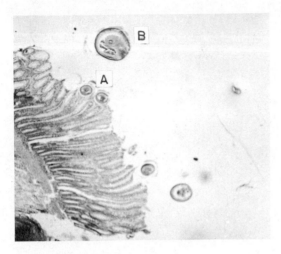

Figure 6-5. Large intestine showing sections through esophagus (A) and body of *Trichuris* (B).

Trichuris from a pregnant woman who had a hemoglobin of 7 gm. Not infrequently, the *Trichuris* infection is accompanied by malnutrition or hookworm or *E. histolytica* infections, making it impossible to determine the exact role of *Trichuris* in the anemia and symptomatology. Studies indicate that children with light and moderate infections have hemoglobin values essentially identical to those of noninfected children. The white blood cell count and differential are usually normal. Eosinophilia is encountered rarely in uncomplicated *Trichuris* infections. *Trichuris* may attach to the appendiceal mucosa and provide an entrance for pathogenic bacteria and subsequent acute or subacute inflammatory processes.

Diagnosis. Clinical trichuriasis cannot be differentiated from infections with other intestinal nematodes, although eosinophilia is present somewhat more consistently. Diagnosis is made by finding the characteristic lemon-shaped eggs in the feces. Light infections may necessitate the use of concentration methods (see Chapter 18).

Treatment. Before mebendazole was introduced, the only effective treatment for trichuriasis was the messy, cumbersome, and emo-tionally traumatic (for doctor and nurse as well as for patient) hexylresorcinol enema. Fortunately, mebendazole, a poorly absorbed and well tolerated oral drug, was developed and found to be very effective. The dose is 100 mg b.i.d. for 3 days. Thiabendazole is not effective. There is probably no need to treat light asymptomatic infections.

Prevention. Infection in highly endemic areas may be prevented by (1) treatment of infected individuals, (2) sanitary disposal of human feces, (3) washing of hands before meals, (4) instruction of children in sanitation and personal hygiene, and (5) thorough washing and scalding of uncooked vegetables; the fifth is especially important in countries using night soil for fertilizer.

Strongyloides stercoralis

Diseases. Strongyloidiasis, Cochin-China diarrhea.

Life Cycle. People are the principal hosts of *S. stercoralis,* but dogs and monkeys have a similar parasite. A similar species, *S. fullerborni,* can infest higher primates and humans. In the parasitic stage, no male form of this organism has been reliably identified, and the female reproduces in a parthenogenetic manner. The parasitic female (Fig. 6-6), 2.20 by 0.04 mm, is a small, colorless, semitransparent filariform nematode with a finely striated cuticle. It has a short buccal cavity and a long, slender, cylindrical esophagus. The paired uteri contain a single file of thin-shelled, transparent, segmented eggs. The parasitic females penetrate the mucosa of the intestinal villi, where they burrow in serpentine channels in the mucosa, depositing eggs and securing nourishment. The worms are most frequently found in the duodenum and upper jejunum, but in heavy infections the pylorus, both the small and large intestines, and the proximal biliary and pancreatic passages may be involved. The eggs of the parasitic form, 54 by 32 μ, are deposited in the intestinal mucosa. They hatch into rhabditiform larvae that penetrate the glandular epithelium and pass into the lumen of the intestine and out in the feces. The eggs

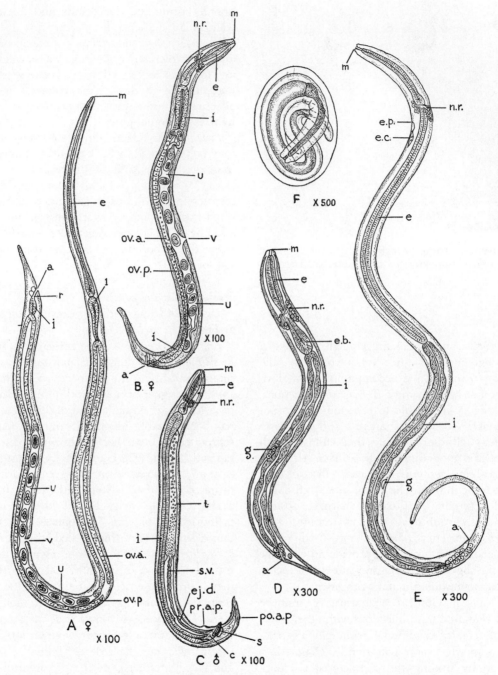

Figure 6-6. *Strongyloides stercoralis.* A. Parasitic female. B. Free-living female. C. Free-living male. D. Rhabditiform larva. E. filariform larva. F. Egg containing mature larva of *S. simiae.* (A–E redrawn or adapted from Looss, 1911. F adapted from Kreis, 1932.)

a, anus; c, cloaca; e, esophagus; e.b., esophageal bulb; e.c., excretory cell; ej.d., ejaculatory duct; e.p., excretory pore; g, genital rudiment; i, intestine; m, mouth; n.r., nerve ring; ov.a., anterior ovary; ov.p., posterior ovary; po.a.p., postanal papilla; pr.a.p., preanal papilla; r, rectum; s, spicules; s.v., seminal vesicle; t, testis; u, uterus; v, vulva.

are seldom found in the stool except after violent purgation.

This parasite has three types of life cycle.

1. DIRECT CYCLE, LIKE HOOKWORM. After a short feeding period of 2 to 3 days in the soil, the rhabditiform larva (Fig. 6-7), 225 by 16 μ, molts into a long, slender, nonfeeding, infective, filariform larva about 700 μ in length. The infective filariform larvae penetrate the human skin, enter the venous circulation, and pass through the right heart to the lungs, where they penetrate into the alveoli. From the lungs the adolescent parasites ascend to the glottis, are swallowed, and reach the upper part of the small intestine, where they develop into adults. Occasionally some larvae pass through the pulmonary barrier into the arterial circulation and reach various organs of the body. During their migration in the host the larvae pass through two molts to become adolescent worms. Mature ovipositing females develop in about 28 days after the initial infection.

2. INDIRECT CYCLE. In the indirect cycle the rhabditiform larvae develop into sexually mature, free-living males and females in the soil. After fertilization the free-living female produces eggs that develop into rhabditiform larvae. These may become infective filariform larvae within a few days and enter new hosts, or they may repeat the free-living generation. The indirect method appears to be associated with the optimal environmental conditions for a free-living existence in tropical countries, while the direct method is more frequently followed in the less favorable, colder regions. Strains may show chiefly one or the other type of development or a mixture of both types.

3. AUTOINFECTION. At times the larvae may develop rapidly into the filariform stage in the intestine and, by penetrating the intestinal mucosa or the perianal skin, establish a developmental cycle within the host. Autoinfection explains persistent strongyloidiases in patients living in nonendemic areas. Several studies indicate that a substantial number of British and Australian veterans of World War II who were exposed in Southeast Asia have carried asymptomatic *Strongyloides* infections for 30

years or more. Autoinfection is also one of the few examples of multiplication of a helminth within the host.

Epidemiology. The distribution of *Strongyloides* infection runs parallel to that of hookworm, but its prevalence is lower in the temperate zones. It is especially prevalent in tropical and subtropical areas, where warmth, moisture, and lack of sanitation favor its free-living cycle. In the United States it occurs in the rural South and in migrant Puerto Ricans. One characteristic of the life cycle that favors transmission is the fact that infective larvae can sometimes be present in the feces or develop rapidly after excretion. Thus, it is not unusual to find cases in mental hospitals or institutions where sanitation is poor. Also, there is evidence that some animals, such as dogs or monkeys, may serve as nonhuman reservoirs of infection, with strains of parasite capable of infecting humans.

Pathology and Symptomatology. Many *Strongyloides* infections are light and go unnoticed by their human host, as they produce no significant symptoms. Moderate infections, with the parasitic females embedded primarily in the duodenal region, may cause a burning, dull or sharp, nonradiating midepigastric pain. Pressure to this area may elicit pain and tenderness. Nausea and vomiting may be present; diarrhea and constipation alternate. Longstanding and heavy infections result in weight loss and chronic dysentery accompanied by malabsorption and steatorrhea. In heavy infections, all the signs and symptoms are more marked, and death may ensue. Pulmonary symptoms, with asthmatic-type wheezing and cough, may predominate in some cases. One of our patients with overwhelming strongyloidiasis had a fatal *E. coli* infection that was probably carried to her bloodstream by the numerous filariform larvae migrating from her intestine. At autopsy, parasitic worms were found embedded in the mucosa, all the way from her stomach to the lower colon, with inflammation of her gastrointestinal tract. Her lungs showed hemorrhage and foci of pneumonia. Filariform larvae were found in most organs of the body. She had moved to New

York from Panama 36 years previously and had never left the city.

In recent years there has been increasing recognition of the association of disseminated, often fatal strongyloidiasis with diseases such as Hodgkin's lymphoma or immunosuppressive therapy for other conditions. The use of corticosteroids especially appears to predispose to disseminated disease.

Diagnosis. Clinical diagnosis is difficult since strongyloidiasis presents no distinctive clinical picture. The sequence of an atypical bronchitis or pneumonitis followed in a few weeks by a mucous or watery diarrhea, epigastric pain,

STRONGYLOIDES STERCORALIS

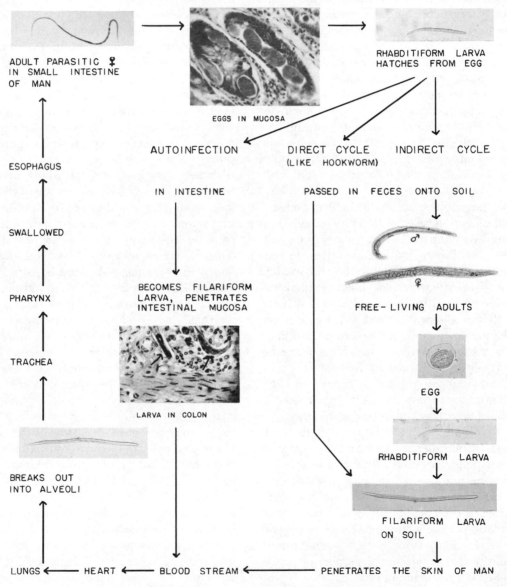

Figure 6-7. Life cycle of *Strongyloides stercoralis.*

and eosinophilia is suggestive. The eosinophilia is moderate, usually ranging from 10 to 20 percent, but is frequently present.

Laboratory diagnosis includes the examination of the feces and duodenal contents by direct or concentration methods. The presence of characteristic motile rhabditiform larvae in fresh feces is diagnostic; in heavy infections they may be found in simple film preparations. The duodenal fluid of suspected subjects should be examined, by aspiration or by the string test, as suggested for giardiasis, if the feces are negative. The duodenal fluid gives slightly higher positive findings. The rhabditiform larvae of *Strongyloides* differ morphologically from those of hookworms, which are rarely found in fresh feces (see Fig. 6-10), while the embryonated *Strongyloides* eggs, slightly smaller than those of hookworms, can only be obtained by a drastic purge or by duodenal intubation. Cultivation of the feces for 48 hours will produce filariform larvae and, depending upon the strain of parasite, may also produce free-living adult *Strongyloides*. Since female worms sometimes become established in the lungs, sputum should be examined for larvae, directly or after concentration.

Most infected individuals have antibodies to *S. stercoralis* or *S. ratti* demonstrable by ELISA and other tests. Relatively few cross-reactions occur with ELISA, which may be especially useful because antibodies decline 6 to 12 months after successful treatment.

Treatment. Thiabendazole (Mintezol) is the drug of choice, 25 mg per kilogram of body weight twice daily for 2 or 3 days. Some resistant cases may require 5 to 7 days of treatment. No special diet or purgation is required. Side effects consisting of anorexia, nausea, vomiting, dizziness, and a prominent garlic taste are common. Less frequent are diarrhea, epigastric distress, pruritis, drowsiness, and headache.

As a second choice, pyrvinium pamoate has some activity against *Strongyloides,* but it must be used at two to three times greater than the usual dosage of 5 to 10 mg per kilogram for 5

days. The maximum daily dosage should be 1.5 gm, and the drug is given after meals to reduce nausea or vomiting

Prevention. The prevention of strongyloidiasis is similar to that of hookworm disease and depends upon the sanitary disposal of human wastes and protection of the skin from contact with contaminated soil. The disease may be self-perpetuating for years because of autoinfection. Autoinfection may be eliminated by treatment. Detection and treatment of subclinical carriers does not appear to be practical, except in family infections.

Human Hookworms

Diseases. Ancylostomiasis, uncinariasis, necatoriasis, hookworm infection.

Species. The species in man include (1) *Necator americanus,* (2) *Ancylostoma duodenale,* and, rarely (3) *A. braziliense,* (4) *A. caninum,* and (5) *A. ceylanicum.*

History. Hookworm infection probably existed among the ancient Egyptians. The disease was described in Italy, Arabia, and Brazil long before *A. duodenale,* the Old World hookworm, was discovered by Dubini in 1838. In 1877, following an epidemic among the laborers at the St. Gotthard tunnel in Switzerland, the metamorphosis of the free-living rhabditiform larva into the infectious filariform larva and the etiopathology, symptomatology, diagnosis, and therapy of hookworm infection were established. During 1905–11 Looss described infection through the skin and the migratory route of the larvae through the body. Although hookworm disease was recognized in the United States as early as 1845, it was not until 1902 that Stiles described the New World hookworm, *N. americanus,* which was brought to the United States from West Africa with the importation of slaves.

Morphology. Adult hookworms are small, cylindrical, fusiform, grayish white nematodes (Fig. 6-8). The females (9 to 13 by 0.35 to 0.6 mm) are larger than the males (5 to 11 by 0.3 to 0.45 mm). *A. duodenale* is larger than *N. americanus.* The worm has a relatively thick cuticle. There are single male and paired female reproductive organs. The posterior end of the male has a broad, translucent, membranous caudal bursa with riblike rays, which is used for attachment to the female during copulation.

The chief morphologic differences in the species are in the shape, buccal capsule, and male bursa. The vulva is located anterior to the middle of the body in *Necator* and posterior in *Ancylostoma*. In the buccal capsule *N. amer-*

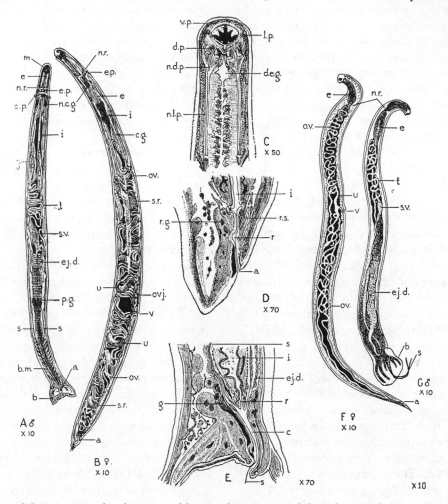

Figure 6-8. Important hookworms of human beings. A. Adult male *Ancylostoma duodenale* from ventral side. B. Young adult female *A. duodenale* from right side. C. Anterior end of *A. duodenale* from dorsal side. D. Longitudinal section through posterior end of female *A. duodenale,* somewhat diagrammatic. E. Longitudinal section through posterior end of male *A. duodenale,* not quite median. F. Female *Necator americanus.* G. Male *N. americanus.* (A-E redrawn from Looss, 1905. F and G redrawn after Placencia from Manson-Bahr, 1936.)

a, anus; b, bursa; b.m., bursal muscles; c, cloaca; c.g., cervical gland; c.p., cervical papilla; d.e.g., dorsal esophageal gland; d.p., dorsal papilla; e, esophagus; e.p., excretory pore; ej.d., ejaculatory duct; g, gubernaculum; i, intestine; l.p., lateral papilla; m, mouth; n.c.g., nucleus of cephalic gland; n.d.p., nerve of dorsal papilla; n.l.p., nerve of lateral papilla; n.r., nerve ring; ov., ovary; ovj., ovejector; p.g., prostatic glands; r, rectum; r.g., rectal ganglion; r.s., rectal sphincter; s, spicules; s.r., seminal receptacle; s.v., seminal vesicle; t, testis; u, uterus; v, vulva; v.p., ventral papilla.

icanus has a conspicuous dorsal pair of semilunar cutting plates, a concave dorsal median tooth, and a deep pair of triangular subventral lancets. *A. duodenale* has two ventral pairs of teeth, *A. braziliense* two ventral pairs, and *A. caninum* three ventral pairs.

The egg (Fig. 6-9) has bluntly rounded ends and a single thin transparent hyaline shell. It is unsegmented at oviposition and in two to eight cell stages of division in fresh feces. The eggs of the several species are almost indistinguishable, differing only slightly in size: *N. americanus* 64 to 76 by 36 to 40 μ and *A. duodenale* 56 to 60 by 36 to 40 μ.

Life Cycle (Fig. 6-9). The life cycles of the several species of hookworm are similar. Humanity is almost the exclusive host of *A. duodenale* and *N. americanus,* although these species have been reported occasionally in primates and other mammals. The adults of *A. braziliense,* a parasite of wild and domestic felines and canines in the tropics, are infrequently found in humans. *A. caninum,* the common hookworm of dogs and cats, is an extremely rare intestinal parasite of humans.

The eggs, passed in the feces, mature rapidly and produce the rhabditiform larvae in 1 to 2 days under favorable conditions and an optimal temperature of 23 to 33 C. Eggs of *A. duodenale* die in a few hours at 45 C and in 7 days at 0 C.

The rhabditiform larvae (Fig. 6-10) of *A. duodenale* and *N. americanus* are somewhat larger, more attenuated posteriorly, and have a longer buccal capsule than the larvae of *S. stercoralis*. The newly hatched larvae, 275 by 16 μ, feed actively upon bacteria and organic debris and grow rapidly to a size of 500 to 700 μ in 5 days. Then they molt for a second time to become slender, nonfeeding, infective filariform larvae (Fig. 6-10), which differ from the filariform larvae of *S. stercoralis* in the absence of notched clefts in the pointed tail and a shorter esophagus. The active filariform larvae, which frequent the upper half-inch of soil and project from the surface, have a strong thigmotaxis that facilitates access to the skin of a new host. Hookworm larvae remain within a few inches of where they are deposited unless carried by floods or animals to other locations.

In heavily infested soil under tropical conditions, practically all the larvae are extremely active, rapidly consume their stored food, and die within 6 weeks. However, constant reinfestation maintains the supply in endemic areas. Although they require little moisture, drying is destructive. They survive best in shaded localities, such as light sandy or alluvial soils or loam covered by vegetation, where they are protected from drying or excessive wetness. At 0 C larvae survive less than 2 weeks, at -11 C less than 24 hours, and at 45 C less than 1 hour.

The filariform larvae gain access to the host through hair follicles, pores, or even the unbroken skin. Damp clinging soil facilitates infection. The usual site of infection is the dorsum of the foot or between the toes. Miners and farmers may acquire the infection on the hands, chiefly in the interdigital spaces, and fishermen have been infected by sitting on infested stream banks. The larvae enter the lymphatics or venules and are carried in the blood through the heart to the lungs, where, because of their size, they are unable to pass the capillary barrier and therefore break out of the capillaries into the alveoli. They ascend the bronchi and trachea, are finally swallowed, and pass down to the intestines. This larval blood and pulmonary migration takes about 1 week. During this period the larvae undergo a third molt and acquire a temporary buccal capsule, which enables the adolescent worm to feed. After a fourth molt at about the thirteenth day, they acquire adult characteristics, and mature egg-laying females are produced in 5 to 6 weeks after infection. Rarely, infection may occur by mouth, the larvae being taken into the body through drinking water or contaminated food.

Epidemiology. The present distribution has been brought about by the migration of people and extends in the tropical and subtropical zones between 45 N and 30 S latitude, except for the presence of *A. duodenale* in the northern mining districts of Europe. *N. americanus* is the

NECATOR AMERICANUS   ANCYLOSTOMA DUODENALE

HOOKWORMS

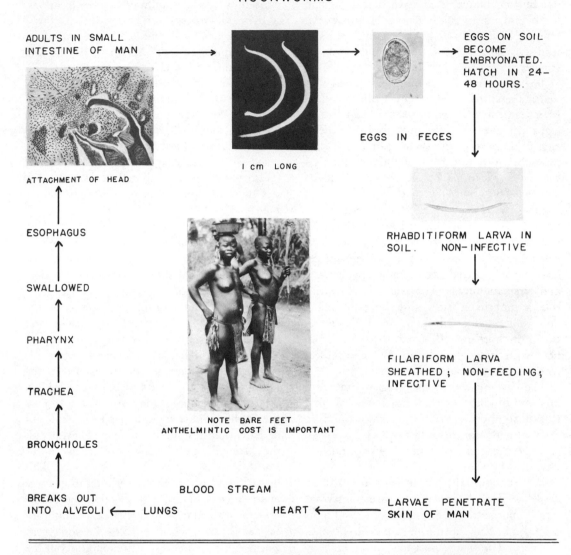

ADULTS IN SMALL
INTESTINE OF MAN

ATTACHMENT OF HEAD

I cm LONG

EGGS ON SOIL
BECOME
EMBRYONATED.
HATCH IN 24–
48 HOURS.

EGGS IN FECES

ESOPHAGUS

SWALLOWED

PHARYNX

TRACHEA

BRONCHIOLES

RHABDITIFORM LARVA IN
SOIL.   NON–INFECTIVE

FILARIFORM LARVA
SHEATHED ; NON–FEEDING;
INFECTIVE

NOTE BARE FEET
ANTHELMINTIC COST IS IMPORTANT

BLOOD STREAM

BREAKS OUT
INTO ALVEOLI ← LUNGS   HEART ←   LARVAE PENETRATE
                                          SKIN OF MAN

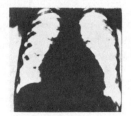

HOOKWORMS   1,498±
Hgb   2.0 g
IRON THERAPY STARTED

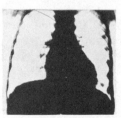

I MONTH AFTER
IRON THERAPY
Hgb 9.0 g

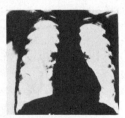

3 MOS. AFTER IRON THERAPY
2 MOS. AFTER C₂Cl₄ THERAPY
HOOKWORMS 120±
Hgb 12 g

CARDIAC ENLARGEMENT CAUSED BY ANEMIA

Figure 6-9. Life cycle of human hookworms.

prevailing species in the Western Hemisphere, in Central and South Africa, southern Asia, Indonesia, Australia, and the islands of the Pacific. *A. duodenale* is the dominant species in the Mediterranean region, northern Asia, and the west coast of South America. It is also found in smaller numbers in areas where *N. americanus* predominates.

It is estimated that throughout the world the hookworms, harbored by 500 million persons, cause a daily blood loss of more than 1 million liters, the total blood of a city the size

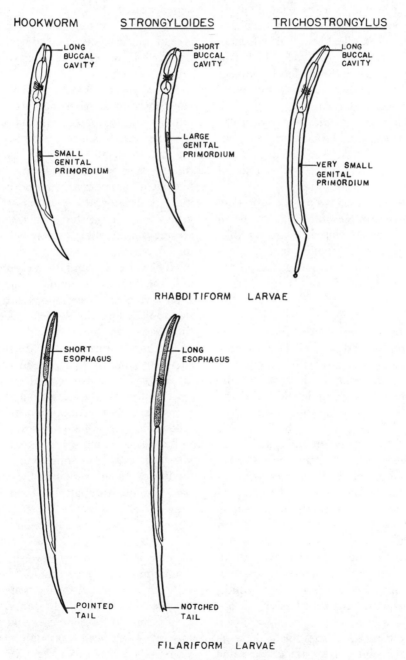

Figure 6-10. Differentiation of nematode larvae from stool.

of Erie, Pennsylvania, or of Austin, Texas.

The following factors favor hookworm maintenance and dispersal:

1. Infected individuals who defecate on the soil in areas frequented by others, fecal concentration in secluded areas near the house. Return to this restricted area by members of the family leads to family infection. The one-room school without sanitary facilities is an excellent source of infection.
2. A shaded sandy or loam soil, which is a favorable culture medium for hookworm larvae. Clay soil, which packs tightly, is unsuitable for the larvae.
3. A warm climate, which favors the development of the eggs and larvae and promiscuous defecation. Cold, snowy climes force people into shelter; hence the widespread use of the privy in such areas.
4. Moisture, 30 to 50 inches of rain, especially during the warm season of the year when egg and larval development are possible.
5. A poor, ignorant population that does not wear shoes. The population of half of the world does not wear shoes, nor can they afford them.

These conditions are found throughout the tropics, subtropics, and parts of the temperate zone. In Egypt, where little effort at concealment is made, defecation is widespread in the unshaded streets, yards, and fields, and the arid winds and sun destroy much of the potential infection. Hence, though hookworm is widespread, the infections are light, and hookworm disease is rare. In China, where mulberry trees are grown for the leaves to maintain silkworms, human night soil is used to fertilize the trees. In this sandy, moist, shady environment as many as 10,000 hookworm infective larvae were recovered from a soil sample. Picking of the mulberry leaves falls to the lot of women, and, as would be expected, they are heavily infected. Cultivation of coffee, sweet potatoes, and bananas offers similar opportunities for infection.

Black people are less susceptible to *N. americanus* than are whites living under the same unsanitary conditions. The reasons for this are not clear. Since this parasite appeared early in Africa there may have been some natural selection. Possibly the thicker skin of black people offers more resistance to the larva's penetration. Nutrition may play some part, since black people appear to be better nourished than their poor-white neighbors. It has been demonstrated that dogs fed a protein- and vitamin-deficient diet fail to develop the degree of immunity to repeated hookworm infection that is acquired by their well-nourished litter mates.

Pathology and Symptomatology. When the larvae penetrate the skin they produce maculopapules and localized erythema. Itching is often severe, and as it is related to contact with the soil, especially on dewy mornings when the moisture permits the larvae to be at the surface, it is known as "ground itch" or "dew itch." If considerable numbers of larvae migrate through the lungs at one time or in sensitized individuals, a bronchitis or pneumonitis may result.

Hookworm is essentially a chronic infection, and the infected individual often shows no acute symptoms. Symptoms attributable to the adult worm usually do not develop until the onset of anemia.

The hookworms attach to the mucosa of the small intestine by their buccal capsules. The favorite site is the upper small intestine, but in heavy infections the worms may be present as far as the lower ileum. They suck the host's blood and mucosal substances by the tractile pull of the contracting and expanding esophagus (Fig. 6-9). An anticoagulating secretion facilitates blood sucking. Since the blood passes rapidly through the worm, it is possible that simple diffusible substances are consumed. As much as 0.03 ml *(N. americanus)* and 0.15 to 0.26 ml *(A. duodenale)* of blood may be withdrawn by a worm in 24 hours. Approximately 50 percent of the red blood cells are hemolyzed during passage through the worm's intestine. *A. duodenale* infections may persist for 6 to 8 years and longer. The majority of *N. americanus* disappear within 2 years; others live 4 to 5 years. An experimental infection in an American scientist persisted for 14 years. The maximum daily egg output by a mature female has been estimated at 20,000 for *A. duodenale* and 10,000 for *N. americanus*. Egg production is relatively constant. Thus, the number of female worms may be calculated from the egg count, and there are usually an equal number of males.

Light infections produce no recognized symptoms, but elimination of the worms sometimes increases the vigor of children. The most prominent characteristic in moderate or heavy chronic hookworm infection is a progressive, secondary, microcytic, hypochromic anemia of the iron-deficiency type. Clinical and experimental evidence indicates that anemia is primarily due to the continuous loss of blood. The pathology and symptomatology are proportional to the number of worms and the iron intake of the patient. A combination of iron deficiency and hookworm infection appears necessary for the establishment of anemia, since it may be offset by the administration of iron. Depending on the degree of anemia, which may be as low as 2 gm of hemoglobin per 100 ml of blood, the patient experiences dyspnea on exertion, weakness, and dizziness, yet is up and about, demonstrating what the human body can withstand if the blood loss is minimal although chronic. This is the "germ of laziness" of Stiles, who left the South secretly after making this comment to the newsmen early in the twentieth century.

The appetite may be enormous or poor and associated with pica. The heart shows hypertrophy; a hemic murmur is present; and the pulse is rapid. There is edema of varying degrees, and albumin is present in the urine. Heavily infected children may be physically, mentally, and sexually retarded. Early in the infection eosinophilia and leukocytosis are marked; as the infection becomes chronic the eosinophilia and leukocytosis both decrease, but the anemia persists. The stools may contain gross blood, and occult blood is readily found.

Diagnosis. The clinical picture, though characteristic, is not sufficiently pathognomonic to permit differentiation from the nutri-

tional deficiency anemias and edemas or from other helminthic infections. Final diagnosis depends upon finding the eggs in the feces. Hookworm eggs may be confused with the root parasite eggs of *Meloidogyne (Heterodera)* or those of *Trichostrongylus*, which are larger, more elongated and have a larger number of blastomeres (see Figure 17-1).

Eggs are found in direct fecal films, but in light infections concentration methods (Chapter 18) may be required. The direct coverglass mount is of value only where there are more than 1200 eggs per gram of feces; cases with fewer than 400 are often missed. The zinc sulfate centrifugal flotation and the formalin-ether concentration methods increase the number of positive findings several-fold. The collection of larvae from eggs hatched on strips of filter paper with one end immersed in water (Harada-Mori culture) is reported to give a high percentage of positive findings. Egg-counting methods, such as the Stoll dilution eggcount (Chapter 18) or Kato's smear method, that indicate the intensity of the infection are useful in surveys, and before and after therapy. It is important to distinguish the rhabditiform larvae of hookworm from those of *Strongyloides*, and *Trichostrongylus*, all of which may be found in stool specimens that are several days old (Fig. 6-10). In fresh stools the eggs of hookworm and *Trichostrongylus* will be found in the early stages of cleavage, and *Strongyloides* as rhabditiform larvae. It must be remembered that the patient may harbor more than one species of parasite.

Treatment. Several effective and safe drugs are now available for treatment of both species of hookworm infections. One of these is mebendazole, used in a dose of 100 mg twice daily for 3 days, for both adults and children. The other drug of equal efficacy, pyrantel pamoate, can be given in a single dose of 11 mg per kilogram, not to exceed 1 gm. While a single dose of pyrantel will greatly reduce the intensity of infection and be convenient for mass treatment programs, there is a greater likelihood of curing the infection by giving pyrantel for 3 days. Neither drug has any special requirements regarding fasting or purgation before or after administration. Both drugs also have the advantage of being effective against *Ascaris*, which is frequently present with hookworm infections.

If significant anemia due to hookworm infection is present, the first consideration is treatment of the anemia. Since hookworm anemia is due to iron deficiency, the hemoglobin level will rise following oral administration of iron even though the hookworm infection is not treated. Antihelminthic treatment can be given after a reticulocyte response occurs. If the hookworms are eliminated without the correction of iron deficiency, the hemoglobin level will not return to normal for months. When hookworm anemia is so severe that transfusion is considered necessary, the patient will tolerate packed red cells better than whole blood because of hypervolemia.

Treatment of light infections in endemic areas, where reinfection is certain and rapid, is of questionable value. However, in individuals not likely to be reexposed even light infections that come to the attention of a physician can probably be treated because the medication is effective, safe, and relatively inexpensive.

Prevention. Hookworm infection may be reduced or even eliminated in a community by (1) the sanitary disposal of fecal wastes, (2) the protection of susceptible individuals, and (3) the treatment of infected individuals. We can go to the moon and return, yet 500 million persons in the world, many in the southern United States, are still hookworm infected.

From a practical standpoint it is most important to treat persons showing clinical evidence of the disease. Mass treatment is advisable when the incidence is greater than 50 percent, the average worm burden greater than 150, and facilities for examining all of the population are not available. Unless mass treatment includes the entire population, is repeated at intervals, and is accompanied by improvements in sanitation, its effect is temporary.

Sanitation is the chief method of control. In rural communities, where sewerage systems are impracticable, promiscuous defecation may be curtailed by the construction of pit privies. Education of the public as to the method of transmission of hookworm infection and the use of privies is as essential as their installation. Attempts to enforce sanitary regulations are less effective than sanitary instruction in the home, publicity campaigns, and training in the schools. The use of night soil as fertilizer in certain countries presents an economic and sanitary problem that may be solved by storage or by chemical disinfection of feces.

The protection of the susceptible individual in an endemic locality is largely an economic and educational problem. It involves the prevention of malnutrition by an adequate diet. Although the wearing of shoes, especially by children, is important, it is economically impossible in the tropics, and to the children it is often unacceptable.

CUTANEOUS LARVA MIGRANS, CREEPING ERUPTION

Disease. Creeping eruption is a dermatitis characterized by serpiginous intracutaneous lesions caused by migration of nematode larvae that normally do not infect the human host. The hookworm of cats and dogs, *Ancylostoma braziliense,* is most commonly incriminated, although other species of hookworms, such as *A. caninum,* are in rare cases the etiologic agents. The infective larvae of other nonhuman helminthic parasites can enter the human skin, or even be ingested, and fail to complete their development in this abnormal host. Some, like the cerceriae of bird schistosomes, can produce annoying skin eruptions known as "swimmer's itch" by allergic sensitization.

Epidemiology. Creeping eruption, which is prevalent in many tropical and subtropical countries of the world and in the United States especially along the Gulf and southern Atlantic states, is caused by the filariform larvae of *A. braziliense,* which lives as an adult in the intestine of humanity's two close animal friends, the dog and the cat. Hence, their feces are ever available to pollute the human environment. Sea and fresh-water bathers who bask in the sun on the beach while their dogs pollute it, plumbers who work in close contact with larva-infested soil, and children whose castles are made in sandboxes that are open to cat and dog pollution are most commonly infected. All of these environments supply the moist, sandy soil required for the development of hookworm larvae.

Pathology and Symptomatology. At the points of larval invasion, indurated, reddish, itchy papules develop, and in 2 to 3 days narrow, lin-

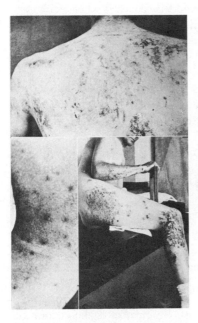
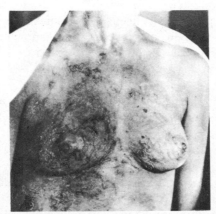
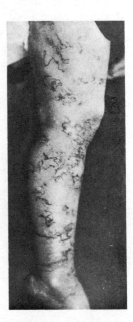

LESIONS SECONDARILY INFECTED AND   UNINFECTED

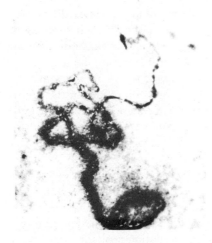
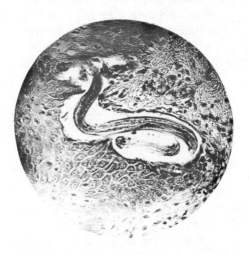

Figure 6-11. Creeping eruption: Cutaneous larva migrans caused by the larva of *Ancylostoma braziliensis*. (After Kirby-Smith, Dove, and White, 1926.)

ear, slightly elevated, erythematous, serpiginous, intracutaneous tunnels, 1 to 2 mm in diameter, are produced by the migratory larvae (Fig. 6-11). They move from a fraction of an inch to more than an inch per day, but rarely pass beyond a few inches from the original site of entry. Vesicles form along the course of the tunnels, and the surface becomes dry and crusty. Local eosinophilia and round-cell infiltration may be present. The itching is intense, especially at night when one has nothing else to distract one's attention, and the resultant scratching may lead to secondary infection. The feet, legs, and hands are most commonly involved, but infection of any portion of the body exposed to infested soil may occur. On babies' faces and buttocks, because of bacterial infections, it may resemble impetigo. Plumbers are most commonly infected on their knees, elbows, buttocks, and shoulders; secondary infection in them may be extensive. The larval infection may persist for weeks or even as long as a year. The senior author, who as a student was given an experimental infection of five larvae by Drs. White and Dove (who unraveled the mysteries of this disease in 1926), noted the decease of the first larva in 2 weeks and the last in 8 weeks, strangers in a strange land, wandering at random. At the site of their demise a red papule was formed. A few patients with cutaneous infections develop a transitory infiltration of the lungs with a high eosinophilia of the blood and sputum, which is the result of pulmonary migration of the larvae and an allergic reaction of the host.

Treatment. Thiabendazole, either topically or systemically, has proven successful. If a 10-percent suspension of thiabendazole can be obtained, it is applied locally to the lesions. Alternatively, the drug is taken orally at 25 mg per kilogram twice daily, not exceeding 3 gm per day, for 2 to 5 days. Light infections with only several larvae may be managed by freezing an area. in the active portion of the lesion with ethyl chloride or carbon dioxide snow. If secondary bacterial infection is present, it should be treated with appropriate antibiotics.

Prevention. Control of creeping eruption of hookworm origin consists of avoiding skin contact with soil that has been contaminated with dog or cat feces. Keeping dogs and cats off beaches and away from the space under houses (where plumbers may work) and anthelmintic treatment of dogs and cats will prevent contamination of the soil. Children's sandboxes should be covered when not in use. Skin infection with *Necator* and *Strongyloides* can be prevented by proper disposal of human excreta.

Enterobius vermicularis

Diseases. Enterobiasis, oxyuriasis, pinworm, seatworm.

Morphology (Fig. 6-12). The small adult female worm (8.0 to 13.0 mm by 0.4 mm) has a cuticular alar expansion at the anterior end, a prominent esophageal bulb, and a long pointed tail. The uteri of the gravid female are distended with eggs. The male, 2 to 5 mm in length with a curved tail and a single spicule, is seldom seen.

Life Cycle (Fig. 6-13). Humanity is the only known host of *E. vermicularis.* The usual habitat of the mature pinworm is the cecum and the adjacent portions of the large and small intestines. Immature females and males occasionally may be found in the rectum and lower part of the colon. At times the worms may travel upward to the stomach, esophagus, and nose. The gravid females, containing from 11,000 to 15,000 eggs, migrate to the perianal and perineal regions, where the eggs are expelled in masses by contractions of the uterus and vagina under the stimulus of a lower temperature and aerobic environment. The eggs mature and are infectious several hours after passage.

Upon ingestion of the egg, the embryonic first-stage larvae hatch in the duodenum. The liberated rhabditiform larvae molt twice before reaching adolescence in the jejunum and upper ileum. Copulation probably takes place in the cecum. The duration of the cycle from the ingestion of the egg to the perianal migration of the gravid female may be as short as 4

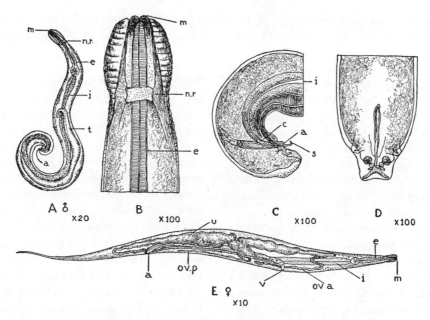

Figure 6-12. *Enterobius vermicularis.* A. Male. B. Anterior end of worm. C. Posterior end of male, lateral view. D. Posterior end of male, ventral view. E. Female. (Redrawn from Leuckart, 1876.)

a, anus; c, cloaca; e, esophagus; i, intestine; m, mouth; n.r., nerve ring; ov.a., anterior ovary; ov.p., posterior ovary; s, spicule; t, testis; u, uterus; v, vulva.

to 6 weeks, but often it is longer. The infection is self-limited and, in the absence of reinfection, ceases without treatment.

Epidemiology. Pinworm has the widest geographic distribution of any helminth, and its success is due to a close association with humans and their environment. Stoll estimated that there are 208.8 million infected persons in the world, and 18 million in Canada and the United States. Surveys have revealed infection rates of from 3 to 80 percent in various groups. An Eskimo village gave a 66 percent infection rate; in tropical Brazil the rate has been 60 percent; and in Washington, D.C., 12 to 41 percent. Although this parasite is more prevalent in the lower economic groups, mental institutions, and orphanages, it is not uncommon in the well-to-do, highly educated, and even in the seats of the mighty. Children are more commonly infected than adults, and the incidence in whites is considerably higher than in black people.

Infection of the same or another person may be effected by (1) the important hand-to-mouth transmission from scratching the perianal areas or from handling contaminated fomites, (2) inhalation of airborne eggs in dust, and (3) rarely, retroinfection through the anus. Eggs hatch in the perianal region and the larvae migrate back into the large intestine. Heavy infections are effected by the transference of eggs from the perianal region to the hands and thence to the mouth directly or through contaminated food. In households with several pinworm-infected members, 92 percent of 241 dust samples collected from floors, baseboards, tables, chairs, davenports, dressers, shelves, picture frames, windowsills, toilet seats, wash basins, bath tubs, bed sheets, and mattresses contained *Enterobius* eggs. The largest number of eggs was found in bedrooms. This study demonstrates how the infection is spread through families or groups living in the same environment. Pinworm eggs have been isolated from the dust of school rooms and the school's cafeteria, which could be the source of a new family infection. Fortunately most of these eggs are dead, as it has been shown that at usual room temperature (20 to 24.5 C) and a relative humidity of 30 to 54 percent, less than 10 percent of eggs survived for 2 days. At hot summer temperatures (36 to 37 C) and a relative humidity of 38 to 41 percent, less than 10 percent of the eggs survived for 3 hours. These data explain why reinfection is not universal in a potentially infected environment. DOGS AND CATS DO NOT HARBOR ENTEROBIUS, yet the eggs from their master's environment may be carried on their fur and serve as a source of infection for their affectionate mistresses and masters.

Parents of infected children may become infected in the bath tub, or on Sunday morning when the small children climb into bed with them with their egg-laden rear ends.

Pathology and Symptomatology. E. vermicularis is relatively innocuous and rarely produces serious lesions. The clinical symptoms are due largely to the perianal, perineal, and vaginal irritation caused by the migrations of the gravid female worm, and less frequently to the intestinal activities of the parasite. The local pruritus and discomfort produce a chain of secondary reflex symptoms that tend to debilitate the patient—this debilitation is due to disturbed sleep.

Various observers have ascribed a number of signs and symptoms to the presence of pinworm, e.g., poor appetite, loss of sleep, weight loss, hyperactivity, enuresis, insomnia, irritability, grinding of the teeth, abdominal pain, nausea, and vomiting, but it is often difficult to prove the causal relationship of pinworm. The gravid females may migrate (and become imbedded and die, with granuloma formation) into the uterus, the fallopian tubes, the peritoneal cavity, and even the urinary bladder. They are frequently found in the appendix but are probably seldom the cause of appendicitis.

Slight eosinophilia has been reported, but it is unusual. As this parasite normally has no tissue-migrating stage and does not attach to the intestine, blood changes would not be expected.

The conscientious housewife's mental distress, guilt complex, and desire to conceal the infection from her friends is perhaps the most important trauma of this persistent, pruritic parasite.

Diagnosis. Pinworm infection is suspected in children who show perianal itching, insomnia, and restlessness. Diagnosis is made by finding the adult worms or eggs. Often the first evidence of infection is the discovery of the adult worms on the feces or in the perianal region. In only about 5 percent of infected persons are eggs found in the feces. They are best obtained by swabbing the perianal region. Graham's Scotch adhesive tape swab (Fig. 6-13) gives the highest percentage of positive results and the greatest number of eggs. In this method, a strip of sticky Scotch tape is applied to the perianal region, removed, and then spread on a slide for examination. The preparation may be cleared by placing a drop of toluol between the slide and tape. A drop of iodine in xylol, which gives a stained background for the eggs as well as clearing, is preferred by some workers. Repeated examinations on consecutive days are necessary because of the irregular migrations of the gravid female worms. A single swabbing reveals only about 50 percent of the infections; three swabbings, about 90 percent. Examinations on 7 consecutive days are necessary before the patient is considered free from infection. The swab for eggs is preferably made in the morning before bathing or defecation. In about one-third of infected children, eggs may be obtained from beneath the fingernails. The eggs are identified by their asymmetrical shape and well-developed embryo.

Treatment. The treatment of a person harboring pinworm is frequently unsatisfactory if other infected members of the household are untreated and remain sources of infection. It is recommended, therefore, if it is not feasible to make several Scotch tape examinations and treat only those found to be infected, that all members of the household be treated simultaneously.

A number of drugs are available for treatment. Mebendazole (Vermox) requires only a single-dose chewable tablet of 100 mg for both adults and children over 2 years of age. A

ENTEROBIUS VERMICULARIS

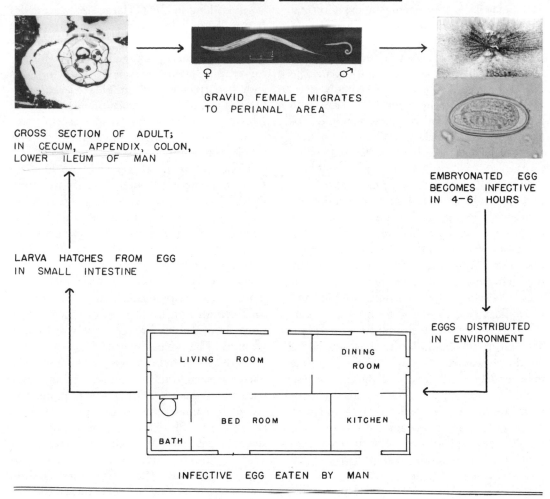

GRAVID FEMALE MIGRATES
TO PERIANAL AREA

CROSS SECTION OF ADULT;
IN CECUM, APPENDIX, COLON,
LOWER ILEUM OF MAN

EMBRYONATED EGG
BECOMES INFECTIVE
IN 4−6 HOURS

LARVA HATCHES FROM EGG
IN SMALL INTESTINE

EGGS DISTRIBUTED
IN ENVIRONMENT

LIVING ROOM

DINING ROOM

BED ROOM

KITCHEN

BATH

INFECTIVE EGG EATEN BY MAN

SCOTCH TAPE DIAGNOSIS

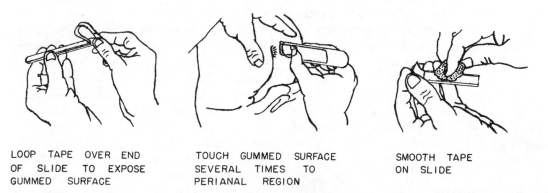

LOOP TAPE OVER END
OF SLIDE TO EXPOSE
GUMMED SURFACE

TOUCH GUMMED SURFACE
SEVERAL TIMES TO
PERIANAL REGION

SMOOTH TAPE
ON SLIDE

Figure 6-13. Life cycle of *Enterobius vermicularis*.

second dose should be given after 2 weeks. Mebendazole is teratogenic in experimental animals, so it should not be given to pregnant women.

Pyrantel pamoate (Antiminth), 11 mg per kilogram orally (maximum 1 gm) as a single dose, repeated after 2 weeks, is equally effective. The drug is in suspension form. Side reactions of headache, dizziness, vomiting, abdominal pain, diarrhea and elevations of liver enzyme (SGOT) levels are mild and transitory.

Pyrvinium pamoate (Povan) is also effective. Both tablets and a liquid preparation are available. The dosage is 5 mg of the base per kilogram (maximum 250 mg). As with the other drugs, a second dose 2 weeks after the first dose is recommended. Pyrvinium colors the stool bright red, and the suspension, if spilled or vomited, will stain garments and bedclothes. Nausea and vomiting may occur.

Prevention. Personal cleanliness is essential. The fingernails should be cut short; the hands should be washed thoroughly after using the toilet and before meals; and the anal region should be washed on rising. A salve or ointment applied to the perianal area will help prevent the dispersal of eggs. Infected children should wear tight-fitting cotton pants to prevent contact of hands with perianal region and the contamination of the bed clothing. Since the bathtub may be a source of infection, the use of a shower bath is suggested. In order to protect others, the infected person should sleep alone, and underwear, night clothes, and bed sheets should be carefully handled and laundered. Food should be protected from dust and from the hands of infected individuals. The difficulty of preventing dustborne and retroinfections may account for the failure of strict hygienic measures. The mother should be informed that it is a self-limited, nonfatal infection, and that neighbors also may harbor it. Kindergarten and play school for the young are fertile sources of *Enterobius*.

Ascaris lumbricoides

Diseases. Ascariasis, ascaris infection, roundworm infection.

Morphology (Fig. 6-14). The white or pink worm is identified by (1) large size, with males 10 to 31 cm and females 22 to 35 cm, (2) smooth, finely striated cuticle, (3) conical anterior and posterior extremities, (4) ventrally curved papillated posterior extremity of male with two spicules, (5) terminal mouth with three oval lips with sensory papillae, and (6) paired reproductive organs in posterior two-thirds of female, and a single long tortuous tubule in male.

The eggs (Fig. 6-14) measure 45 to 70 by 35 to 50 μ. There is an outer, coarsely mammillated, albuminous covering that serves as an auxiliary barrier to permeability but may be absent. The egg proper has a thick, transparent, hyaline shell with a relatively thick outer layer that acts as a supporting structure, and a delicate vitelline, lipoidal, inner membrane that is highly impermeable. At oviposition the shell contains an ovoid mass of unsegmented protoplasm densely impregnated with lecithin granules. The typical infertile eggs (see Figure 17-3), 88 to 94 by 39 to 44 μ, are longer and narrower than fertile eggs, have a thinner shell with an irregular coating of albumin, and are completely filled with an amorphous mass of protoplasm, with refractile granules. Bizarrely shaped eggs without albuminous coating or with abnormally extensive and irregular coating are also found. The infertile eggs are difficult to identify and may be missed by the unwary and untutored. They are found not only in the absence of males but in about two-fifths of all infections, since repeated copulations are necessary for the continuous production of fertile eggs.

Life Cycle (Fig. 6-14). The adult worms normally live in the lumen of the small intestine. They obtain their nourishment from the semidigested food of the host. Male or female worms are found alone in very lightly infected persons. A female worm has a productive capacity of 26 million eggs and an average daily output of 200,000. The eggs are unsegmented when they leave the host in the feces. Under favorable environmental conditions in the soil, infective second-stage larvae, after the first molt, are formed within the egg shell in about 3 weeks. The optimal temperature for development is about 25 C, ranging from 21 to 30 C. Lower temperatures retard development but favor survival. At 37 C they develop only to the eight-cell stage. Since eggs require oxygen, their development in putrefactive material is retarded.

The infective egg, when ingested by humans, hatches in the upper small intestine, freeing its rhabditiform larva (200 to 300 by 14 μ in size), which penetrates the intestinal wall to reach the venules or lymphatics. In the portal circulation larvae pass to the liver and

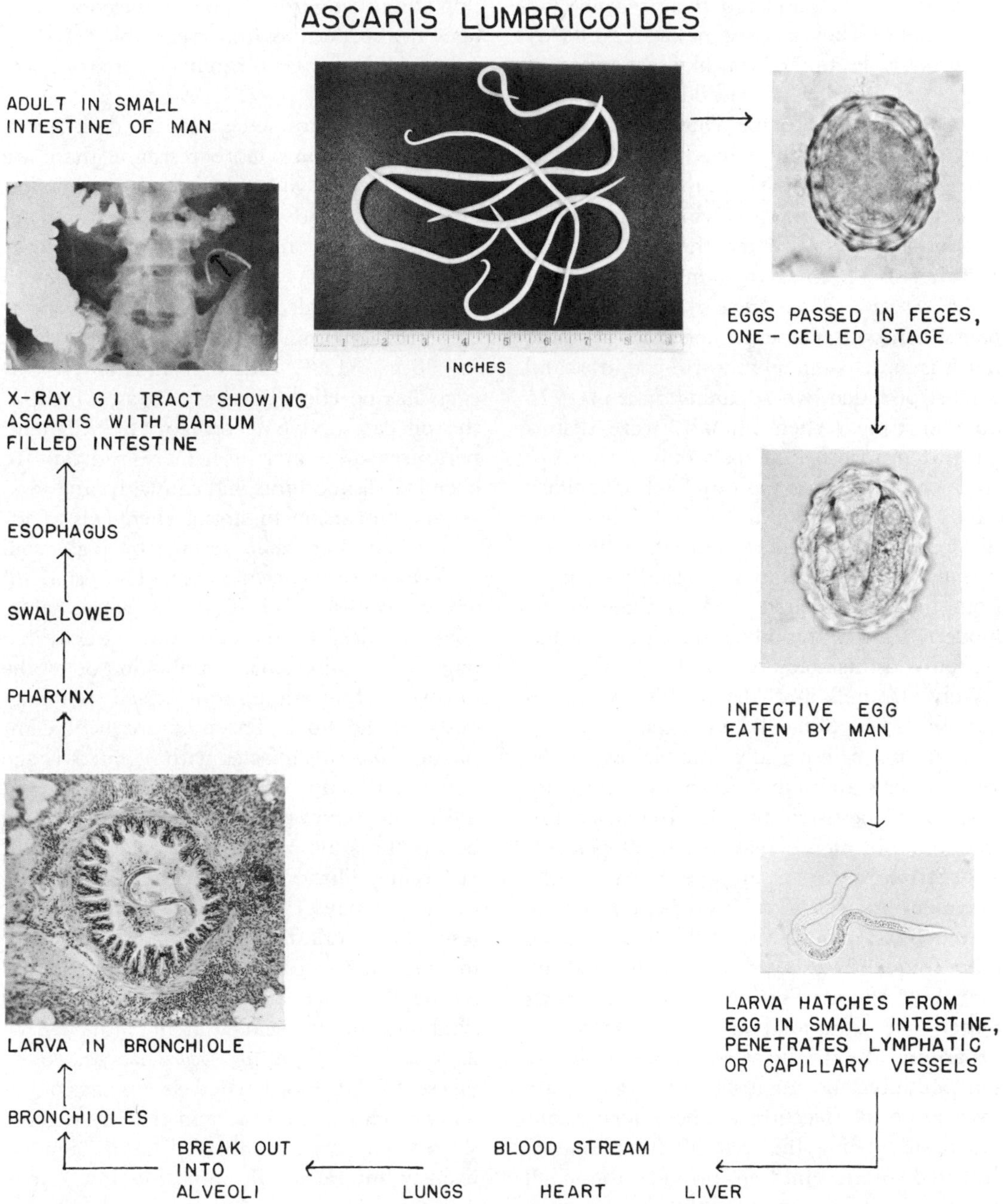

ASCARIS LUMBRICOIDES

ADULT IN SMALL
INTESTINE OF MAN

INCHES

X-RAY GI TRACT SHOWING
ASCARIS WITH BARIUM
FILLED INTESTINE

EGGS PASSED IN FECES,
ONE-CELLED STAGE

ESOPHAGUS

SWALLOWED

PHARYNX

INFECTIVE EGG
EATEN BY MAN

LARVA IN BRONCHIOLE

LARVA HATCHES FROM
EGG IN SMALL INTESTINE,
PENETRATES LYMPHATIC
OR CAPILLARY VESSELS

BRONCHIOLES

BREAK OUT   BLOOD STREAM
INTO
ALVEOLI   LUNGS   HEART   LIVER

Figure 6-14. Life cycle of *Ascaris lumbricoides.*

thence to the heart and lungs. The larvae may reach the lungs 1 to 7 days after infection. Since they are 0.02 mm in diameter and the pulmonary capillaries only 0.01 mm in diameter, they break out of the capillaries into the alveoli. Occasionally some reach the left heart by the pulmonary veins and are distributed as emboli to various organs of the body. In the lungs the larvae undergo their second and third molts. They migrate or are carried by the bronchioles to the bronchi, ascend the trachea to the glottis, and pass down the esophagus to the small intestine. During the pulmonary cycle the larvae increase fivefold, to 1.5 mm in length. On arrival in the intestine they undergo a fourth molt. Ovipositing females develop about 2 to 2½ months after infection, and they live from 12 to 18 months.

Epidemiology. A. lumbricoides is a prominent parasite in both temperate and tropical zones, but it is more common in warm countries and is most prevalent where sanitation is poor. In ancient times when humans were distinguished from other animals only by an upright position rather than by food or sanitary habits, the vast majority probably harbored this parasite. Over the centuries, as humanity's habits and sanitation gradually changed from those of a quadruped to those of the modern stance, this ubiquitous parasite has partially lost its hold on us, although approximately 900 million of the earth's population harbor Ascaris. Some 1 million people in the United States, especially inhabitants of the mountainous and hilly areas of the South, are hosts of this persistent parasite. In many countries the prevalence may reach 80 percent.

Ascariasis occurs at all ages, but it is most prevalent in the 5- to 9-year-old group of preschool and young school children, who are more frequently exposed to contaminated soil than are adults. The incidence is approximately the same for both sexes. The poorer urban and the rural classes, because of heavy soil pollution and unsatisfactory hygiene, are most afflicted. Infection is a household affair, the family being the unit of dissemination. Infected small children provide the chief source of soil contamination by their promiscuous defecation in dooryards and earthen-floored houses, where the resistant eggs remain viable for long periods.

The infective eggs are chiefly transmitted hand-to-mouth by children who have come in contact with contaminated soil directly, through playthings or through dirt eating. In districts of Europe and in the Far East, where night soil is extensively used for the fertilization of market gardens, human infection in all ages is also derived from vegetables (Fig. 6-16). Drinking water is rarely a source of infection.

Ascaris eggs are susceptible to desiccation, although they are more resistant than are *Trichuris* eggs. A moist, loose soil with moderate shade provides a suitable environment. Dryness is unfavorable for survival. The eggs are destroyed by direct sunlight within 15 hours and are killed at temperatures above 40 C, perishing within an hour at 50 C. Exposure to −8 to −12 C, although fatal to *Trichuris* eggs, has no effect on *Ascaris* eggs, which, in the soil, can survive the ordinary freezing temperatures of winter. Eggs are resistant to chemical disinfectants and can withstand temporary immersion in strong chemicals. They survive for months in sewage or night soil.

Pathology and Symptomatology. The usual infection, consisting of 10 to 20 worms, often goes unnoticed by the host, and is discovered only on a routine stool examination or by the discovery of an adult worm passed spontaneously in the stool. The most frequent complaint of patients infected with *Ascaris* is vague abdominal pain. An eosinophilia is present during the larval migration, but patients harboring the adult worms may exhibit little or no eosinophilia. During the lung migration, the larvae may produce host sensitization that result in allergic manifestations, such as pulmonary infiltration, asthmatic attacks, and edema of the lips. Some instances of Loeffler's syndrome and tropical eosinophilia have been attributed to migrating *Ascaris* larvae. Koino ingested 2000 embryonated *Ascaris* eggs of human source at one time and thereby demonstrated that large numbers of larvae simultaneously migrating through the lungs may cause a serious hemorrhagic pneumonia (Fig. 6-15). In Nigeria, Fiske attributes the high bronchopneumonia rate in children of over 5 months of age to the migration of *Ascaris* larvae.

Serious and sometimes fatal effects of ascariasis are due to the migrations of the adult worms. They may be regurgitated and vomited, escape through the external nares, or, rarely, be inhaled into a bronchus. Many instances of invasion of the bile ducts, gallbladder, liver, and appendix have been reported. They may occlude the ampulla of Vater and cause acute hemorrhagic pancreatitis. The worms may carry intestinal bacteria to these sites and stimulate the production of abscesses. The worms may penetrate the intestinal wall, migrate into the peritoneal cavity, and produce peritonitis. Continuing their migration, they may come out through the body wall, usually at the umbilicus in children and the inguinal region in adults. Intestinal volvulus, intussusception, and obstruction may also result from *Ascaris* infection. Fever and certain drugs are two of the causative factors of *Ascaris* migration.

Even when the worms cause little or no traumatic damage, the byproducts of living or dead worms may rarely produce marked toxic manifestations in sensitized persons, such as edema of the face and giant urticaria, accompanied by insomnia and loss of appetite and weight.

Young pigs infected with *Ascaris* do not gain weight normally, and it is likely that the human *Ascaris* may affect undernourished children similarly. This action may be due to the food actually consumed by the worms or to the trypsin-inhibiting substance they produce that interferes with the host's protein digestion. It has been shown that 20 adult worms consume 2.8 gm of carbohydrate and 0.7 gm of protein daily. Hence, heavy infections, running into the hundreds, would consume a significant proportion of their host's meager diet.

Diagnosis. The clinical symptoms of intestinal ascariasis are indistinguishable from those of other intestinal helminthic infections. Diagnosis is made by finding the eggs in the feces. The numerous eggs are detected in the direct coverglass mount. If direct examination is negative, concentration technique may be employed. Infertile eggs are easily missed by the examiner. Egg production is fairly constant and egg-counting methods (Chapter 18) give a fairly reliable index of the number of worms. The adult worm may be detected radiologically (Fig. 6-14). This is obviously the only way an infection with only immature and male worms can be detected.

Treatment. Piperazine citrate is safe and very effective in ascariasis; a single dose will cure 75 to 85 percent of the infections. A dose on 2 consecutive days will eliminate approximately 95 percent of the infections. Piperazine can be given at any time of day, since the presence of food in the digestive tract has little, if any, effect on its activity against *Ascaris*. Purgation is not required. The dosage schedule is a two-day course of 75 mg per kilogram orally (maximum 3.5 gm), daily.

Piperazine acts on the transmembrane potential of *Ascaris* muscle, temporarily relaxing it. The worm thereby loses its urge to move upstream and to press against the sides of its host's intestine in order to maintain its position. Peristalsis carries the worm out while it is relaxed.

Piperazine citrate syrup has been used successfully for the medical treatment of partial intestinal obstruction due to ascariasis, combined with abdominal decompression with a Levin tube and supportive therapy. If, in addition to *Ascaris,* hookworms are also present, mebendazole or pyrantel pamoate may be used, since they are effective against both parasites.

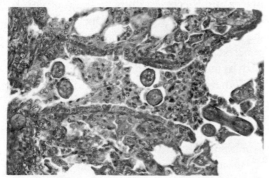

Figure 6-15. *Ascaris* larvae in lung. Note extensive hemorrhagic verminous pneumonia. (× 200)

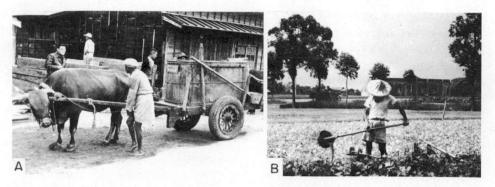

Figure 6-16. Use of night soil as fertilizer. A. Collection from homes. B. Diluted night soil applied to vegetables, with T.L.C.

Pyrantel pamoate has recently been introduced and is very effective as a single oral dose of 11 mg per kilogram (maximum 1 gm). Another useful drug for ascariasis is mebendazole, at 100 mg twice daily for 3 days. The same dose is used for children over 2 years of age.

Prevention. Since ascariasis is essentially a household and dooryard infection and is intimately associated with family hygiene, prophylaxis depends upon the sanitary disposal of feces and upon health education. Anthelmintic treatment is ineffective because of repeated reinfection in endemic areas. Control is difficult because of ignorance, poverty, and inertia among the people most afflicted. The installation of a latrine, 4 to 6 feet deep, is ineffective unless accompanied by an educational campaign designed to promote its use, especially by children. This educational program calls for the concerted efforts of schools, civic organizations, home economics educators, and public health workers. Night soil should not be used as fertilizer unless treated by compost manuring or chemicals (Fig. 6-16).

VISCERAL LARVA MIGRANS

Toxocara canis and *T. cati*

Disease. Toxocariasis, or visceral larva migrans (VLM), is a clinical syndrome resulting from the invasion of human visceral organs by nematode larvae of the genus *Toxocara*. These parasites are ascarids of the dog and cat, but puppies especially are epidemiologically most important as the cause of human infection.

Life Cycle. The dog and cat *T. canis* and *T. cati* are widely distributed throughout the world, and undetected human infections with their larvae are probably more widespread than the reports from many countries would indicate. The adult female worms are 10 to 12 cm in length and pass numerous eggs into their host's feces. In moist soil the eggs become embryonated in several weeks. When ingested by puppies or cats, the larvae hatch in the small intestine, migrate through the intestinal mucosa, and by way of the bloodstream reach the liver, lungs, bronchial tree, and trachea. They are swallowed again and mature in the small intestine of these animals. In adult dogs the larvae do not always complete the cycle but encyst in various tissues to be stimulated to migrate in pregnant bitches and cross the placenta to become adults in the puppies. In humanity, an aberrant host, the larvae hatching from ingested embryonated *Toxocara* eggs penetrate the intestinal mucosa and are carried by the bloodstream to the liver, lungs, and other organs. Here they wander for weeks and months, or become dormant, strangers in a strange land, causing inflammation and stimulating the production of eosinophilic granulomas.

Pathology and Syptomatology. The characteristic lesion has most frequently been encountered in the liver and consists of a gray, elevated, circumscribed area approximately 4 mm in diameter. Microscopically, these granulomatous lesions consist of eosinophils, lymphocytes, epithelioid cells, and giant cells of foreign-body type surrounding the larvae. Extensive hepatic parenchymal necrosis may be present, and Charcot-Leyden crystals may be seen. Eosinophilic granulomatous lesions without larvae are numerous and are encountered in practically every organ of the body. They may be due to larval migration through the area or represent the site of the death and disintegration of the larva. Lesions containing *Toxocara* larvae have been found in the liver, brain, eye, spinal cord, lungs, cardiac muscle, kidney, and lymph nodes. (Fig. 6-17).

To date the disease has been recognized largely in children from 1 to 4 years of age. A history may be elicited of close contact with the soil, dogs, or cats and of dirt eating. The disease frequently follows a benign course characterized by a marked persistent eosinophilia of 20 to 80 percent and hepatomegaly. Intermittent pain, dermatitis, and neurologic disturbances may be present in more severe infections. Pneumonitis is often present, and pulmonary infiltration may be seen in roentgenograms of the chest. The liver and spleen may be enlarged. Skin rashes on the lower extremities have been reported. Clinical manifestations may persist for two years, probably because of reinfections.

A number of the children have exhibited anemia accompanied by a high white blood cell count. There is usually a marked increase in blood globulins, largely gamma globulin. The liver function tests are often normal. The erythrocyte sedimentation rate is usually elevated, and there may be albuminuria.

An adult given 100 to 200 *T. canis* eggs had only an eosinophilia of 20 to 60 percent for 4 months without other definite symptoms. This suggests that light infections may often go unnoticed. The varied clinical manifestations are related to the number of embryonated eggs ingested, the location of the migrating larvae, and the individual patient's allergic response to their presence. One patient with a severe infection that ended fatally was found to harbor 60 larvae per gram of liver, five per gram of skeletal muscle, and four per gram of brain tissue. Repeated infections of abnormal hosts with larval nematodes frequently result in the development of allergic reactions. Hence, the infection may become more severe in hypersensitive individuals. Death would likely be due to cardiac and/or central nervous system involvement, but few fatalities have been reported.

The larvae of several nematodes, including

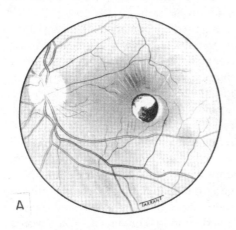 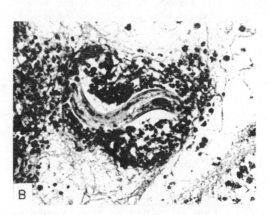

Figure 6-17. Visceral larva migrans (*Toxocara canis*) in eye. A. Tension lines radiating from granuloma. (From Duguid: Br J Ophthalmol 45:793, 1961.) B. Larva surrounded by eosinophils in vitreous chamber. (From Wilder: Trans Am Acad Ophthalmol Otolaryngol 55:99, 1950.)

Toxocara, can lodge in the eye, causing choroiditis, iritis, or hemorrhage. Studies of the eyes of children (aged 3 to 13 years), removed because of a clinical diagnosis of retinoblastoma, a malignant tumor with definite hereditary prediposition, revealed nematode larvae in a number of them, primarily *Toxocara,* usually unilateral and in the macular area. Furthermore, in contrast to VLM, the patients with eye involvement are somewhat older children and frequently exhibit only a slight eosinophilia.

Diagnosis. The diagnosis of larval *Toxocara* infections is usually established on clinical grounds with the triad of marked eosinophilia, hepatomegaly, and hyperglobulinemia. Because the great majority of cases occurs in children, a history of exposure to dogs and of dirt eating are helpful points in diagnosis. Actual demonstration of the larvae is the only definitive method of proving the diagnosis, but they are not numerous enough to be found in needle biopsy specimens of the liver with any regularity. While finding the typical eosinophilic granulomatous lesions is suggestive, such lesions are not diagnostic. An ELISA test, using *Toxocara* larval antigen and absorption of serum with *Ascaris* antigen appears to detect specific antibodies to *Toxocara* antigen. This test with specific *Toxocara* antigen has also been reported to be positive in some of the patients with *Toxocara* endophthalmitis. English workers have reported a *Toxocara* skin test to be useful, but the specificity of the skin test has not been confirmed. Elevated antibody levels to A and B blood-group antigens, because of cross reactivity with larval antigen, commonly occurs in VLM patients. They also have elevated serum IgE levels.

The differential diagnosis may include trichinosis, eosinophilic leukemia, Loeffler's syndrome, idiopathic hypereosinophilic syndromes, asthma, polyarteritis nodosa, retinoblastoma, and liver invasion by *Capillaria hepatica,* an animal nematode. Stool examination is useless since *Toxocara* never completes its life cycle in human beings.

Treatment. Because the clinical course of VLM is so variable, it is very difficult to evaluate efficacy of any treatment. In addition, since the infection is usually self-limited, only severe cases need to be treated. Thiabendazole, 25 mg per kilogram b.i.d. for 5 days, appears to shorten the course of the disease. In severe cases, especially with prominent allergic manifestations, or when the eye is involved, corticosteroids for a limited period of time can be used in addition to thiabendazole.

Prevention. Small children should be protected against contact with infected dogs and cats, especially kittens and puppies, which are more commonly and heavily infected and may carry *Toxocara* eggs on their fur. Animals under 6 months should be dewormed with piperazine every month, and older ones every 2 months. Worms passed as a result of treatment should be destroyed. Dog and cat stools passed in children's play areas should be buried, and sandboxes, which offer an attractive defecating area to cats, should be covered when not in use. There is no satisfactory chemical for killing the eggs in soil.

Anisakis spp.

Disease. Anisakiasis, herring disease.

History. Anisakiasis is a recently recognized parasitic infection of humans; the first case was described from the Netherlands in 1955. The causative nematode is a parasite of a wide variety of planctonic crustacea, sea fish, and sea mammals.

Ingested by humans as the third-stage larva in the flesh of raw fish, it may invade the stomach or intestine and produce an inflammatory response of varying severity. Thus, the infection is a human zoonosis, with people as accidental hosts. Humans were more likely to escape infection as long as fisherman were required to "gut," i.e., eviscerate, the fish at sea soon after catch—undoubtedly a cold and unpleasant task. After storing fish on ice began, so that they could be eviscerated later on shore, cases of "herring disease" began to be noted among Dutchmen who savored their herring raw. The reason is that in some fish, notably herring, there is a migration of *Anisakis* larvae from the viscera into the musculature after the death of the fish. Such migrations can be prevented and the larvae can be killed by freezing the fish at -20 C and storing them on board ship for 24 hours. Since the introduction in 1968 of freezing regulations for green herring in the Netherlands, the number of reported cases has decreased greatly. Anisakiasis is very common in Japan, and sporadic cases have been reported from European countries, Korea, and from the United States (seven cases).

Life Cycle and Morphology. Some features of the life cycle of Anisakine nematodes are still uncertain because several species of *Anisakis,* and a related genus of nematode, *Phocanema,* have been involved in human infections. In addition, many fish found harboring larvae have probably acquired infection by eating other infected fish and are therefore "transport," or paratenic, hosts. The life cycle is believed to involve marine crustaceans and fish as intermediate hosts for the larvae, with marine mammals, such as the whale, dolphin, and propoise harboring the adult parasites. Seals are also definitive hosts, especially for the genus *Phocanema.* The adult worms, about 3.5 to 7.0 cm in length for males and 4.5 to 15.0 cm in length for females, are found attached to the stomach wall of their definitive hosts. The eggs pass out in the feces of their host and produce larvae that infect marine crustaceans. When the larvae are ingested by fish, they migrate to the body cavity, the liver, or the muscles, depending upon the species of fish, and then encapsulate. Larvae recovered from fish are 2 to 3 cm in length and 0.5 to 1.0 mm in width.

Epidemiology. Anisakiasis is determined by the food habits of different ethnic groups that eat raw or partly raw fish or squid containing the larvae. In northern Europe, the source is usually raw or "green" herring, even if marinated with vinegar and salt or smoked, while in Japan the vehicle is likely to be *sashimi,* prepared from squid, cod or mackerel. With most human cases reported from Japan and northern Europe, one might expect that fish of northern waters are more commonly infected, but anisakine larvae have been found in fish from the Indian Ocean, New Zealand, the Philippines, and the South Atlantic. Alas, even "ceviche" from red snapper has been implicated. The larvae escape notice within the flesh because they are colorless and tightly coiled. Cases tend to occur more commonly in adult males, perhaps reflecting the association of eating raw marine food with alcoholic beverages.

Pathology and Symptomatology. Signs and symptoms will depend upon the site of the lesion. Larvae may attempt to penetrate the gastrointestinal tract anywhere from the pharynx to the small bowel. Most commonly the stomach or upper small bowel are involved, with a severe inflammatory reaction surrounding the larva. The local tissue response varies from a granulomatous, foreign-body type reaction to massive eosinophilic infiltration with hemorrhage, fibrinous exudate, and edema of the intestinal wall that produces intestinal obstruction. If sought for, a larva can often be found in the center of the lesion.

Gastric involvement will produce epigastric or midabdominal pain, nausea, and vomiting. The course can be acute or chronic over a period of weeks or months. Involvement of the small bowel is more likely to present as partial intestinal obstruction within 7 days of ingestion of raw seafood. These signs, plus peritoneal irritation, often lead to surgical exploration. Although eosinophilic infiltration of the involved tissue is prominent, peripheral eosinophilia of a significant degree is often absent.

Immunodiagnostic tests are still under investigation. Removal of gastric larvae by gastroscopy has been reported. If surgical intervention is not required for obstruction or perforation of the bowel, or to rule out malignancy, the patient with anisakiasis can be managed conservatively.

FAMILY TRICHOSTRONGYLIDAE

The members of the family TRICHOSTRONGYLIDAE are thin worms in which the buccal capsule is absent or rudimentary. The male bursa has two large lateral lobes and a small dorsal lobe with well-developed rays. These worms are intestinal parasites of ruminants and, less frequently, of humans and other mammals. The species parasitic in humanity belong to the genera *Trichostrongylus* and *Haemonchus*.

Several species of the genus *Trichostrongylus* are natural parasites of mammals. They are small nematodes, 4 to 7 mm, that inhabit the jejunum and upper ileum of humans. At times the biliary passages may be invaded. The parasites have a more-or-less cosmopolitan distribution in people in Africa (Egypt), Asia Minor, Asia, Japan, Indonesia, Australia, and, rarely, the United States. Their prevalence is variable, being frequently reported in selected groups in Asia and the Far East. The several species include *T. colubriformis,* with a high frequency in Indonesia and Iraq, and *T. orientalis,* common in Japan and Korea. The rhabditiform larvae (Fig. 6-10), characterized by a minute knob at the tip of the tail, develop into pseudofilariform larvae in 3 to 4 days in the soil. A high humidity, warm temperature, abundant shade, and grass or carpet vegetation are necessary for their extracorporeal development. Ingested with contaminated green vegetation, the larvae burrow into the intestinal wall and then erupt as adolescent worms into the intestinal lumen to become adults in about 21 days. Infections are usually so light that no clinical symptoms are produced. Heavy infections may cause a secondary anemia, as a result of the worm's bloodsucking, and signs of cholecystitis. Eosinophilia is transient. Diagnosis is based upon finding in the feces or duodenal contents ellipsoidal greenish eggs (see Figure 17-1) that are larger and more pointed at one end than are hookworm eggs.

Thiabendazole (Mintezol) and pyrantel pamoate are effective against *Trichostrongylus* (see hookworm therapy, earlier in this chapter). Some reported therapeutic failures in hookworm infection may be due to mistaking *Trichostrongylus* eggs for those of hookworm. Prevention depends upon avoiding the consumption of raw plants.

The sheep wireworm, *Haemonchus contortus,* a cosmopolitan parasite of economic importance

in sheep, cattle, and other ruminants, has been reported as an incidental parasite of humans in Brazil and Australia. It measures 10 to 30 mm in length and has an attenuated anterior end. The elongated eggs resemble those of *Trichostrongylus* and can only be differentiated by cultivation of the larvae. Development is direct, with a single host and a free-living larval stage. Infection takes place through the digestive tract. Heavy infections produce an anemia resembling that of hookworm infection.

FAMILY STRONGYLIDAE

The members of the family STRONGYLIDAE are parasites of the digestive tracts of mammals. The well-developed buccal capsule is without teeth or cutting plates but bears a crown of chitinous leaflike processes. The male has two prominent copulatory spicules; the vulva is located in the posterior half of the female. People are incidental hosts of three species.

Ternidens deminutus, which resembles the hookworm, is found in monkeys. It has been reported in natives of Africa and Asia. The worm, which may be found in the colon, at times produces cystic nodules or ulcers but gives rise to no particular symptoms other than anemia during heavy infection. Therapy with piperazine and bephenium hydroxynaphthoate is effective. *Oesophagostomum apiostomum,* a common parasite of monkeys and gorillas, has been reported from humans in Africa and Indonesia. The encysted larvae produce exudative and proliferative nodular fibrous tumors in the cecum, from which the immature worms emerge to complete their growth. *O. stephanostomum* was found once in humans in Brazil. The immature worms form fibrous nodules in the ileum, cecum, and colon.

FAMILY PHYSALOPTERIDAE

The members of the family PHYSALOPTERIDAE have a cuticular cephalic collar, two large triangular denticulated lips, and no buccal capsule. The caudal end of the male has pedunculated papillae and large asymmetrical alae that join ventrally. The female deposits smooth, transparent, thick-shelled embryonated eggs. The life cycle probably involves intermediate arthropod hosts. Various species are parasitic in the digestive tracts of birds, reptiles, and mammals.

Physaloptera caucasia, the only species parasitic in humans, was discovered in the Caucasus. *P. mordens,* recorded from Africa, is believed to be the same species. It is a natural parasite of monkeys and sometimes of humans. It is found attached to the walls of the esophagus, stomach, and small intestine. The maximum length of the male is 5 cm, and that of the female 10 cm.

ACANTHOCEPHALA

The ACANTHOCEPHALA, or thorny-headed roundworms, form a unique group by reason of their structure and extreme parasitic habits. These worms are common parasites of fish and birds and, less frequently, of other vertebrates. Although superficially resembling the roundworms, they differ in several fundamental characteristics from the NEMATODA, and perhaps more nearly resemble the CESTOIDEA. These distinctive features are absence of digestive tract, a more-or-less flattened body, a spinous retractile proboscis, a protonephridial excretory system, and embryonic hooklets. These parasites are included here with intestinal nematodes merely for convenience.

The worms are mostly small, but range from a few millimeters to over 60 cm in length. The elongate, nonsegmented body is roughly cylindrical or spindle-shaped. The surface is irregularly roughened by transverse ridges. There is a sheathed retractile proboscis armed with rows of recurved hooks. The sexes are separate, the male being distinguished by its much smaller size and muscular copulatory bursa. The life cycle of the ACANTHOCEPHALA involves alternation of hosts. The parasites of aquatic animals probably have crustaceans or larval insects as intermediate hosts, and those of terrestrial animals have various insects. Two species have been found in humans, with the adult form of the worm presumably embedded in the intestinal wall.

Macracanthorhynchus hirudinaceus has a cosmopolitan distribution. The worm has a rugose appearance, with pseudosegmentation and a retractile proboscis with five to six rows of spines. The length of the female is 20 to 65 cm, and that of the male 5 to 10 cm. The eggs are fully embryonated at oviposition. The larva is enclosed in three embryonic envelopes and has hooklets in the anterior end. The natural definitive hosts are hogs, wild boars, peccaries, and, less frequently, dogs and cats. People are accidental hosts. The intermediate hosts are species of larval beetles. Human infections, possibly spurious, have been reported once in Bohemia and once in southern Russia, diagnosis being made from eggs in the feces.

Moniliformis moniliformis, too, has a cosmopolitan distribution. The adult worm resembles a confluent beaded chain of pseudosegments. The length of the female is 10 to 27 cm, and that of the male 4 to 5 cm. The cylindrical proboscis has 12 to 15 rows of recurved hooks. The ellipsoidal eggs, 85 to 118 μ, have three envelopes and four hooklets. The definitive hosts are rats, mice, hamsters, dogs, and cats. Humanity is an incidental host. The intermediate hosts are beetles and cockroaches. Single cases of natural infection in humans have been reported from Italy, the Sudan, and British Honduras. Experimental infection in humans indicates that the parasite, when present in considerable numbers, may produce acute abdominal pain, diarrhea, and exhaustion. Prevention involves the protection of food from beetles and cockroaches.

NEMATODE PSEUDOPARASITES OF HUMANS

Other rhabditoid worms have been reported as pseudoparasites or accidental parasites of humanity. *Meloidogyne (Heterodera) radicicola,* a root parasite of vegetables, once attained considerable prominence as a human parasite under the name *Oxyuris incognita,* because its eggs were confused with those of *Enterobius,* hookworm, and *Trichostrongylus* (see Figure 17-3) and were found in human feces. The adult worm is digested by a human being; the undigestible eggs are found in the stool.

Three species of the genus *Rhabditis* and *Turbatrix aceti,* the vinegar eel, are accidental food contaminants.

REFERENCES

Trichinosis

Barret-Connor, et al: An epidemic of trichinosis after ingestion of wild pig in Hawaii. J. of Infect Dis 133: 473–477, 1976.

Kazura: Host defense mechanisms against nematode parasites: Destruction of newborn *T. spiralis* larvae by human antibodies and granulocytes. J Infect Dis 143: 712–718, 1981.

Gould (ed): Trichinosis in man and animals. Springfield, Ill., Charles C. Thomas, 1970.

Trichuriasis

Jung and Beaver: Clinical observations on *Trichocephalus trichuris* (whip worm) infestation in children. Pediatrics 8: 548–557, 1951.

Mathan and Baker: Whipworm disease—Intestinal structure and function of patients with severe *Trichuris trichuria* infestation. Am J Dig Dis 15: 913–918, 1970.

Wolfe and Wershing: Mebendazole—treatment of trichuriasis and ascariasis in Bahamian children. JAMA 230: 1408–1411, 1974.

Strongyloidiasis

Burke: Strongyloidiasis in childhood. Am J Dis Child 132: 1130–1136, 1978.

Grove: Strongyloidiasis in Allied ex-prisoners of war in Southeast Asia. Br Med J 1: 598–601, 1980.

Igra-Siegman et al: Syndrome of hyper-infection with *Strongyloides stercoralis.* Rev Infect Dis 3: 397–407, 1981.

Neva, et al: Comparison of larval antigens in an Elisa assay for strongyloidiasis in humans. J Infect Dis 144: 427–432, 1981.

Hookworms and Creeping Eruption

Kirby-Smith, et al: Some observations on creeping eruption. Am J Trop med IX: 179–193, 1929.

Rhoads, et al: Observations on the etiology and treatment of anemia associated with hookworm infection in Puerto Rico. Medicine, 13: 317–375, 1934.

Roche and Layrisse: The nature and causes of "hookworm anemia". Am J Trop Med Hyg 15: 1031–1102, 1966 (a separate Nov. Issue—Part 2).

Pinworm

Brooks, et al: Pelvic granuloma due to *Enterobius vermicularis.* JAMA 179: 492–494, 1962.

Kropp, et al: *Enterobius* vermicularis (pinworms), introital bacteriology and recurrent urinary tract infection in children. J Urol 120: 480–482, 1978.

Symmers: Pathology of Oxyuriasis. Arch Pathol 50: 475–516, 1950.

Weller and Sorenson: Enterobiasis: Its incidence and symptomatology in a group of 505 children. N Engl J Med 224: 143–146, 1941.

Ascariasis and Visceral Larva Migrans

Glickman, et al: *Toxocara*—specific antibody in the serum and aqueous humor of a patient with presumed ocular and visceral toxocariasis. Am J Trop Med Hyg 28: 29–35, 1979.

Huntley, et al: Visceral larva migrans syndrome. Clinical characteristics and immunological studies in 51 patients. Pediatrics. 4: 523–536, 1965.

Jelliffe and Jung: Asceariasis in children. West Indian Med J 6: 113–122, 1957.

Vogel and Minning: Beiträge zur Klinik der Lungen-Ascariasis und zur Frage der flüchtigen eosinophilen Lungeninfiltrate. Beitr Klinik der Tuberculose. 98: 620–654, 1942.

Waller and Othersen: Ascariasis: surgical complications in children. Am J Surg 120: 50–54, 1970.

Anisakiasis

Smith and Wooten: *Anasakis* and Anasakiasis. In Lumsden (ed): Advances in Parasitology. Muller and Baker. Vol. 16, New York, Academic Press, 1978.

Van Thiel: Review-The present state of *Anasakis* and its causative worms. Trop. Geog. Med 28: 75–85, 1076.

7

Blood and Tissue Nematodes of Human Beings

The parasitic nematodes of the blood and tissues may be arranged in two groups: (1) the filarial worms and the guinea worm and (2) parasites that normally infect other hosts but occasionally visceralize in humans.

FILARIAL PARASITES OF HUMAN BEINGS

Filariae

The slender filarial worms of the family FILA-RIIDAE are arthropod-transmitted parasites of the circulatory and lymphatic systems, muscles, connective tissues, or serous cavities of vertebrates. The principal species parasitic in humans are *Wuchereria bancrofti, Brugia malayi, Onchocerca volvulus, Loa loa, Dipetalonema perstans,* and *Mansonella ozzardi.* Candau (WHO) estimated that 200 million persons around the world are infected. Microfilariae identical with those of *Dipetalonema streptocerca,* a parasite of the chimpanzee, have also been found in humans. Increasing instances of infection

with *Dirofilaria* of animals have been reported in humans.

The filiform, creamy white worms (Fig. 7-1) range from 2 to 50 cm in length, the female being twice the size of the male. The simple mouth is usually without definite lips, and the buccal cavity is inconspicuous. The esophagus is cylindrical, has no cardiac bulbus, and is usually divided into an anterior muscular and a posterior glandular portion. In some species the males possess caudal alae; in others they are absent. There are two copulatory spicules.

A distinctive feature of filarial worms is that the viviparous female gives birth to prelarval microfilariae (Fig. 7-2). Their morphology, location in the host, and type of periodicity are of value in differentiating species. A sheath is present in *W. bancrofti, B. malayi,* and *Loa loa.* It is a delicate, close-fitting membrane that is derived from the original eggshell and is only detectable as it projects beyond the head or tail. The cuticle has transverse striations. A column of cells with deeply staining nuclei, which represents the rudiments of the intestine

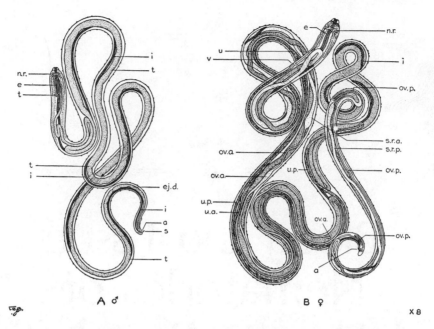

Figure 7-1. Morphology of *Loa loa*. A. Male. B. Female.
a, anus, e, esophagus; ej.d., ejaculatory duct; i, intestine; o.v.a., anterior ovary; ov.p., posterior ovary; n.r., nerve ring; s, spicules; s.r.a., anterior seminal receptacle; s.r.p., posterior seminal receptacle; t, testis; u, uterus; u.a., anterior uterus; u.p., posterior uterus; v, vulva. (Redrawn from Looss, 1904.)

and perhaps other organs, extends nearly the whole length and occupies almost the entire width of the body. Its absence or presence at the tip of the tail varies in the different species. Size is so variable that it cannot be used alone for the differentiation of species. A fungus conidia of the genus *Helicosporium,* which when airborne may contaminate blood smears, resembles a microfilaria, although it is much smaller and has a capsule. This may confuse the unwary and untutored (Fig. 7-3).

The microfilariae do not appear in the host until some months after infection, the latent, or prepatent, period corresponding to the growth of the worms to maturity and to the birth and escape of the microfilariae into the blood and tissues. Approximately 6 months after infection, the microfilariae of *W. bancrofti* are found in appreciable numbers in the blood. These microfilariae reach the blood by migration through the walls of the lymphatics to the neighboring small blood vessels, or by

way of the thoracic duct. They remain for several months in the host after the destruction of the adult female worms by chemotherapeutic agents or surgical removal. When microfilariae are injected intravenously into an uninfected nonimmune host, their survival varies with the species, from weeks to years. Of course they develop no further unless ingested by the insect vector.

The periodicity of microfilariae in the peripheral blood varies with the species. Nocturnal periodicity is a prominent characteristic of the microfilariae of *W. bancrofti* in the Western Hemisphere, Africa, and Asia. They are found in the blood chiefly at night, the number increasing to a maximum about midnight and then decreasing to a minimum about midday. Nocturnal periodicity is only relative, since a few microfilariae are present in the blood during the day. In the islands of the South Pacific east of longitude 170 E they are nonperiodic, present both by day and night. In the Philip-

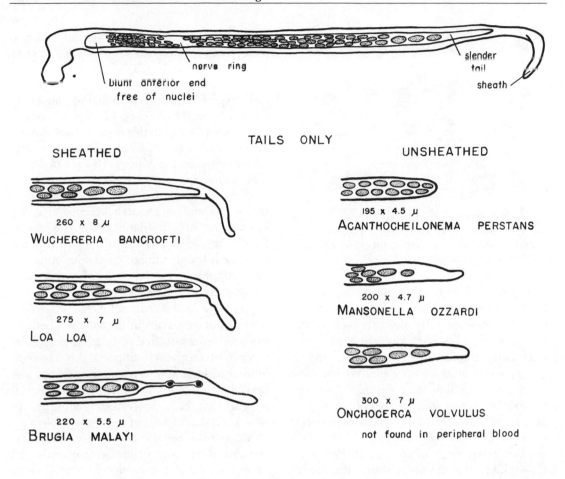

Figure 7-2. Microfilariae of humans: diagnostic characteristics.

pines there is a modified periodicity, the number during the day being about one-third that during the night.

The nocturnal periodicity of the microfilariae of *W. bancrofti* was first described by Manson in Amoy, China. The experimental infection of monkeys and dogs with mammalian species of filariae that show nocturnal periodicity indicates that the microfilariae are concentrated in the small blood vessels of the lungs during the day and are liberated into the peripheral circulation at night. The stimulus that initiates this migration has not yet been identified. Increased oxygen pressure by hyperventilation or exercise is one stimulus that causes the microfilariae of *W. bancrofti* to leave the lungs for the peripheral circulation. Hawking suggests an inborn periodicity plus changes in the venous-arterial tensions during the day and night. *Loa loa*, with a diurnal periodicity, is not affected by changes in oxygen pressure. Periodicity in a patient with *W. bancrofti* has been reversed by altering the sleeping hours. Periodicity is a phenomenon associated with species; the microfilariae, when transfused into a new host, show the same periodicity as in the donor.

The life cycle of the filarial worm involves (1) the ingestion of the microfilaria from the blood or tissues by a bloodsucking insect, (2) the metamorphosis of the microfilaria in the arthropod vector first into a rhabditoid and

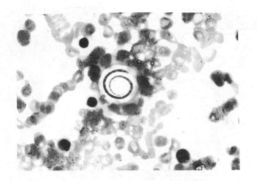

Figure 7-3. *Helicosporium* sp., filiform-coiled conidia (helicospore) of airborne fungus, occasionally found contaminating blood smears and confused with microfilariae. ($\times$ 500)

then into an infectious filariform larva, and (3) the transference of the infective larva to the skin of a new host by the proboscis of the biting insect and the development of the larva, after entry through the bite wound, into a mature worm at its selective site. Within a few hours after ingestion by a suitable insect, the microfilaria penetrates the wall of the midgut and makes its way to the thoracic muscles, where it undergoes metamorphosis. In 1 to 3 weeks it reaches the infective stage. When the insect bites the definitive host, the larvae probably escape from the tip of the proboscis to the skin near the bite wound, through which they enter the body.

Immune Response to Filarial Infections. The issue of acquired immunity to filarial infections of humans is confusing, but new insights are emerging that link immune responses to the clinical outcome of the infection. Observations on susceptible population groups with relatively short but heavy exposure to filariasis indicate that they commonly experience acute episodes of lymphatic inflammation. Without further exposure such individuals rarely exhibit microfilariae in the blood. This suggests that the immune response is often able to destroy the microfilariae that are produced. Support for this hypothesis comes from the demonstration of either antimicrofilarial antibody or cell-mediated immune responses to filarial antigens, or both findings, in amicrofi-

laremic individuals living in filarial endemic areas. Similar patterns of immune response have been noted in filarial infections of animals. The most striking evidence of immunologic hyperresponsiveness to filarial antigens is seen in "occult" filariasis, or tropical eosinophilia (see p. 159). In this situation individuals are infected with a filarial parasite but trap microfilariae in the lungs or lymph nodes so they do not appear in the circulation.

With continued exposure to filarial infection in endemic areas, it is believed that the immune response to filarial antigens is modulated. This "damping down" of the immune response is brought about by various immunologic suppressor mechanisms, involving both humoral and cellular elements. While such a sequence of events has not been proven by repeated observations in the same individual, study of representative population groups by several investigators supports this concept. Similar loss of immune responsiveness has also been shown in human schistosomiasis. Thus, it appears that the presence of circulating microfilaria in the blood represents a "tolerant" immune state on the part of the host. The patients with microfilaremia frequently are asymptomatic and show no evidence of filarial disease. Appreciation of these immunologic correlates of filariasis make one wonder whether our usual concept of this infection is actually the reverse of reality, i.e., that lymphangitis and the absence of microfilaremia is the "normal" host response, while the asymptomatic, microfilaremic state represents "failure" of the normal host response.

Much remains to be sorted out as to how the immune response in filariasis relates to the pathology associated with this infection. Multiple antigens are involved, from adult worms as well as the microfilariae. The presence of circulating immune complexes is commonly present in patients with filariasis, and free circulating antigen may also be present. These patients also show prominent manifestations of immediate hypersensitivity. They often have very high IgE levels; eosinophilia is common; and their basophils can be shown to be sensitized with specific reaginic antibody (IgE). How all these immunologic events function in the course of filarial infection and whether they in fact actually contribute to the disease need more study.

The evidence suggests that the disease of filarial infections is immunopathologic in nature. The lymphangitis appears to be related to presence of the developing worms in the lymphatics. Exactly how the perilymphatic inflammatory reaction develops and the role of adult worm antigens or death of the worms for such reactions can only be surmised. Why this process progresses in some to lymphatic obstruction, collagen deposition, and ultimate elephantiasis is still unknown. The immunopathology associated with trapping of microfilariae in the tissues is more clearly understood. Allergic responses are prominent in this situation, with bronchoconstriction and an asthmatic-type syndrome resulting when the lungs are the shock organ (see tropical eosinophilia, p. 159). The cellular response to the microfilariae in the tissues is a virtual eosinophilic abscess. It is likely that some of the pathologic changes in the skin of patients with onchocerciasis involve similar immunologic mechanisms.

The interpretation of serologic and skin tests in the diagnosis of filariasis is confounded by the complex nature of antigens associated with the parasite, as well as by the fact that presumably infected people are often without microfilaremia. With respect to serologic tests for filarial antibodies, common antigens from other helminthic parasites frequently elicit cross-reacting antibodies, so low titers are not reliable in the diagnosis of filarial infection. Very high levels of antifilarial antibody may, however, be indicative of infection with a filarial parasite, especially in one without circulating microfilariae. The immediate-type skin test should probably be reinvestigated, in conjunction with other immunologic assessment of immediate hypersensitivity, such as the histamine-release reaction from IgE sensitized basophils. Such tests may be found to be more helpful than has been appreciated, now that

there is greater understanding of filarial infection without microfilaremia. The skin-test antigen developed by Sawada seems to be less cross-reactive than earlier antigens.

Wuchereria bancrofti

Diseases. Bancroftian filariasis, wuchereriasis, elephantiasis.

Life Cycle. Humanity is the only known definitive host. Transmission of infection requires a suitable species of mosquito (Fig. 7-4). The adult worms, with females 8 to 10 cm long, are located in the lymphatics, and the microfilariae are found in the blood and lymph. Adults of both sexes lie tightly coiled in the nodular dilations of the lymphatic vessels and sinuses of the lymph nodes. The length of life of *W. bancrofti* in the human host is considered to be about 5 years, as estimated from the duration of the microfilariae in the blood of persons after departure from endemic regions.

The microfilariae ingested by the mosquito along with its blood meal migrate to its muscles. After 6 to 20 days of development, the larvae force their way out of the muscles, causing considerable damage, and migrate to the proboscis. Observers have found that 3 microfilariae per cubic millimeter of blood will produce optimal infections in the mosquito; that 0.5 will fail to infect; and that 10 will kill the mosquito. Perhaps individuals with heavy microfilaremia should not be treated; rather, they could be allowed to serve as sources of lethal meals for mosquitoes! During the blood meal the developed larvae emerge from the proboscis onto the skin of the new host. On penetrating the skin through the bite wound, the larvae pass to the lymphatic vessels and nodes, where they grow to maturity in 6 or more months. The adult worms tend to frequent the varices of the lymphatic vessels of the lower extremities, the groin glands and epididymis in the male, and the labial glands in the female. The microfilariae migrate from the parent worm through the walls of the lymphatics to the neighboring small blood vessels or are carried in the lymphatic circulation to the bloodstream.

WUCHERERIA BANCROFTI

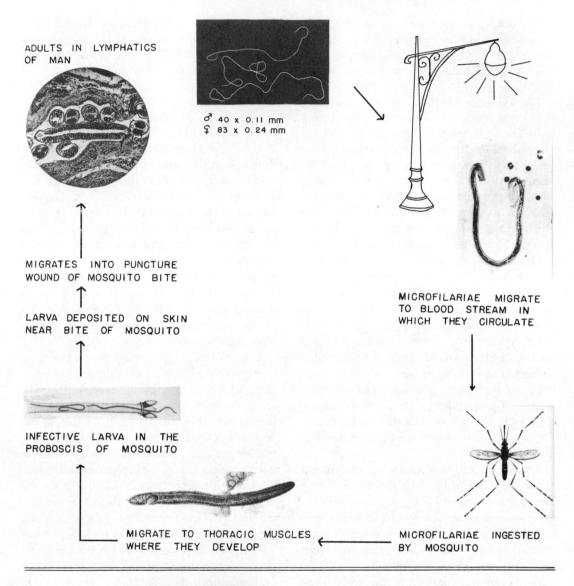

ADULTS IN LYMPHATICS
OF MAN

♂ 40 x 0.11 mm
♀ 83 x 0.24 mm

MIGRATES INTO PUNCTURE
WOUND OF MOSQUITO BITE

LARVA DEPOSITED ON SKIN
NEAR BITE OF MOSQUITO

INFECTIVE LARVA IN THE
PROBOSCIS OF MOSQUITO

MICROFILARIAE MIGRATE
TO BLOOD STREAM IN
WHICH THEY CIRCULATE

MIGRATE TO THORACIC MUSCLES
WHERE THEY DEVELOP

MICROFILARIAE INGESTED
BY MOSQUITO

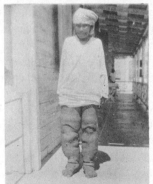

ELEPHANTIASIS

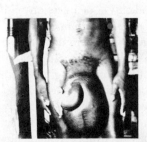

Figure 7-4. Life cycle of *Wuchereria bancrofti*.

148

Epidemiology. The parasite has a worldwide range in tropical and subtropical countries, extending as far north as Spain and as far south as Brisbane, Australia. In the Eastern Hemisphere it is present in Africa, Asia, Taiwan, the Philippines, Indonesia, and the islands of the South Pacific. In the Western Hemisphere the distribution is more limited and focal, being found in some Caribbean islands, the Atlantic coast of Costa Rica, and northern South America. The infection in the United States, which was introduced by African slaves to Charleston, South Carolina, died out more than 50 years ago. The prevalence of periodic filariasis is correlated with density of population and poor sanitation, since *Culex quinquefasciatus,* the principal vector, breeds mainly in water contaminated with sewage and decaying organic matter. In the South Pacific the incidence of nonperiodic filariasis in the rural districts is as high as or higher than in the large villages, since its chief vector is *Aëdes polynesiensis,* a brush mosquito. Prevalence varies with race, age, and sex, largely due to environmental factors. Europeans, who are better protected against mosquitoes, have a much lower incidence than natives.

The principal vector in the Western Hemisphere is *C. quinquefasciatus* (= *fatigans*), and in the South Pacific *A. polynesiensis.* The former is a night-biting, domesticated, urban mosquito, and the latter is a day-biting, sylvatic, nondomesticated mosquito. At least 48 species of mosquitoes, including *Aëdes, Anopheles, Culex,* and *Mansonia,* are natural or experimental vectors.

The designation of the specific name *W. pacifica* for the nonperiodic filaria of the South Pacific by Manson-Bahr led to an academic controversy as to whether this form should be considered a separate species or a variety of *W. bancrofti.* In the South Pacific, nonperiodic filariasis differs from the periodic in its geographic distribution, e.g., Fiji and Samoa vs Micronesia and Melanesia, in its sylvan instead of urban foci, in its vector *A. polynesiensis,* as opposed to *C. quinquefasciatus, Anopheles farauti,* and *A. punctulatus,* and in somewhat questionable minor morphologic differences in the adult worms. Periodicity is reported to be retained even when infected populations are transferred to nonperiodic regions. Also, a Fijian strain of *C. quinquefasciatus,* susceptible to periodic microfilariae, has proved refractory to nonperiodic microfilariae.

Pathology and Symptomatology. Filarial symptoms are caused mainly by the adult worms, living as well as dead and degenerating. Microfilariae apparently cause less pathology, although they have been associated with tropical pulmonary eosinophilia, granulomas of the spleen, and allergic reactions following their destruction by drugs. The adult worms lie in the dilated lymphatics or in the sinuses of the lymph nodes. The pseudotubercular granulomatous reaction around the trapped worms becomes pronounced on their death. It occludes the small lymphatics, narrows the larger ones, and ultimately walls off the necrotic tissues surrounding the degenerating worms. The early cellular reactions and edema give way to vascular and lymphatic hyperplasia, fibroblastic proliferation, and caseation. Finally, there is absorption and replacement of the parasite by hyalinized, or even calcified, scar tissue. The lymphatics become varicose; collateral branches open up; and lakes of lymph develop in the sinuses of the lymph nodes. The living and dead worms and microfilariae evoke an infiltration of eosinophilic leukocytes in the inflamed tissues.

Because bancroftian filariasis may run its course over many years, it varies greatly in its clinical manifestations. It is possible to classify broadly the results of filarial infection into the asymptomatic, inflammatory, and obstructive types.

ASYMPTOMATIC FILARIASIS. In endemic areas children are exposed to infection at an early age, and by the age of 6 years they exhibit microfilariae in their blood without experiencing symptoms referable to their infection. On physical examination the patient may exhibit a moderate generalized enlargement of lymph nodes, especially of the inguinal region. Blood examination discloses numerous microfilariae and a low-grade eosinophilia. In time the adult worms die, and the microfilariae disappear without the patient's being aware of the infection.

INFLAMMATORY FILARIASIS. The inflammatory filarial infection is an allergic phenomenon due to sensitivity to the products of the living and dead adult worms. Superimposed streptococcal infections may be involved. Recurrent attacks are characterized by funiculitis, epididymitis, orchitis, retrograde lymphangitis of the extremities, and localized areas of swelling and redness of the arms and legs. Fever, chills, headache, vomiting, and malaise may accompany these attacks, which last from several days to several weeks. The lymphatics of the legs and genitalia are chiefly affected. In males acute lymphangitis of the spermatic cord (funiculitis), with tender, thickened cord, epididymitis, orchitis, and scrotal edema, are common. The red blood cells, hemoglobin, and sedimentation rate are unchanged. There is a leukocytosis of up to 10,000, and an eosinophilia of 6 to 26 percent. Yet most of these patients do not have microfilaremia. Somewhat similar acute attacks may occur at monthly or longer intervals in patients with or without elephantiasis. Usually the affected extremity becomes red, hot, and very painful. Therapy with antimicrobial drugs is usually unsuccessful, suggesting a verminous rather than bacterial etiology. Abscesses of the pelvis of the kidney, epididymis, retroperitoneal tissues, inguinal nodes, and iliopsoas muscles may result from the dead and degenerating worms. These abscesses may be sterile, but frequently pyogenic bacteria are present. The acute granulomatous reaction in the lymphatics due to the worms and their toxic products, which is manifest by local inflammation and systemic allergic symptoms, gradually merges into a chronic proliferative overgrowth of fibrous tissue around the dead worms that produces lymphatic obstruction, recurrent attacks of lymphangitis, and, at times, elephantiasis.

OBSTRUCTIVE FILARIASIS. Elephantiasis is the dramatic end result of filariasis (Fig. 7-4). Many mistakenly believe that it is the inevitable termination of every filarial infection, but, fortunately, the grossly enlarged scrotum, breast, or leg is the exception rather than the

rule. Elephantiasis probably does not develop in more than 10 percent of infected populations in various parts of the world, many of whom are exposed to infective mosquitoes from birth. Obstructive filariasis develops slowly, usually follows years of continuous filarial infection, and is preceded by chronic edema and often by repeated acute inflammatory attacks. In the chronic stage the cellular reaction and edema are replaced by fibroblastic hyperplasia. There is absorption and replacement of the parasite by proliferative granulation tissue, and extensive lymph varices are produced. The high protein content of the lymph stimulates the growth of dermal and collagenous connective tissue, and gradually, over a period of years, the enlarged affected parts harden, producing chronic elephantiasis. The site of the obstructive inflammation determines the parts of the body affected. Obstruction of the thoracic duct or the median abdominal lymph vessels may affect the scrotum and penis of the male and the external genitalia of the female, while infection of the inguinal glands may involve the extremities and external genitalia. Elephantiasis is uncommon in persons under 30 years of age. There is little correlation between the presence of microfilariae in the blood and elephantiasis, since microfilariae disappear after the death of the worms. Rupture of the lymphatics of the urinary bladder or kidney may produce chyluria, those of the tunica vaginalis, hydrocele or chylocele, and those of the peritoneum, chylous ascites. The most common features are hydrocele and lymphangitis of the genitalia and recurrent attacks of lymphangitis with fever and pain. Recurrent lymphangitis, and even elephantiasis, may be accentuated or in some cases even produced by superimposed streptococcal infections.

Prognosis is good in light infections. Once elephantiasis has developed, the prognosis is poor unless surgery is successful.

Diagnosis. The diagnosis of filariasis depends upon a history of exposure to mosquitoes in an endemic area, in conjunction with the clinical findings discussed above. The blood should be examined for microfilariae by placing a drop, obtained at night, on a slide and examining it under the low power of the microscope for actively moving microfilariae. To determine the species of microfilariae, thin or thick blood smears stained with Wright or Giemsa stain will bring out the diagnostic characteristics. To detect light infections, 1 ml of night blood is laked in 10 ml of a 2-percent formalin solution. The sediment is examined directly or may be allowed to dry on a slide and then stained (Chapter 18). A slightly more sensitive method for detection of microfilariae is filtration of 1 to 5 ml of heparinized blood through a 5 μ Nucleopore filter and examination of the stained filter on a slide. The blood of patients with clinical filariasis does not always contain microfilariae. Approximately 6 to 12 months may elapse from the time of infection until the worm matures and produces microfilariae. Hence, during the early months of clinical inflammatory filariasis, microfilariae will not be found in the blood. Likewise, late in the disease, by the time elephantiasis has developed, the adult worms and the microfilariae may both have died. The intradermal test using *Dirofilaria* antigen, and the complement-fixation, hemagglutination, and flocculation tests may be of diagnostic value when microfilariae cannot be found in the blood. The microfilariae of *W. bancrofti*, which may occur in the urine when chyluria is present, are easily separated by centrifuging.

Treatment. Diethylcarbamazine (Hetrazan), which is given orally, is quickly lethal to microfilariae and may also damage the adult worms, especially if larger than usual doses are used. The dosage is 2 mg per kilogram of body weight t.i.d., for 14 days—occasionally for as long as 30 days. Headache, dizziness, nausea, and fever may be encountered during therapy and are at least partially due to disintegration of the microfilariae. Antimicrobial drugs are useful in recurrent lymphangitis caused by secondary streptococcal infection.

The massive edema that precedes and accompanies elephantiasis of the legs may be alleviated by pressure bandaging. Administration of steroids to patients with elephantiasis may be followed by diuresis and an increased number of microfilariae in the bloodstream. Both effects are ascribed to a lessening of the inflammatory reaction around the adult worms, which allows freer lymphatic drainage from the smaller limb. Various operative measures have been tried in elephantiasis. The removal of the enlarged scrotum is usually successful and results in permanent cure. The repair of enlarged legs, attempting to provide anastomosis between the deep and superficial lymphatics, is not entirely satisfactory.

Prevention. The prevention of wuchereriasis in endemic areas includes the control of mosquitoes and human sources of infection. The residual spraying of houses and the use of larvicides, successful against *C. quinquefasciatus* and other domesticated mosquitoes (p. 271), are not effective against sylvan mosquitoes such as *A. polynesiensis*. The mass administration of Hetrazan to destroy the microfilariae in the blood of carriers and the use of insecticides to control the mosquitoes have proven successful on St. Croix, the Virgin Islands, and Tahiti. The protection of the individual by screened quarters, bed nets, mosquito repellents, and protective clothing is an educational and economic problem.

Brugia (Wuchereria) malayi

Disease. Malayan filariasis.

Life Cycle. Humanity is usually the only definitive host, but there is another variety of *B. malayi* that infects monkeys and felines. The fine, white, threadlike adult worm closely resembles *W. bancrofti*, the female being 55 by 0.16 mm and the male 23 by 0.09 mm. The nocturnal periodicity of the morphologically distinct, sheathed microfilariae (Fig. 7-2) is less absolute than that of *W. bancrofti*. The intermediate hosts are *Mansonia, Anopheles, Aëdes,* and *Armigeres*. The microfilaria in the mosquito develops into an infective larva in 6 to 12 days.

Epidemiology. The extensive geographic distribution of this parasite includes Sri Lanka, Indonesia, the Philippines, Southern India, Asia, China, Korea, and a small focus in Japan. Its distribution in the flat alluvial areas along the coast corresponds to that of its principal insect hosts, *Mansonia* mosquitoes. It is most prevalent in low regions, where numerous ponds are infested with water plants of the genus *Pistia,* which are essential for the breeding of these mosquitoes. When *Mansonia* mosquitoes are the vectors, the disease is essentially rural in distribution, with cats and monkeys as reservoirs and the microfilariae having a subperiodic appearance. When *Anopheles* mosquitoes are the vectors, it tends to be urban or suburban, with nocturnal periodicity of the microfilariae.

Pathogenicity. The parasite, like *W. bancrofti,* produces lymphangitis and elephantiasis. It differs from *W. bancrofti* in that persons with clinical filariasis show a much higher microfilarial rate than those without symptoms. In Malaya there are about five times as many symptomless carriers as those suffering from elephantiasis. Malayan filariasis is characterized by superficial lymphadenopathy and a high eosinophilia (7 to 70 percent).

Diagnosis. Diagnosis is made by identification of microfilariae in the blood (Fig. 7-2). The "knotting" of the microfilaria, an agonal phenomenon during drying of the film, may be prevented by adding chloroform or menthol to the blood.

Treatment. Similar to *W. bancrofti* (see preceding section on treatment).

Prevention. The principal means of prevention is the control of *Mansonia* mosquitoes by destruction or removal of the water plant *Pistia stratiotes.* Phenoxylene 30 (sodium and ammonium salts of methyl chlorphenoxyacetic acid) is a cheap, satisfactory herbicide.

Onchocerca volvulus

Diseases. Onchocerciasis, onchocercosis, river blindness.

Life Cycle. Humanity is the only definitive host, although closely allied species occur in other mammals. The adult worms are found in the subcutaneous tissues, usually encapsulated in fibrous tumors, within which the worms are intricately coiled. The tumors contain a variable number of worms and microfilariae. Occasionally, the unencapsulated

worms migrate in the tissues. The liberated microfilariae (Fig. 7-2) are present in the nodules, subcutaneous tissues, and skin, rarely in the blood or internal organs.

The principal intermediate hosts are the black flies of the genus *Simulium.* The metamorphosis to an infective larva in *S. damnosum* requires 6 to 10 or more days in the thoracic muscles, from which the mature larvae migrate to the proboscis of the fly. When the infected black fly bites, larvae escape to the skin of the new host and penetrate the bite wound. The worm becomes an adult in less than a year and lives for at least 5 years.

Epidemiology. In Africa, onchocerciasis occurs on the west coast from Sierra Leone to the Congo Basin, extending eastward through Zaire, Angola, and the Republic of the Sudan to East Africa. In the Volta River basin it is estimated that 1 million are infected, with eye defects in 60,000. In the Americas it is found in the highlands of Guatemala, in the states of Oaxaca and Chiapas in Mexico, in Colombia, Brazil, and in northeastern Venezuela. A special strain is found in the Yemen. Endemic areas in Central America are confined to the highlands, usually at 1000 to 4000 feet above sea level, along streams and river courses where black flies are abundant. In Africa the infection is common below 1000-foot elevation. The disease is confined to the neighborhood of rapidly flowing small streams, where the insects breed. The incidence falls markedly after a distance of 5 miles, owing to the distribution of the insect vectors, which rarely travel over 2 to 3 miles from the water courses (although they will travel farther when windblown). People are the only source of infection. On clear days the female bites most frequently in the early morning and evening, but she bites at all hours in the shade or when the sky is overcast.

The disease is more prevalent in men than in women because of greater occupational exposure. It is less prevalent in Europeans in Africa than in the natives because of better protection against black flies.

Pathology and Symptomatology. Onchocerciasis is a chronic infection of the subcutaneous tissues, skin, and eyes. Its lesions are produced by the adult worms and microfilariae, augmented by the allergic response of the host. The nodules, 5 to 25 mm in size, may appear in any part of the body, but in Africa they are seen most commonly on the trunk, thighs, and arms (Fig. 7-5) and in the Americas on the head and shoulders. The cause of this distribution may be partially explained by the practice of exposure of the whole unclothed body in tropical Africa, and of only the head, feet, and hands in the cool upland endemic areas in the Americas. The number of nodules per patient is usually 3 to 6, although as many as 150 have been reported.

The histologic appearance of the tumor varies according to age and size. The early nodules show an initial inflammatory reaction with vascular dilatation and later a foreign-body granulomatous reaction around the worms, with granulocytes, endothelial cells, small round cells, and, occasionally, plasma cells and lymphocytes. Microfilariae are present in the nodule and neighboring tissues. The late nodules contain fibroblasts, endothelial cells, and often giant cells. There is a fibrous capsule with a grayish white, collagenous periphery and a soft, yellowish, grumous, inner portion. The nodules gradually undergo caseation, fibrosis, and calcification.

In Africa the first manifestation of the disease, especially in children, is often involvement of the skin with pruritus, which may disappear or persist throughout life. The earliest change is a diminution of the subepidermal elastic fibers; that is followed by a progressive reduction in the subepidermal and dermal elastic fibers. The final burned-out stage is characterized by the absence of elastic fibers, depigmentation, thickening of epidermis, and proliferation of connective tissue in the subepidermal layers. The chronic cutaneous manifestations take the form of xeroderma, lichenification, achromia, atrophy, and pseudoichthyosis, with thick, wrinkled skin, leading in some instances to "hanging groin" (genital elephantiasis). Superimposed on this condition may be a pruriginous dermoepidermitis, the so-called filarial itch (Fig. 7-6). It may start as an acute febrile erysipelas or as a

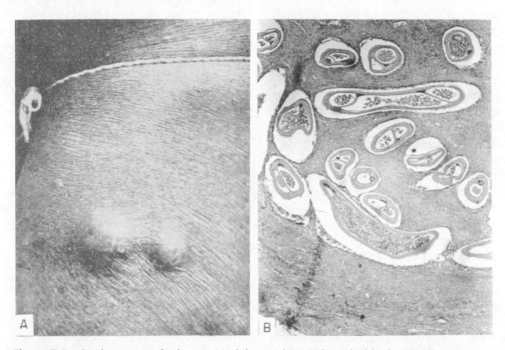

Figure 7-5. *Onchocerca volvulus.* A. Nodules on hip. (After Blacklock, 1926.) B. Section through nodule showing adults containing microfilariae. ($\times$ 30)

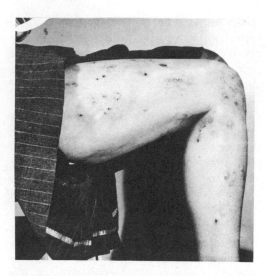

Figure 7-6. Onchocercal skin lesions. Microfilariae were found in scrapings from the lesions. (Patient is a missionary from Angola.)

slowly progressive myxedematous thickening of the skin, at times accompanied by keratitis and iritis. The second type chiefly affects the face but may also involve the arms and, less often, the legs. The skin is thickened and hyperpigmented, and there is intense itching. In the third type there are papulovesicular excoriated lesions sometimes impetiginous, or there may be papillomatous, verrucose, and hyperkeratotic patches on the arms, hands, and neck. Microfilaria may be found in scrapings from these lesions.

During the incubation period of several months to a year, there is an eosinophilia of 15 to 50 percent and transient urticaria. The tumors are well tolerated although at times painful. A slight fever may be present.

Ocular involvement represents the most serious clinical manifestations of the disease, is responsible for much blindness, and is related to the site, intensity, and duration of the infection. The eye acts as a trap for the penetrating microfilariae, which may be found in all the ocular tissues but seem to have a predilection for the cornea, choroid, iris, and anterior chambers. Numerous living and dead microfilariae may be observed in the vitreous humor of the posterior chamber. They can always be found in any ocular lesion and not infrequently are observed in eyes without lesions. The production of ocular pathology has been variously attributed to (1) the mechanical action or secretory products of the living microfilariae, (2) toxins from dead microfilariae, (3) toxins from the adult worm, and (4) supersensitivity of the patient. The first ocular symptoms are photophobia, lacrimation, blepharospasm, and sensation of a foreign body.

The conjunctiva contains many microfilariae, especially at the limbus. Some persons show no reaction and others a chronic conjunctivitis with small nodules, dilated blood vessels, and brown spots on the limbus. The ocular changes are due to a slow and insidious sclerotic process that first manifests itself clinically 7 to 9 years after the initial infection. The earliest and most typical corneal lesion is a superficial punctate keratitis that is visible by the corneal microscope. Later refractile, snowflake opacities, 1 to 2 mm in diameter and composed of corneal infiltrations of leukocytes or dead microfilariae, may be observed, and still later superficial and deep vascularization. The lesions become serious when a diffuse plastic iritis that affects vision develops. The iris becomes thickened, and adhesive synechiae give the pupil an irregular pear shape. Finally, the iris becomes adherent to the anterior surface of the lens capsule and undergoes atrophy, with depigmentation and pumice stone appearance. Lesions of the posterior eye are poorly understood, but chorioretinitis and even optic atrophy can occur. Except in patients with serious ocular involvement, prognosis is favorable. Chemotherapy and early surgical removal of nodules may check the progress of ocular lesions. There is no evidence of the existence of natural or acquired immunity.

Diagnosis. The presence of subcutaneous nodules, eosinophilia, cutaneous manifestations, and ocular lesions in persons in endemic regions is suggestive of onchocerciasis. The development of allergic symptoms, especially of the eyes and pruritus, following the administration of diethylcarbamazine is of diagnostic value. The microfilariae may be obtained by teasing slices of skin on a slide in a drop of physiologic sodium chloride solution, or in the dermal lymph collected by pressing a fold of skin between the blades of a forceps until pitted, and puncturing the middle of the fold to a depth of 1 mm with a fine needle. Microfilariae may be found when no nodules are detectable and may be present in clinically healthy skin. Repeated examination may be necessary. The scapular region is the area of choice for obtaining specimens.

Treatment. Surgical removal of the encysted adult parasites is an established procedure, but it is difficult to locate all the parasitic nodules. It is only partially effective treatment for ocular onchocerciasis, since the microfilariae may survive for 4 to 8 months after the destruction of the adult worms. Diethylcarbamazine destroys the microfilariae; however, it has little effect on the adult worm, since the microfilariae and the skin lesions reappear in 2 to 4 months. The destruction of the microfilariae produces pronounced allergic reactions that take the form of intense pruritus, dermatitis, edema, conjunctivitis, adenopathy, and fever. The allergic symptoms are so pronounced that the use of diethylcarbamazine as a diagnostic agent has been advocated, and careful administration of the drug is required in ocular onchocerciasis. An initial dose, orally, of 25 mg daily for 3 days, 50 mg daily for 5 days, 100 mg daily for 3 days, and 150 mg daily for 12 days, and at the same time steroids and antihistaminics should be administered to reduce inflammation. This treatment should be followed by Suramin,° which acts upon the adult worm, and the microfilariae begin to disappear in about 4 months, while in 2 months the nodules show degenerated worms. The initial dose is 100 to 200 mg intravenously, and then 1 gm is given at weekly intervals for 5 weeks. Suramin is toxic and may produce severe vomiting and loss of consciousness; it is contraindicated in patients with severe ocular involvement. The logical approach is to treat first with surgery to eliminate the adult worms if nodules are present, then with diethylcarbamazine to destroy the microfilariae, and with Suramin if microfilar-

iae persist, indicating that living adults still persist.

A recent study indicates that mebendazole in very large doses—1 gm twice daily for 28 days—affects developing microfilariae in the worm and thereby has a long-lasting effect.

Prevention. Prevention of onchocerciasis includes the removal of nodules, the source of infection, control of the vector, and the protection of susceptible persons. Treatment of the infected persons is important. A combination of surgical removal of the adult worms and the destruction of the microfilariae by diethylcarbamazine reduces the infectivity of carriers, but this method of control alone is not completely effective. Control of the vectors depends upon the destruction of the aquatic larvae by larvicides, especially during the dry seasons, and the spraying of riparian vegetation with insecticides, since residual spraying of houses is ineffective because *Simulium* does not invade them. The individual may be protected by fly-proof clothing, headnets, and especially by repellents.

Loa loa

Diseases. Loasis, eye worm, fugitive swellings, Calabar swellings.

Life Cycle. Humans and, possibly, monkeys are the only definitive hosts. The adult, threadlike cylindrical worms (Fig. 7-1) inhabit the subcutaneous tissues. The sheathed microfilariae (Fig. 7-2) usually have a diurnal periodicity in the blood. The length of life of the worm in humans has been variously reported as 4 to 17 years. The principal intermediate insect hosts are *Chrysops silacea* and *C. dimidiata.* The ingested microfilaria passes through a cyclic development in these flies in 10 to 12 days. A person, when bitten by the fly, is infected by the escape of the infective larvae from the membranous labium to the skin near the bite wound. Within an hour the larvae penetrate to the subcutaneous and muscular tissues, where they become adult worms in about 12 months.

Epidemiology. Loasis is limited to the African equatorial rain forest and its fringe. Prevalence in endemic areas varies greatly (from 8

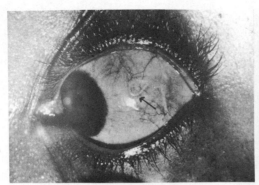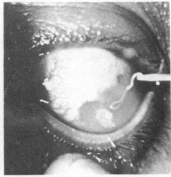

Figure 7-7. *Loa loa* in the eye. (From Fenton and Smith: Arch Ophthalmol 76:877, 1966.)

to 75 percent), depending on the prevalence of and exposure to *Chrysops* flies, which breed in muddy streams and swamps. It is found in tropical West Africa from Sierra Leone to Angola, the watershed of the Congo River, the Congo Republic, Cameroon, and Southern Nigeria. Occasionally Europeans are infected, but usually they are well protected from the flies. The frequency of natural infection in flies is from 1 to 35 percent in the various localities. Humans are usually bitten during the daytime by the flies, which shun bright sunlight and frequent woodland, particularly forest swamp land.* In the tropical rain forests a complex host-parasite-vector relationship may exist between humans, monkeys, and several species of *Chrysops*.

Pathology and Symptomatology. The parasite usually causes no serious damage to the host. The adult worms migrate through the subcutaneous tissues, the maximal recorded rate being an inch in 2 minutes. They have been removed from all parts of the body, but they are particularly troublesome when passing in the orbital conjunctiva or across the bridge of the nose. Involvement of the eye (Fig. 7-7) causes irritation, congestion, pain, tumefaction of the eyelids, and impaired vision. Temporary inflammatory reactions, known as *fugitive* or *Calabar swellings,* are characteristic of the infection. These slightly painful, pruritic, non-

pitting, subcutaneous swellings, which may reach the size of a hen's egg, are most frequently observed on the hands, forearms, and in the vicinity of the orbit. They appear spontaneously at irregular intervals, disappear in about a week, and are probably manifestations of allergic reactions to the parasite or its products.

The experimental injection of a minute amount of *Dirofilaria* antigen into the skin of a patient with *Loa loa* results in the production of a large Calabar swelling. At times the skin shows papules, becomes infiltrated, and later is lichenified. Aggregations of microfilariae may produce an eosinophilic inflammation and fibrosis in the spleen. During the incubation period of 1 or more years, there may be vague symptoms of slight fever, pain in limbs, paresthesia, pruritus, and sometimes urticaria. Infected persons include symptomless carriers and patients with allergic manifestations, including edema, pruritus, and eosinophilia, with or without demonstrable adult worms or microfilariae. The first signs of the disease may be the development of Calabar swellings or the appearance of the worm under the conjunctiva. Infected persons have a wide variety of clinical symptoms attributable to the wandering worm. There may be an urticarial dermatitis, soreness from indurated tendon sheaths, and abscesses from secondary pyogenic infection. There is an eosinophilia of 12 to 70 percent.

* See Chapter 15.

Diagnosis. Diagnosis is based on observing the worm under the conjunctiva, Calabar swellings, eosinophilia, and finding the characteristic microfilariae in the blood during the day (Fig. 7-8). Microfilariae are detectable only in 20 to 30 percent of patients. Intracutaneous and complement-fixation tests with *D. immitis* antigen are helpful when other diagnostic methods fail.

Treatment. Surgical removal of the adult filarial worms, when they are accessible, is an accepted method of treatment. A favorable time is during their migration across the nose or conjunctiva. Chemotherapy with diethylcarbamazine (see preceding sections) is effective, but several courses of treatment may be needed. Antihistaminics and corticosteroids reduce the allergic reactions common to this therapy.

Prevention. Protective measures include the control of *Chrysops* with larvicides as far as practicable, the elimination of carriers by treatment with diethylcarbamazine, and the protection of persons from the flies by nets, screens, and repellents.

Dipetalonema perstans

Diseases. Dipetalonemiasis, acanthocheilonemiasis.

Life Cycle. The adult female worm is 80 mm in length; the male, 45 mm. The adult is found in the mesentery, the retroperitoneal tissues, the pleural cavity, and the pericardium. The microfilariae (Fig. 7-2) are found in the peripheral blood and capillaries of the lungs. In different places they show either a diurnal or, more commonly, a nocturnal periodicity, but they are essentially nonperiodic.

Humanity is the chief definitive host. The same species, or closely related ones, have been found in the chimpanzee and the gorilla. The intermediate hosts are the bloodsucking midges of the genus *Culicoides*. After a 7-to-10-day metamorphosis in the midge, the infective larva is transferred to the skin of a new host by the biting insect.

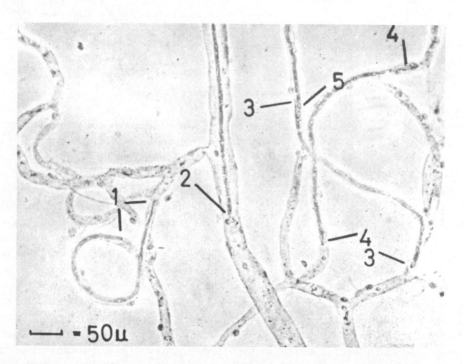

Figure 7-8. Five microfilariae of *Loa loa* in capillaries of the retina. (From Toussaint and Danis: Arch Ophthalmol 74, 1965.)

Epidemiology. This parasite is found mainly in tropical Africa, although it has been reported in North Africa and also in Panama and South America. Human infection is very common in endemic areas where intermediate hosts are abundant. The incidence is much lower in Europeans, who are better protected than the natives against the night-biting *Culicoides.*

Pathogenicity. The encysted worms usually occur singly and cause little tissue reaction. The incubation period is unknown. Usually there are no symptoms other than minor allergic phenomena, although edema, Calabar swellings, and lymphatic varices have been attributed to its presence. Microfilariae have been found in enlarged painful livers. Diethylcarbamazine therapy as used against *W. bancrofti* (see preceding sections) is the treatment of choice.

Diagnosis. Diagnosis is made by finding the characteristic microfilariae in the blood.

Prevention. Preventive measures include the control of the vector, protection of the individual, and residual spraying of houses.

Mansonella ozzardi

Diseases. Mansonelliasis ozzardi, Ozzard's filariasis.

Life Cycle. The adult worm inhabits body cavities, mesentery, and visceral fat. The sharp-tailed microfilaria is unsheathed and nonperiodic (Fig. 7-2). Humanity is the only known definitive host. *Culicoides* are the vectors in which the larvae become infective by the sixth day; by the eighth day they migrate to the proboscis.

Epidemiology. This parasite is found in parts of Central and northern South America and some of the islands of the West Indies.

Pathogenicity. The adult worms cause little damage to the connective tissue of the peritoneum. Occasionally a hydrocele or enlarged lymph node is noted. No particular symptoms are attributed to this worm. Although microfilariae are normally in the blood, it is not unusual to find them outside vessels in the dermis as well. However, no cutaneous pathology has been noted in such instances.

Prevention. Prophylaxis depends on the control of the vectors and protection of persons from their bites.

Dipetalonema streptocerca

Epidemiology. D. streptocerca is found in Ghana, Cameroon, Nigeria, and the Republic of the Congo in Africa.

Pathogenicity. The adult worm has been found in the connective tissues of chimpanzees and in papules of human skin after treatment with diethylcarbamazine. The unsheathed microfilariae, which are found in the skin of humans and chimpanzees, have the appearance of a walking stick with a crooked handle. Humans and chimpanzees are definitive hosts. The intermediate insect host is *Culicoides,* in which infective forms are produced by the eighth day. The worm is usually nonpathogenic, but it may cause cutaneous edema and elephantiasis. Most infected persons are symptomless. Diethylcarbamazine, at a dose of 150 mg per day will kill adult worms as manifested by formation of skin papules within 3 to 5 days of therapy. The effect of the drug on microfilariae is less evident.

DIROFILARIAL INFECTIONS OF HUMAN BEINGS

Human infections with various animal *Dirofilaria* were reviewed by Beaver and Orihel in 1965. More than 40 of these have been reported from the United States; the majority are from southern and eastern states, but they are cosmopolitan in distribution. Additional cases undoubtedly occur, some coming to the attention of the authors, but go unreported because they are no longer a novelty. Most human *Dirofilaria* infections are caused by *D. immitis,* a very common filarial parasite of dogs. In the dog the adult worms—25 and 15 cm in length for the female and male, respectively—live in the right ventricle and pulmonary artery. These parasites have been encountered frequently by medical students in their physiology lab classes. *D. immitis* microfilariae are unsheathed and exhibit partial nocturnal periodicity, several species of mosquitoes can serve as vectors for this parasite. The dog filaria has served as a very useful model for immunologic studies of human filariasis.

Almost all human infections with *D. immitis* come to medical attention as solitary, peripheral nodules in the lung ("coin lesions"), or as subcutaneous nodules. The pulmonary nodules may turn up as incidental findings on x-ray examination of the chest or may be associated with minimal pulmonary symptoms of cough, chest pain, and, rarely, hemoptysis. Such findings often ultimately lead to surgical exploration and excision of a reasonably well-circumscribed lesion, 1 to 3 cm in diameter. Peripheral blood eosinophilia is usually absent in such patients. The chest lesions are found to be sharply defined infarcts of small pulmonary arteries. On sectioning the lung or subcutaneous lesion, the central area is often necrotic, and histologic examination reveals a worm on cross-section, in various states of degeneration. Surrounding the central necrotic area is a granulomatous zone composed of epithelioid and giant cells, lymphocytes, macrophages, and eosinophils. The worm can usually be identified, sometimes to species, on the basis of size of the worm, internal structure, and cuticular features. There are only four recorded instances in which adult worms of *D. immitis* have been found in the heart or great vessels of humans.

Dirofilaria tenuis and D. repens

D. tenuis and *D. repens* occur in humans as subcutaneous nodules of a few weeks' or months' duration, occurring on the extremities or body and the conjunctiva or eyelid. Filarial parasites found in the area of the eye have been reported as *D. conjunctivae* in the literature, but those occurring in the United States are now believed to be *D. tenuis,* a filarial parasite of the raccoon. The other filaria, *D. repens,* which infects cats and dogs, does not occur in the United States.

Unfortunately, these patients do not have antifilarial antibodies by usual tests, which would permit presurgical diagnosis of human *Dirofilaria* infections. Treatment, therefore, is surgical removal.

Tropical Eosinophilia

Tropical eosinophilia is a clinical syndrome characterized by pulmonary symptoms, extreme eosinophilia ($> 3000/mm^3$), elevated serum IgE and antibody levels to filarial antigens, and therapeutic response to diethylcarbamazine. Although findings and treatment response implicate filarial infection, microfilariae are not found in the blood. The condition has, therefore, also been termed occult filariasis. Originally believed due to infection with a nonhuman filarial parasite, it has become increasingly clear that tropical eosinophilia is an exaggerated immunologic host response to infection with human filaria. It occurs most commonly where *W. bancrofti* and *B. malayi* are prevalent, as in India, Sri Lanka, the Malay peninsula, and other Southeast Asian countries. There may be some genetic predisposition involved, since certain population groups appear to be disproportionately affected.

There are two main clinical pictures, the most common resembling asthma, with episodic dyspnea, wheezing and cough, malaise, and loss of appetite and weight. The lungs show transient, variable types of pulmonary infiltrates. The other clinical picture may include some or all of the pulmonary signs and symptoms described above, but also exhibits generalized lymphadenopathy and hepatomegaly, especially if occurring in children. If enlarged lymph nodes are biopsied, microfilariae can often be found in the eosinophilic abscesses that the nodes display. Both clinical syndromes are associated with leukocytosis and 30 to 80 percent eosinophilia, elevated serum IgE and antifilarial antibody levels, and an increased sedimentation rate. Microfilariae are absent from the blood.

Laboratory studies have shown that the basophils of patients with tropical eosinophilia are sensitized by specific antifilarial IgE antibodies. Thus, peripheral leukocytes release larger amounts of histamine when exposed to microfilarial antigens from human, rather than from nonhuman, filarial parasites. In some instances in which lung tissue has been removed from these patients, microfilariae have been found.

Additional evidence for the filarial etiology of tropical eosinophilia is the prompt and beneficial effect of treatment with diethylcarbamazine. The drug is given at 2 mg per kilogram t.i.d. for 7 to 10 days. If symptoms recur, a second course of treatment may be given.

Dracunculus medinensis

Diseases. Dracontiasis, dracunculosis, dracunculiasis, fiery serpent of the Israelites.

Life Cycle. The female is 500 to 1200 by 0.9 to 1.7 mm; the male, 12 to 29 by 0.4 mm. The adult worm inhabits the cutaneous and subcutaneous tissues and attains sexual maturity as early as 10 weeks. The life span of the female is 12 to 18 months. The fate of the male is unknown. In about a year the gravid female migrates to the subcutaneous tissues of the leg, arm, shoulders, and trunk, parts most likely to come in contact with water. When ready to discharge the larvae, the cephalic end of the worm produces an indurated cutaneous papule, which soon vesiculates and eventually forms an ulcer. When the surface of the ulcer comes in contact with water, a loop of the uterus, which has prolapsed through a rupture

in the anterior end of the worm, discharges the motile larvae into the water. Repeated contacts with water evoke successive discharges of larvae (Fig. 7-9).

The slender rhabditiform larvae move about in water and are ingested by species of *Cyclops*, in which they metamorphose in the body cavity into infective forms within 3 weeks. Numerous species of *Cyclops* are suitable hosts. The infective larva is actively motile in the body cavity of *Cyclops* during the first month and then becomes inactive and tightly coiled. Ordinarily only one to three larvae are present, and more than five cause the death of the crustacean. The cycle is completed when the infected copepods are ingested in drinking water by susceptible definitive hosts, such as human beings or domesticated and wild fur-bearing animals. The larvae penetrate the wall of the human digestive tract and migrate to the loose connective tissues. Multiple infections occur.

Epidemiology. Stoll estimates that 48 million persons are infected. In humans the parasite is found in North, West, and Central Africa; southwestern Asia; northeastern South America; and the West Indies. *D. insignis* is present in fur-bearing animals in North America and China.

In western India a high percentage of the inhabitants, mostly under the age of 20 years,

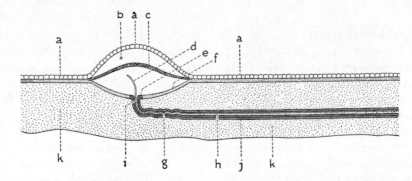

Figure 7-9. Diagram illustrating relationship of *Dracunculus medinensis* to blister and sheath.

a, skin; b, blister fluid; c, fibrogelatinous layer; d, filamentous coil of uterus; e, central eschar; f, granulomatous base; g, convoluted portion of worm; h, straight portion of worm; i, anterior end of worm; j, connective tissue sheath; k, subcutaneous tissues. (Adapted from Fairley and Liston, 1924.)

have been infected by drinking water from step wells. These wells are not provided with a bucket and rope; people stand ankle or knee deep while filling containers. During this time the parent worm ejects her larvae, and at the same time previously infected *Cyclops* are withdrawn with water.

Pathology and Symptomatology. If the worm fails to reach the skin, it dies and either disintegrates, is absorbed, or becomes calcified (Fig. 7-10). The presence of worms in the mesenteric tissues may explain certain pseudo-peritoneal syndromes and allergic manifestations.

When the worm reaches the surface of the body, it liberates a toxic substance that produces a local inflammatory reaction in the form of a sterile blister with serous exudation. The worm lies in a subcutaneous tunnel with its anterior end beneath the blister, which contains a clear yellow fluid (Fig. 7-9). Its course may be marked by induration and edema. The blisters may appear at any location that favors the escape of the larvae to the water, the usual distribution being legs, ankles, and feet (especially between the toes), and less frequently the arms and trunk. The contamination of the ruptured blister may produce abscesses, cellulitis, extensive ulceration, and necrosis.

The onset of symptoms occurs just previous to the local eruption of the worm. The early

manifestations of urticaria, erythema, dyspnea, vomiting, pruritus, and giddiness are of an allergic nature. Symptoms usually subside with the rupture of the worm, but sometimes they recur during the operative removal of the worm, probably from the escape of the secretions into the tissues. There is a slight-to-moderate increase in eosinophils. If the worm is broken during extraction and the larvae escape into the subcutaneous tissues, a severe inflammatory reaction ensues, with disabling pain, and secondary bacterial infection may result in abscess formation and sloughing of the tissues.

Diagnosis. Diagnosis is made from the local lesion, worm, or larvae. The outline of the worm under the skin may be revealed by reflected light. Calcified worms may be located by roentgenologic examination (Fig. 7-10). The discharge of larvae may be stimulated by cooling the ulcerated area.

Treatment. The drug of choice is metronidazole, 200 mg t.i.d. for 7 days. One mechanism of action is the antiinflammatory effect of metronidazole, as well as its action upon the worm itself. In any event, it causes a high percentage of worms to be eliminated spontaneously, or eases their manual removal. Niridazole, 25 mg per kilogram orally daily (maximum 1.5 gm) for 7 days, or thiabendazole, 25 mg per kilogram b.i.d. for 2 days have also shown effectiveness against *Dracunculus*.

The ancient method of rolling up the worm on a stick so as to remove a few centimeters per day is still employed in Asia and Africa. Severe inflammation and sloughing result if the worm is ruptured during this procedure. Surgical removal under procaine anesthesia by multiple incisions after localization of the worm by radiograph and collargol injections is also possible.

Prevention. Lack of education makes it difficult to institute prophylactic measures in many localities. The native religious practice of ablution favors contamination of the water, with resulting infection of *Cyclops*. In order to protect the sources of drinking water, wells and springs should be surrounded by cement curbings, and bathing and washing in these

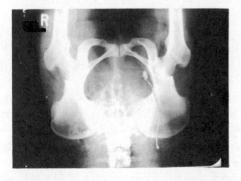

Figure 7-10. Radiograph showing calcified *Dracunculus medinensis* in abdominal wall of an African studying in New York City. There were numerous scars on her feet from removal of worms.

waters should be prohibited. Suspected water should be boiled, and, whenever possible, supplies should be taken from running water, a source relatively free from *Cyclops*. The destruction of *Cyclops* may be achieved by treating water supplies with chlorine or copper sulfate, or by planting fish that are destructive to these crustaceans. Immature worms are destroyed by diethylcarbamazine when this drug is used prophylactically.

Larva Migrans of Gnathostoma spinigerum

Disease. Gnathostomiasis.

Life Cycle. The adult worm, which lives in tumors of the intestinal wall in fish-eating mammals, is a large, reddish nematode, the male being 11 to 25 mm, and the female, 25 to 54 mm. The egg, 69 by 37 μ, has a sculptured shell with a transparent knob at one end.

People are unnatural hosts in whom the worms do not reach maturity. The life cycle involves two intermediate hosts, *Cyclops* and a fish, reptile, or amphibian. The eggs, which erupt into the mammal's intestinal tract and are passed in the feces, in water produce motile larvae, which are ingested by species of *Cyclops*. In order to become infective to the definitive hosts the larvae require further development in a second intermediate host, such as a fresh-water fish, frog, or snake. But, the third-stage larva in this second host may be transferred to other hosts (i.e., paratenic hosts). If domestic chickens, ducks, or pigs are fed with infected fish wastes, the larva simply remigrates and encysts in the skeletal muscles of the fowl or pig. When an appropriate natural host (i.e., domestic cat or dog) ingests infected muscle, the larva is digested free of its cyst wall and undergoes a long migration through the abdominal cavity and muscles. It eventually returns to the stomach wall to complete its development nearly a year later.

Epidemiology. This parasite is found in many countries of the Orient, but the most important foci for human infections are Japan and Thailand. Other species of gnathostomes occur in the Americas, Africa, and the Middle East, but there are no reports of human infec-

tion in these areas. A person acquires infection by eating raw, marinated, or poorly cooked fish; these are common delicacies in Japan and Thailand. Third-stage larvae have been found in pork. It is suspected that food prepared from poorly cooked meat of paratenic hosts, such as the hog or chicken, may be important sources of human infection. There is the possibility that infective larvae liberated from dead aquatic intermediate hosts can be ingested in drinking water.

Pathology and Symptomatology. In the natural hosts the adult worms are enclosed in indurated nodules in the wall of the stomach or intestine. In humans, however, the larvae cannot complete their development, so the partially developed worms migrate aimlessly in the internal organs or near the skin. They produce local, transitory, inflammatory swellings. In the early stages of migration there may be abdominal pain and allergic manifestations. Within several weeks the migrating larva tends to make its way to the subcutaneous tissues of the body. Movement of larvae through the dermal tissues is facilitated by spines on the head and body and secretions of the worm. The trail of a moving parasite is marked by edema, small hemorrhages, and relatively few inflammatory cells, but a stationary worm elicits an intense inflammatory reaction containing many eosinophils. Peripheral blood eosinophilia is present. Cases reported from Japan tend to be relatively benign, with intermittent subcutaneous swellings, while reports from Thailand have featured more serious manifestations, such as involvement of the eye and spinal cord.

Diagnosis. The subcutaneous swellings, associated eosinophilia, residence in an endemic area, and the partaking of local foods suggest the possibility of infection. Definitive diagnosis is very difficult unless the larva or developing worm, 1 cm or less in length, can be found.

Biopsy of a subcutaneous swelling is usually disappointing, for it usually marks the place where the larva has been and shows only an inflammatory reaction with eosinophils. Skin test for immediate hypersensitivity with *Gna-*

thostoma antigens have been described as being useful, but they are not commercially available or standardized.

Treatment. If location of the worm can be identified with reasonable certainty and is accessible, surgical removal can be undertaken. Otherwise, the treatment is symptomatic.

Prevention. In endemic areas thorough cooking of fish, pork and chicken, and drinking of potable water are recommended.

Angiostrongylosis

Disease. Two species of *Angiostrongylus* nematodes, *A. cantonensis* and *A. costaricensis,* which normally live in pulmonary or mesenteric arterioles of rats, can cause human infections. When infective larvae of *A. cantonensis* are ingested by a person, they migrate to the brain and spinal cord, producing an eosinophilic meningoencephalitis. The other species, *A. costaricensis,* causes an acute abdominal syndrome with an inflammatory lesion of the ileocecal region when it infects humans.

Life Cycle. In the case of the rat lungworm, *A. cantonensis,* the adult female worms discharge eggs into the pulmonary vessels, which lodge as emboli in the smaller vessels. These eggs develop and their larvae break into the respiratory tract, migrate up the trachea, are swallowed and pass out in the rat's feces.

Molluscan intermediate hosts, snails of the genera *Achatina* and *Pila,* as well as slugs, planaria, and fresh-water prawns, either eat the larvae or are penetrated by them. The larvae undergo several molts to reach the infective third stage and remain viable for a long time. When rats or humans eat these infected molluscs, the larvae migrate to the brain or spinal cord. In the normal host for this parasite, the rat, the larvae leave the nervous system and migrate via the venous system to the lungs to complete their development. In the infected human host, the larvae probably remain in the brain for a longer period, and do not develop to the adult stage.

A. costaricensis has a somewhat similar life cycle, involving a snail or slug as intermediate host and usually the cotton rat *(Sigmodon hispi-*

dus) as the definite host. When infective larvae are ingested by the rat, they migrate to the mesenteric arterioles of the ileocecal region. Eggs are deposited in the intestinal wall, where they embryonate, hatch as first-stage larvae, and migrate to the intestinal lumen to be excreted in the feces. Contrary to development in the rat, however, in humans the eggs deposited in the gut wall do not hatch; instead, they degenerate and provoke a severe inflammatory reaction.

Epidemiology. Although the life cycle of *A. cantonensis* in the rat and its intermediate hosts has been defined, the way in which human infection occurs is not entirely clear. Transfer of infective larvae from snails to paratenic hosts, such as fresh-water prawns, which are used for certain dishes, may be an important way in which people become infected. Contamination of water or vegetables by infective larvae is another possible route of infection.

Human eosinophilic meningitis and the parasite causing it have a wide geographic distribution. It has been documented in Taiwan, Thailand, Cambodia, Vietnam, Indonesia, and a number of the Pacific Islands, including Hawaii and Tahiti. The parasite has not been found on the U.S. mainland, but several cases have been reported from Cuba in 1981.

Abdominal angiostrongylosis was first described in 1971 by Morera and Céspedes in Costa Rica. Since then human cases have been reported more widely in the Western Hemisphere, from Mexico to Brazil, with the greatest concentration in Central America. The parasite in cotton rats has recently been found in Texas, but there have been no human cases. In Costa Rica the disease caused by *A. costaricensis* mainly involves children in the 6-to-13-year age group. Male patients were twice as common as females; socioeconomic status did not seem to be a predisposing factor. In one study, involving 116 cases seen over a decade at a children's hospital, patients were encountered more frequently during the wettest months of the year. This correlated with the period of the greatest number and the activity of the slugs that serve as the intermediate host *(Vaginulus plebeius)*.

Pathology and Symptomatology. Central nervous system angiostrongylosis originally came to notice because sporadic cases of acute meningoencephalitis had eosinophils in their spinal fluid. Hence the name *eosinophilic meningitis.* The clinical picture is one of acute onset of severe headache, nuchal rigidity, and low-grade fever. Surprisingly, most of the findings seem to reflect systemic signs and symptoms, rather than localizing neurologic signs. Nausea and vomiting are commonly present. Of neurologic abnormalities, the most frequent are paresthesias and cranial-nerve involvement, such as diplopia and strabismus. Weakness or paralysis of an extremity is relatively uncommon. The spinal fluid is often under increased pressure and frequently contain 500 or more cells per mm^3, with 10 to 90 percent being eosinophils.

Even though a patient may exhibit striking neurologic deficits and be very sick at the height of illness, complete recovery can occur, or only minimal neurologic sequelae may remain. This is presumably because the larvae or developing worms have migrated out of the central nervous system. This aberrant, incidental parasite of humans has also been found in the eyes and no doubt will be found elsewhere in the body.

There have not been many fatal cases of eosinophilic meningitis, so observations on pathology caused by *A. cantonensis* are limited. Immature male and female worms have been found in the brain substance and meninges. Infiltration around living worms consisted of eosinophils, monocytes, and foreign-body giant cells, while dead worms were surrounded by areas of tissue necrosis (Fig. 7-11).

The clinical picture of human *A. costaricensis* infection is one of an "acute abdomen," with abdominal pain and tenderness localized to the right lower quadrant, and low-grade fever. The duration of illness is usually about 2 to 4 weeks, and often a painful tumorlike mass is palpable. Leukocytosis and eosinophilia are frequent laboratory findings. The terminal ileum, cecum, and ascending colon show edema and thickening of the bowel wall, with mesenteric adenitis. Histologically, the findings are those of a granulomatous, eosinophilic inflammatory reaction with adult worms and eggs in the tissue.

Diagnosis. Since both varieties of clinical angiostrongylosis have a relatively restricted geographic distribution, history of travel to or residence in an endemic area is a useful diagnostic feature. Inquiry into eating habits and food eaten may also provide clues. Leukocytosis and peripheral blood eosinophilia occur in both clinical syndromes, and are especially prominent in *A. costaricensis* infections.

The key feature in diagnosis of eosinophilic meningitis is the examination of cells in the CSF for presence of eosinophils. Unless specifically requested, clinical laboratories may not do a differential count on cells in the spinal fluid. Only rarely have the larvae been found in the CSF. While a low level of eosinophils may sometimes occur in the CSF in some infections, such as fungal meningitis, along with malignancy, their presence in a proportion of 10 percent or more will exclude the more common causes of meningitis, e.g., viral or bacterial. However, other parasitic infections that can affect the central nervous system, such as cerebral cysticercosis, trichinosis, visceral larva migrans, schistosomiasis, and gnathostomiasis, must be ruled out.

The most common differential diagnoses for abdominal angiostrongylosis involve acute appendicitis, granulomatous disease of the bowel, and tumor. If a G.I. series or barium enema are done, the findings are reduced lumen and inflammatory changes in the terminal ileum and filling defects of the cecum or ascending colon. These radiographic changes are not, of course, specific. Examination of the stool does not help particularly in diagnosis since the patients frequently harbor other parasites and because *A. costaricensis* eggs and larvae are trapped in the bowel wall and not excreted in the feces.

A skin test with *A. cantonensis* antigens has been described but is not commercially avail-

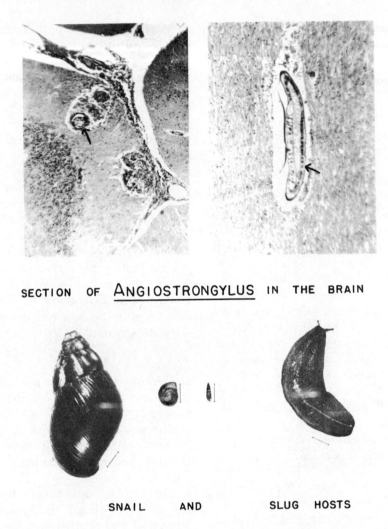

SECTION OF ANGIOSTRONGYLUS IN THE BRAIN

SNAIL   AND   SLUG   HOSTS

Figure 7-11. *Angiostrongylus cantonensis* and molluscan hosts. (From Rosen et al: JAMA 179:620, 1962.)

able and has not been critically evaluated. Precipitin and latex-agglutination tests for abdominal angiostrongylosis are under study, but more experience is needed with their clinical usefulness and specificity.

Treatment. No anthelminthic treatment can be recommended at present. In fact, it is possible that drugs that damage or kill the parasite could increase the tissue reaction around them and exacerbate the disease. While this might theoretically be controlled by anti-inflammatory agents, such medical therapy would require careful evaluation. Many cases of eo-

sinophilic meningoencephalitis will recover completely, or with only minor disability. On the other hand, abdominal angiostrongylosis often may necessitate surgical intervention, especially if perforation or obstruction of the bowel has occurred. Surgery may be needed to rule out other diseases. Thiabendazole has been used in treatment, but no controlled evaluation of its effectiveness has been done.

Prevention. Boiling infected snails or prawns for 2 minutes kills the larvae, as does refrigeration at −15 C for 24 hours. Careful washing and cooking of vegetables and attention to hygienic practices of hand washing and the drinking of safe water should be stressed.

Minor Nematodes of Human Beings

Capillaria hepatica

C. hepatica is a cosmopolitan parasite, primarily of the rat, and also of other rodents, dogs, cats, peccaries, monkeys, and, rarely, of humans. The adult worm, which is named for the organ in which it lives, the hepar, resembles Trichuris trichiura. The lemon-shaped eggs, 51 to 68 by 30 to 35 μ, have outer shells that are pitted like a golf ball. The adult female worm deposits eggs in the liver, where they remain undeveloped. When the infected liver of a rat is eaten through cannibalism by another rat, the eggs escape in the feces to become embryonated in the soil from which infective eggs are ingested. In rodents and humans the accumulations of eggs cause an inflammatory reaction in the liver with the production of fibrous connective tissue and, in heavy infections, extensive tissue destruction and hepatic cirrhosis. A fatal infection in a child was characterized by enlarged liver, ascites, anemia, and eosinophilia.

Diagnosis is possible only by microscopic examination of a liver biopsy. Numerous observers have reported eggs in human feces, but these are spurious cases contracted from eating infected but cooked, animal livers.

Capillaria philippinensis

C. philippinensis was first described in 1964 from a male patient from Ilocos Norte, Philippines, who, after a year of recurrent ascites, emaciation, and cachexia, died after months of intractable diarrhea. The worms, embedded in both the small and large intestines, measured 2.5 to 4.3 mm for the female and 2.3 to 3.17 mm for the male. In the next five years, more than 1200 cases and 100 deaths were reported, many with a malabsorption syndrome. Apparently all the victims have unusual food habits, especially that of eating uncooked fish. However, the life cycle of this parasite still has not been elucidated. The female worm is unusual in that it contains normal Trichuris-like eggs, some with thin-shelled eggs and embryos and some with developing larvae, which suggests that autoinfection is possible. Fluid and electrolyte replacement is important because of the extreme and persistent diarrhea. There is rapid weight loss, muscle wasting, and weakness, with abdominal distention and edema. Hypotension and other cardiac abnormalities occur. Death due to cardiac failure or intercurrent infection may occur in 2 to 8 weeks after the onset of symptoms. In 1973 Cross reported a marked decline in the number of new infections, possibly because of the general use of thiabendazole. Studies by the same author several years later indicate that mebendazole, 200 mg b.i.d. for 20 days, is the drug of choice. Thiabendazole must be given for 30 days, at a dosage of 25 mg per kilogram daily.

Dioctophyme renale

D. renale, the kidney worm, is found in Europe, North and South America, and China. The female, 20 to 100 cm by 5 to 12 cm, is a large, reddish nematode. The male measures 14 to 40 cm by 4 to 6 cm. The brownish yellow, barrel-shaped eggs, 66 by 42 μ, have thick, pitted shells.

The parasite is most frequently found in the dog and mink, but it has been observed in other wild and domesticated fish-eating animals. Our studies demonstrated it to be common in dogs in North Carolina. The eggs, passed in the urine, are ingested by annelids parasitic on fresh-water crayfish. When the oligochetes, with their encapsulated embryos, are eaten by fish, the larvae pass through a third and fourth stage in their mesentery. Mammals acquire the adult worms by consuming infected fish.

The parasite is usually found in the right kidney, less frequently in the abdominal cavity of mammals. It destroys the kidney substance, leaving an enlarged cystic shell containing the coiled worm and purulent material. If both kidneys were invaded, the host would die, and the worm would become extinct. All 11 cases of human infection have been of the renal type, and the symptoms have been those of renal dysfunction or ureteral obstruction. The only treatment is removal of the infected kidney. Diagnosis is made by finding the eggs in the urine.

Gongylonema pulchrum

This is a cosmopolitan parasite of the upper digestive tract of ruminants, equines, hogs, and other mammals, and, accidentally, of the human buccal cavity. The variously named species reported in humans have been grouped under *G. pulchrum.* Some 20 human infections have been recorded, 9 in the United States. The long, slender, yellowish white female nematode is 14.5 cm long. The males attain a maximal length of 6.2 cm. The eggs, 60 by 30 μ, have thick, transparent shells. The embryonated eggs, passed in the feces, are ingested by a species of dung beetles or by the cockroach, *Blattella germanica.* The liberated larvae develop within 4 weeks in the body cavity of the insect into infective forms about 2 mm in length. Upon ingestion by the definitive mammalian host, they probably burrow into the wall of the stomach or duodenum and then migrate to the esophagus and oral cavity, where they become adult worms in the mucosa or submucosa.

In humans the threadlike worm has been found only in the mucosa and subdermal connective tissues in the vicinity of the mouth, where its migrations produce local irritation, inflammation, and reflex nervous symptoms. Surgical removal is the only therapy available.

Since humans are infected through the accidental ingestion of the insect host or through contaminated food or water, prophylaxis depends largely upon personal and household hygiene, especially roach control.

Syngamus laryngeus

The members of the genus *Syngamus,* commonly known as gapeworms, are parasites of the respiratory tract of birds and mammals.

Humans are accidental hosts of *S. laryngeus,* a parasite of the upper respiratory passages of ruminants. Some 25 cases of human infection have been reported, most from Puerto Rico, the Caribbean islands, and Brazil. The exact life cycle and the manner in which a person becomes infected with this parasite is not known. Infection may occur from accidental ingestion of eggs, or possibly even developing adult worms, present on vegetation. Some suspect that an intermediate host may be involved. The adult worms, attached to the mucosa of the larynx or upper respiratory tract, produce coughing and sometimes hemoptysis. Commonly, the adult worms, characteristically joined together in copula, about 1.5 cm in length, are spit up in a fit of coughing. The eggs, which measure about 65 by 90 μ, may also be found in the sputum, or possibly in the feces if they have been swallowed. Treatment is removal of the worms. One case has been reported that was treated with thiabendazole and presumably cured.

Thelazia callipaeda

The members of the family THELAZIIDAE are parasites of the orbital, nasal, and oral cavities of mammals and birds. The life cycles are incompletely known but probably involve an arthropod intermediate host. The species that have been reported from humans, *T. callipaeda* and *T. californiensis,* are parasites of the eyes of dogs and other mammals, the former in the Orient and the latter in California. The slender, creamy white adult worms are 5 to 17 mm in length, and the embryonated eggs are 57 by 35 μ. The adult worms inhabit the conjunctival sac and frequently crawl across the corneal conjunctiva, giving rise to lacrimation and severe pain and paralysis of the ocular muscles. Diagnosis depends upon the identification of the worm after removal from the anesthetized eye. No method of prevention is known, other than the avoidance of ingesting arthropods and contaminated water.

Metastrongylus elongatus

Species of the family METASTRONGYLIDAE are parasites of the respiratory and circulatory tracts of mammals.

M. elongatus, the porcine lungworm, is a filariform, flesh-colored nematode, 12 to 50 mm in length. It is a common parasite of hogs and, at times, of deer, sheep, and cattle; it has been reported three times in humans. The eggs are evacuated in the sputum or swallowed and passed in the feces. The larvae are ingested by earthworms, in which they develop to the infective stage. The definitive host is infected by the ingestion of infected earthworms or, less frequently, contaminated soil. Diagnosis is made from the eggs in the sputum or feces.

REFERENCES

Filarial Parasites and Dracontiasis

Beaver and Orihel: Human infection with filariae of animals in the United States. Am J Trop Med Hyg 14: 1010–1029, 1965.

Duke: Onchocerciasis. Br Med Bull 28: 66–71, 1972.

Edeson: Filariasis. Br Med Bull 28: 60–65, 1972

Kale: Mebendazole in the treatment of dracontiasis. Am J Trop Med Hyg 24: 600–605, 1975.

Neva and Ottesen: Tropical (filarial) eosinophilia. N Engl J Med 298: 1129–1131, 1978.

Ottesen: Immunopathology of lymphatic filariasis in man. Springer Seminars in Immunopath. 2: 373–385, 1980.

Wartman: Filariasis in American armed forces in World War II. Medicine 26: 333–394, 1947.

Gnathastoma, Angiostrongylus, Capillaria and Other Nematodes

Chin-Yun Yu: Clinical observations on eosinophilic meningitis and meningo-encephalitis caused by *A. cantonensis* on Taiwan. Am J Trop Med Hyg 25: 233–249, 1976.

Loria-Cortes and Francisco: Clinical abdominal angiostrongylosis—a study of 116 children with intestinal eosinophilic granuloma caused by *A. costaricensis*. Am J Trop Med Hyg 29: 538–544, 1980.

Punyagupta: Radiculomyeloencephalitis associated with eosinophilic pleocytosis—report of 9 cases. Am J Trop Med Hyg 17: 551–560, 1968.

Singson, et al: Mebendazole in the treatment of intestinal capillariasis. Am J Trop Med Hyg 24: 932, 1975.

Weinstein and Molavi: *Syngamus laryngeus* infection (Syngamosis) with chronic cough. Ann Intern Med 74: 577–580, 1971.

THE CESTODA, OR TAPEWORMS

8

Cestoda

The tapeworms are parasitic worms of the class CESTODA of the phylum PLATYHELMINTHES. The adults inhabit the intestinal tract of vertebrates, and the larvae inhabit the tissues of vertebrates and invertebrates. These elongated, ribbonlike adults, generally flattened dorsoventrally, have no alimentary or vascular tracts and are usually divided into segments or proglottides that, when mature, contain both male and female sets of reproductive organs. The anterior end is modified into an organ of attachment, the scolex, armed with suckers and often with hooks. The important pathogenic species are *Diphyllobothrium latum, Hymenolepis nana, Taenia saginata, T. solium, Echinococcus granulosus,* and *E. multilocularis.*

Morphology. The adult tapeworm consists of (1) a *scolex* equipped for attachment, (2) a *neck,* the posterior portion of which is the region of growth, and (3) the *strobila,* a chain of progressively developing segments, or *proglottides.* The length of the different species varies from 3 mm to 10 meters, and the number of proglottides from 3 to 4000.

The globular or pyriform scolex has one of three types of organs for attaching the worm to the intestinal wall of the host: (1) two elongated suctorial grooves or bothria *(D. latum),* (2) four cuplike sucking discs *(T. saginata),* and (3) in addition to suckers a rostellum armed with chitinous hooks *(T. solium).*

Each proglottid is essentially a functioning individual, a member of a colonial chain or strobila. They originate in the posterior part of the neck and become progressively more mature. Thus, the anterior, undifferentiated segments gradually merge into large, mature proglottides with completely formed sexual organs (see Figure 9-9), and these in turn into gravid proglottides, which consist essentially of a uterus distended with eggs (Fig. 9-9). The gravid proglottides either break off from the strobila or disintegrate while still attached.

The white body is covered with a homogenous, elastic, resistant cuticle, or tegument, which is continuous from one segment to another. Electron microscopic studies have shown that the tegument contains mitochon-

169

dria, membranes, vacuoles, inclusion bodies, and hydrolytic and oxidative enzymes; it is connected by protoplasmic tubes to cells lying deep in the parenchyma. Pore canals extend from the surface to the base of the tegument (Fig. 8-1). The surface is covered with microtriches, microvilluslike structures. Beneath the tegument is a single layer of circular muscles and a thin layer of longitudinal muscles. Two layers of transverse fibers extend from side to side, enclosing a medullary portion that contains most of the organs. Dorsoventral fibers also pass from one surface to the other. The parenchyma fills the spaces between the organs and the muscular layers.

Usually dorsal and ventral longitudinal excretory canals extend along the lateral margins of the segments, from their anastomoses in the scolex to their openings at the posterior border of the terminal proglottid. A transverse canal connects the ventral longitudinal trunks in the posterior part of each proglottid. The main canals receive branches formed by the collecting tubules from the terminal flame cells distributed throughout the parenchyma.

In the scolex there are cephalic ganglia with commissures and several anterior ganglia that are connected by commissures to form a rostellar ring—the brain(?). The sensory and motor peripheral nerves of the anterior end of the worm arise from these ganglia. A main lateral and two accessory longitudinal nerve trunks extend on each side from the cephalic ganglia through the entire series of proglottides. In each proglottid these lateral trunks are connected by transverse commissures.

Most cestodes are hermaphroditic. Each mature proglottid contains at least one set of male and female reproductive organs. The vas deferens of the male and the vagina of the female have a common genital pore that opens on the ventral surface or on the lateral margin of the proglottid. The genital opening may be on the same side of each proglottid (*Hymenolepis*), irregularly alternate (*Taenia*), or bilateral when two sets of reproductive organs are present (*Dipylidium*).

The male reproductive organs (Fig. 9-9) are situated in the dorsal part of the proglottid.

The minute ducts, *vasa efferentia*, which lead from the 3 (*Hymenolepis*) to 500 or more (*Taenia, Diphyllobothrium*) testes, join to form the *vas deferens*, which follows a convoluted course to the *cirrus*, a protrusile, muscular organ enclosed in a thick-walled cirral pouch. The lower part of the vas deferens is often dilated to form the seminal vesicle. The cirrus opens anterior to the vagina into a common cup-shaped genital atrium.

The female reproductive organs (Fig. 9-9) lie toward the ventral surface of the proglottid. The *vagina*, a thin, straight tube, extends inward and downward from its opening into the genital atrium, often expanding to form the *seminal receptacle*. The *ovary*, usually bilobed, is situated in the posterior part of the proglottid. The ova are discharged into the oviduct, which joins the *spermatic duct* from the seminal receptacle to form a common passage leading to the *ootype*, where the egg is formed. The *vitellaria* are concentrated in a single or bilobed mass or are diffusely distributed as discrete follicles throughout the proglottid. Their contents enter the ootype through the vitelline duct. Surrounding and opening into the ootype is a cluster of unicellular shell glands, *Mehlis' gland*, which is absent in some species. The *uterus* extends from the anterior surface of the ootype as a central tube of variable form.

Physiology. Tapeworms lie in the intestinal lumen of the host, with the scolex attached to the mucosa. The usual site is the ileum, but the worms may be present in the jejunum and occasionally in the colon. They have been reported also from extraneous sites such as the gallbladder.

Evidently, cestodes must possess some form of anaerobic metabolism that enables them to live in a relatively oxygen-free intestinal tract. Under aerobic conditions oxygen is consumed, but the quantitative formation of acids is the same in both aerobic and anaerobic environments. Glycogen, which apparently plays the major role in metabolism, is evidently synthesized from dextrose.

Adult tapeworms obtain a good share of their nourishment by absorbing easily diffusible substances from the semidigested food of

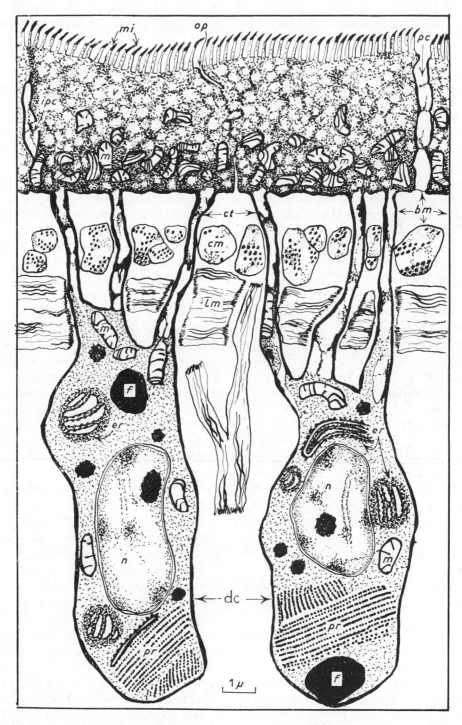

Figure 8-1. Diagrammatic representation of a section through the tegument and neighboring structures of *Dipylidium.*

mi, microtriches; m, mitochondria; v, vacuoles; pc, pore-canal; bm, basement membrane; ct, connecting tube between dark cell (dc) and tegument; cm, circular muscle; lm, longitudinal muscle; n, nucleus; er, endoplasmic reticulum; pr, protein crystalloid; f, inclusions of fat or glycogen; op, opposed membranes; ipc, incomplete pore-canal. (From Threadgold: Quart J Micr Sci 103:139, 1962.)

the host, but apparently part of their nourishment is derived directly from the host. The tegument is thought to be the main absorptive structure of cestodes, with the microtriches greatly increasing the surface area for absorption. Various enzymes that are present in the tegument participate in food absorption. The proximal portions of the microtriches probably serve for absorption of food materials, some by simple diffusion, others by active transport. The distal portions of the microtriches may serve for attachment by interdigitating with the microvilli of the intestinal mucosa or may possibly be abrasive, thus freeing tissue fluids for absorption. Evidently, proteins are obtained largely from the intestinal mucosa of the host, whereas the greater part of the carbohydrates are absorbed from the intestinal contents. Thus, tapeworms are sensitive even to partial reduction of carbohydrates in the diet of the host. Starvation of the host and lack of vitamin B complex in the diet reduces the number of tapeworms, retards their growth, and curtails the production of eggs. Larval cestodes absorb nourishment from the surrounding host's tissues.

The reproductive organs have obtained an excessive development in order to overcome the hazards of completing the life cycle. Hermaphroditism and self-fertilization ensure fertility, although cross-fertilization between segments of the same or of other worms may take place. Asexual reproduction in the intermediate host *(Echinococcus)* further increases the progeny.

Adult tapeworms such as *T. solium, T. saginata,* and *D. latum* have a life span of 20 to 25 years, while some species are short-lived.

Life Cycle. With the exception of *H. nana,* for which a single host suffices for both larva and adult, the common tapeworms of humans require one or more intermediate hosts in which the larval worm develops after the ingestion of the egg. The definitive host acquires the adult worm by ingesting flesh containing the larva. In most cestodes there is a high degree of species selectivity in both intermediate and definitive hosts; e.g., the definitive host of *T. solium* is humanity, and the intermediate host

is the hog. The egg of *T. solium,* however, when accidentally ingested by a person, may develop into the larval *Cysticercus cellulosae.* Humans are intermediate hosts of *E. granulosus,* dogs and other canines being the definitive hosts.

There are two main classes of larvae: (1) solid and (2) vesicular, or bladder. The characteristic solid form is seen in *D. latum.* Characteristic vesicular larvae are seen in the other tapeworms of humanity. There are two types: the *cysticercoid* and the *cysticercus,* or true bladder larva. The cysticercoid (Fig. 8-2C) has a slightly developed bladder that is usually reabsorbed or cast off and a solid posterior portion *(Diplylidium caninum).* The simple cysticercus (Fig. 8-2D) is formed by the enlargement of the central cavity, the invagination of the proliferating wall, and the production of a scolex at the apex of the invaginated portion *(T. solium).* When a number of scolices develop from the germinal layer of the cyst wall, the cyst is known as a *coenurus* (Fig. 8-2E). When the germinal layer produces daughter cysts, or brood capsules, which give rise to numerous scolices, the larval form is termed *echinococcus,* or hydatid cyst (Fig. 8-2F). In the coenural and echinococcal forms, a single cyst, through asexual development, may give rise to numerous progeny, each capable of producing an adult worm.

Pathogenicity. In spite of their great size, the adult tapeworms produce minimal intestinal irritation and few if any definite systemic effects. All manner of vague gastrointestinal and nervous symptoms have been attributed to toxic products of the worm and to the host's being deprived of food. But the same frequency of similar indefinite and nonspecific symptoms can be elicited from uninfected individuals. After patients see a few segments of a tapeworm that they have passed, all sorts of symptoms may develop! With *D. latum,* however, a specific vitamin B_{12} deficiency has been thoroughly studied; the vitamin is absorbed by the worm, thereby depriving the host. The larval stages of tapeworms, in contrast, may produce serious disease. Cysticerci of *T. solium* in the brain may cause symptoms similar to

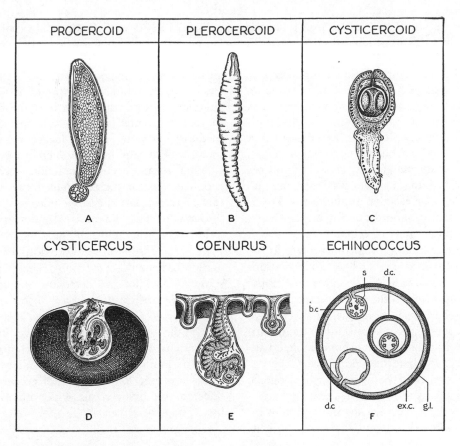

PROCERCOID	PLEROCERCOID	CYSTICERCOID
A	B	C
CYSTICERCUS	COENURUS	ECHINOCOCCUS
D	E	F

Figure 8-2. Larval forms of tapeworms.
 b.c., brood capsule; d.c., daughter cyst; ex.c., external laminated cuticula; g.l., germinal or inner nucleated layer; s, protoscolex.

brain tumors. Echinococcal cysts, which often attain diameters of from 10 to 20 cm, or coenurus cysts, behave as space-occupying lesions.

Resistance and Immunity. Our knowledge of the immunity of cestode infections has been chiefly obtained from studies of the cestodes of lower animals. The adult tapeworms, which are not tissue invaders and as a rule do not cause appreciable intestinal damage, seldom evoke demonstrable immune reactions. On the other hand, intermediate hosts develop definite immunologic responses against the tissue-invading larval cestodes. In experimental animals the degree of immunity may be determined by the number and rate of growth of the surviving larval worms.

Probably the most important factor deter-mining susceptibility or resistance to infection with either the egg or larval stage of tapeworms is the physiochemical environment of the gut. Certain proteolytic enzymes are required for the hatching of the egg, and surface active substances such as bile are needed to "activate" the released oncosphere. The composition of bile salts and bile acids is also important in determining whether an adult tapeworm can develop in a particular host. For example, biles from unsuitable hosts for *Echinococcus* are rich in deoxycholic acid, whereas biles from suitable carnivorous hosts, such as the dog and fox, are relatively poor in this bile acid, which would lyse the cuticle of the evaginated protoscolices. Under some circumstances the size of individual worms and possibly their number may be inversely related to the number of worms present in the gut. Possibly this "crowding effect" operates in some human tapeworm infections.

There is no clear understanding as yet of the immunologic host response in the tissues to the larval stages of different tapeworms. A sequence of changes, including cellular infiltration and eosinophilia has been described in intestinal villi harboring cysticercoids of *H. nana*. But cysticerci of *T. solium* and echinococcal cysts in human tissues generally have no striking cellular reaction around them. This is said to occur around dead or dying cysticerci, and irregular areas of cellular reaction with tissue eosinophilia are sometimes found at the edge of hydatid cysts. These observations might be explained by the presence of the hydatid cyst wall in the latter instance and, in the case of *H. nana*, by the lack of an effective barrier around the cysticercoids in the intestinal villi. But the barrier is not complete with hydatid cysts since host proteins can be detected in cyst fluid. Some leakage of antigenic material probably occurs in the other direction as well, to account for the antibody response to larval antigens that most patients exhibit. Larval cyst fluids of several tapeworms have been shown to consume complement, but the significance of this finding is not clear. It has been postulated that local consumption of complement around the larval cestode assists in evading an immune inflammatory response. However, a complement-mediated immune reaction locally could also increase permeability of the membrane to antibodies. In any event, interaction of parasite products and complement may be an important feature of larval cestode infections.

Diagnosis. The diagnosis of intestinal cestodes depends upon identifying the parasite by the characteristics of the proglottides, eggs, and, occasionally, the scolex. There are no serologic tests for the detection of infections with adult tapeworms, probably because there is little or no immune response to their presence in the lumen of the gut. However, human infection with larval stages of cestodes provokes an immune response. Several larval antigens are used for diagnosis of echinococcal infection and cysticercosis, which involves the larval stage of *T. solium*.

9

Intestinal Tapeworms of Human Beings

Diphyllobothrium latum

Diseases. Diphyllobothriasis, bothriocephaliasis, dibothriocephalus anemia, fish tapeworm infection, broad tapeworm infection.

Life Cycle. The definitive hosts are humans, the dog, the cat, and, less frequently, at least 22 other mammals, including the mongoose, the walrus, the seal, the bear, the fox, and the hog.

The ivory or grayish yellow adult tapeworm (Fig. 9-1), the longest tapeworm of humans, ranges from 3 to 10 meters in length and may have more than 3000 proglottides. The usual habitat of the worm is the ileum and sometimes the jejunum. It is attached to the mucosa by two suctorial grooves. Its life span covers up to 20 years. Self-fertilization is the rule, but cross-fertilization between segments may occur.

The small, almond-shaped scolex (Fig. 9-3), 2 to 3 by 1 mm, has two deep dorsoventral suctorial grooves. The mature segments are broader than long—hence the name *latum*—and contain both male and female reproductive organs (Fig. 9-2). The male organs terminate in a muscular cirrus at the common genital pore. The female organs are characterized by a symmetrically bilobed ovary, a vagina that extends from the common genital pore, and a uterus that opens through the uterine pore in the midventral line a short distance behind the common genital pore. The dark, rosettelike, coiled uterus in the middle of the mature proglottid is a diagnostic characteristic. Daily, 1 million yellowish brown eggs are discharged into the intestine from the distended uteri of the gravid proglottides, which disintegrate when egg laying has been completed. The egg, 55 to 76 by 41 to 56 μ, has a single shell with an inconspicuous operculum at one end and often a small knoblike thickening at the other. The life cycle (Fig. 9-3) involves two intermediate hosts. The first intermediate hosts are fresh-water copepods of the genera *Cyclops* and *Diaptomus*. The second are some of our finest fresh-water fishes: pike, salmon, trout, whitefish, and turbot. This complex life cycle was worked out by Janicki and Rosen.

At a favorable temperature the eggs hatch

175

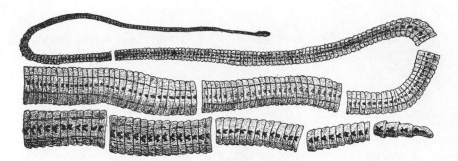

Figure 9-1. Adult *Diphyllobothrium latum.* (Redrawn from Leuckart, 1863).

in 9 to 12 days after reaching water, the embryo in its ciliated embryophore escaping through the opercular opening. The free-swimming, ciliated coracidium is ingested within 1 to 2 days by a suitable species of fresh-water crustacean, *Diaptomus* or *Cyclops,* in which it loses its cilia, penetrates the intestinal wall aided by its hooklets, and gains access to the body cavity. Here it increases in size from 55 to 550 μ to form an elongated procercoid larva.

When the infected copepod is ingested by a suitable species of fresh-water fish, it is digested, and the procercoid larva penetrates the fish's intestinal wall and enters the body cavity, viscera, fatty and connective tissues, and muscles. In 7 to 30 days it is transformed into a pleroceroid larva, an elongate, chalky, spindle-shaped, pseudosegmented organism,

10 to 20 by 2 to 3 mm. Carnivorous fishes may also obtain the plerocercoid larva by ingesting small infected fishes, but in such transport hosts the plerocercoid larva undergoes no further development. A fish may contain numerous plerocercoids. When raw or insufficiently cooked fish is eaten by a susceptible mammalian host, the larva attaches to the intestinal wall and grows at an estimated rate of about 30 proglottides per day to reach maturity in 3 to 5 weeks.

Epidemiology. The parasite is prevalent in regions of the temperate zones where fresh-water fish form an integral part of the diet. It is present in Europe in the Baltic countries, the lake region of Switzerland and adjoining countries, and Rumania and the Danube Basin; in Asia it is found in Russian Turkestan, Israel, northern Manchuria, and Japan; in

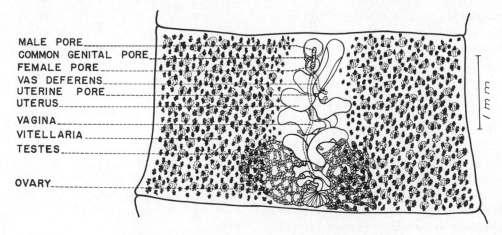

Figure 9-2. *Diphyllobothrium latum* proglottid.

DIPHYLLOBOTHRIUM LATUM

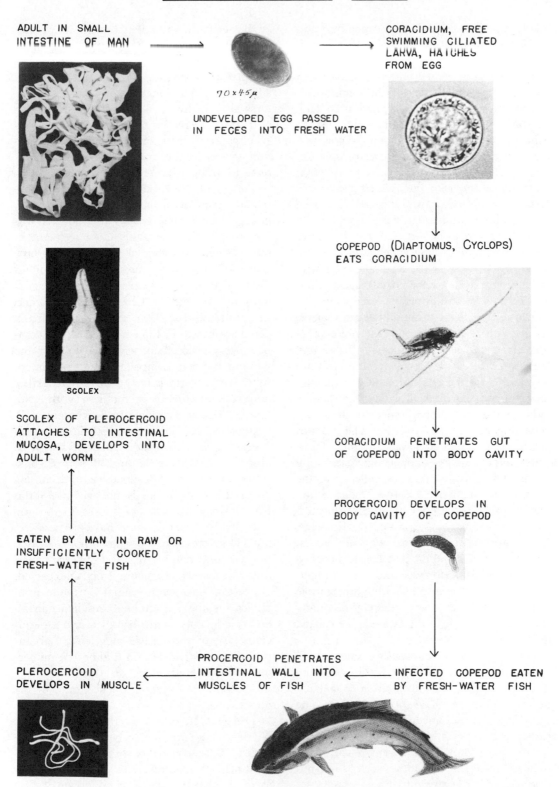

ADULT IN SMALL
INTESTINE OF MAN

70 × 45μ

UNDEVELOPED EGG PASSED
IN FECES INTO FRESH WATER

CORACIDIUM, FREE
SWIMMING CILIATED
LARVA, HATCHES
FROM EGG

COPEPOD (DIAPTOMUS, CYCLOPS)
EATS CORACIDIUM

CORACIDIUM PENETRATES GUT
OF COPEPOD INTO BODY CAVITY

PROCERCOID DEVELOPS IN
BODY CAVITY OF COPEPOD

SCOLEX

SCOLEX OF PLEROCERCOID
ATTACHES TO INTESTINAL
MUCOSA, DEVELOPS INTO
ADULT WORM

EATEN BY MAN IN RAW OR
INSUFFICIENTLY COOKED
FRESH-WATER FISH

PLEROCERCOID
DEVELOPS IN MUSCLE

PROCERCOID PENETRATES
INTESTINAL WALL INTO
MUSCLES OF FISH

INFECTED COPEPOD EATEN
BY FRESH-WATER FISH

Figure 9-3. Life cycle of *Diphyllobothrium latum.*

South America, in Chile and Argentina; and in North America, in Michigan, Minnesota, California, Florida, Alaska, and central and western Canada. A few infections have been reported in Australia (mostly in immigrants), in East Africa and Malagasy, and in Ireland. The development of endemic foci in North America through infected immigrants, first recognized in 1906, illustrates the transplantation of an Old World parasite to a new environment. A separate but related species, *D. pacificum*, acquired from marine fish, has been found to infect humans in Peru.

Humans are chiefly responsible for establishing and maintaining endemic foci. In endemic areas, dogs, cats, and, at times, wild fish-eating mammals are heavily infected but are relatively unimportant except in the spread of the infection in uninhabited regions. Inadequate sewage disposal, the presence of suitable fresh-water intermediate hosts, and the custom of eating raw or semiraw fish are responsible for the establishment and maintenance of endemic areas. Epidemiologic studies indicate that the North American areas are becoming increasingly infected. The practice of allowing untreated sewage to enter freshwater lakes is the most important contributing factor. The fish of the lakes, other than the Great Lakes in north Central United States and Canada, are frequently highly infected. The infection is most prevalent in Russians, Finns, and Scandinavians, who are accustomed to eating raw or insufficiently cooked fish. The Jewish housewife and her daughter, in training, in preparing Gefüllte fish, sample it as they add condiments, thereby becoming infected. Her family, who later eat the cooked dish, do not become infected.

Pathology and Symptomatology. Infection is usually limited to a single worm, although instances of intestinal obstruction by a large number of worms have been reported. The blood shows no significant eosinophilia. Many persons suffer no ill effects from the fish tapeworm. Some, however, present a variety of minor clinical manifestations, such as nervous disturbances, digestive disorders, abdominal discomfort, loss of weight, weakness, malnutrition, and anemia. A woman who passed 5 feet of the worm in the toilet thought it was her intestines. The indefinite digestive symptoms include hunger pains, epigastric fullness, loss of appetite, anorexia, nausea, and vomiting. The vague, questionable, and varied symptoms are usually attributed to the absorption of the toxic secretions or byproducts of degenerating proglottides, or to the mucosal irritation caused by the worm and are most common in those who know they are infected.

The anemias associated with *D. latum,* particularly the pernicious hyperchromic type, have received considerable attention. It was first noted that anemia is more frequent in patients with a history of vomiting proglottides, and this in turn was shown to be due to the attachment of the worm high in the small intestine. As noted in Chapter 8, it has been demonstrated that *Diphyllobothrium* attached in the jejunum within 145 cm of the mouth competes very successfully with the host for the vitamin B_{12} that is ingested, and anemia results. If the worm is forced to retreat farther down the intestine by chemotherapy, the anemia is relieved. The vitamin B_{12} content of *D. latum* is reported to be over 50 times that of *Taenia saginata. D. latum* has been shown to absorb as much as 80 to 100 percent of a single oral dose of radioactive vitamin B_{12} given the host. There is no evidence for a hemotoxin.

In North America there have been no reports of severe anemia in autochthonous cases, but the total number of infections is so small that the absence of anemia is not unexpected.

Diagnosis. Diagnosis cannot be made from clinical symptoms, although residence in an endemic locality, a raw-fish diet, and a pernicious type of anemia are suggestive. Laboratory diagnosis is based on finding the numerous operculated eggs or the evacuated proglottides in the feces or, at times, in the vomitus.

Treatment. In order to effect a cure, it is necessary that the scolex be expelled. If the scolex is not recovered or seen in the feces after treatment, it is necessary to wait 3 months to ascertain that the patient is no longer passing proglottides or eggs. Niclosamide° (Yomesan) is the drug of choice, 4 tablets (2 gm) chewed thoroughly in a single dose after a light meal. A few patients experience nausea and abdominal pain. Unfortunately, use of niclosamide produces a macerated and partly digested worm, so it is usually impossible to identify a scolex in the material passed after treatment.

Paramomycin, a poorly absorbed antibiotic, is also effective. The dose is 1 gm every 4 hours for 4 doses. There may be side-effects of mild gastrointestinal disturbance.

Another drug for the treatment of tapeworms is quinacrine hydrochloride (Atabrine). One advantage of this drug is that it permits recovery of the worm largely intact (stained yellow) to verify whether the scolex was expelled. But quinacrine has its disadvantages also. The relatively large dose given at one time can cause nausea and vomiting. Preparation of the patient is necessary: a liquid diet on the day preceding treatment and the omission of the evening meal, except for liquids. The drug is given the next day on an empty stomach, and 2 hours later a saline purgative should be given to flush out the worm. If recovery of the worm and scolex is an important issue, an additional measure that will make recovery easier is to have the patient take a soap-suds enema the evening before treatment to reduce the amount of fecal material examined. The dose of quinacrine for adults is 0.8 gm given over a half-hour interval. For children up to 34 kg the dose is 0.4 gm; for those 34 to 45 kg, 0.6 gm; the adult dose of 0.8 gm is given to those over 45 kg.

Prevention. The prevention of fish tapeworm infection in an endemic region depends upon controlling the source of infection, the disposal of sewage, and the marketing of fish. Animal reservoir hosts may complicate the problem of controlling the sources of infection. The disposal of untreated sewage into bodies of fresh water should be prohibited. In spite of administrative difficulties, the sale of fish from heavily infested lakes should be prohibited. Freezing at -10 C for 24 hours, thorough cooking for at least 10 minutes at 50 C, and proper drying and pickling of the fish will kill the larvae. The public should be educated about the danger of eating raw or imperfectly cooked fish.

Hymenolepis nana

Disease. Dwarf tapeworm infection.

Morphology. The short worm (Fig. 9-4), averaging 20 by 0.7 mm, may have as many as 200 proglottides. The small, globular scolex

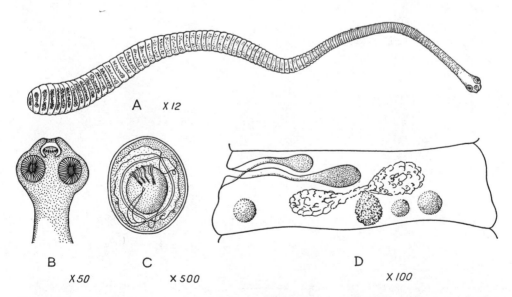

Figure 9-4. *Hymenolepis nana.* A. Adult worm. B. Scolex. C. Egg. D. Mature proglottid showing reproductive organs. (A redrawn from Leuckart, 1863. B redrawn from Blanchard, 1886. C redrawn from Stiles, 1903. D redrawn from Leuckart, 1886.)

bears a short, retractile rostellum with a single ring of small hooks and four cup-shaped suckers. The mature trapezoidal proglottid, about four times as broad as long, has a single genital pore on its left side, three round testes, and a bilobed ovary. In the gravid proglottid, the sacculate uterus contains 80 to 180 eggs. The oval or globular egg, 47 by 37 μ, has two membranes enclosing a hexacanth embryo with six hooklets. The inner membrane has two polar thickenings from each of which arise four to eight slender polar filaments.

The habitat of the worm is in the upper two-thirds of the ileum. Its life span is several weeks. The morphologically indistinguishable murine species, *H. nana* var. *fraterna,* is found in rats and mice.

Life Cycle. The natural definitive hosts are humans, mice, and rats. No intermediate host is required for its life cycle (Fig. 9-5). The murine *H. nana* var. *fraterna* uses fleas and beetles as intermediate hosts, and infection of the definitive host results from their ingestion. The gravid proglottides of *H. nana* rupture in the intestine, setting free the eggs, which are immediately infective when passed in the feces. When ingested by a new host, the oncosphere is liberated in the small intestine and penetrates a villus, where it loses its hooklets and, in 4 days, becomes a cercocystis. Then it

HYMENOLEPIS NANA

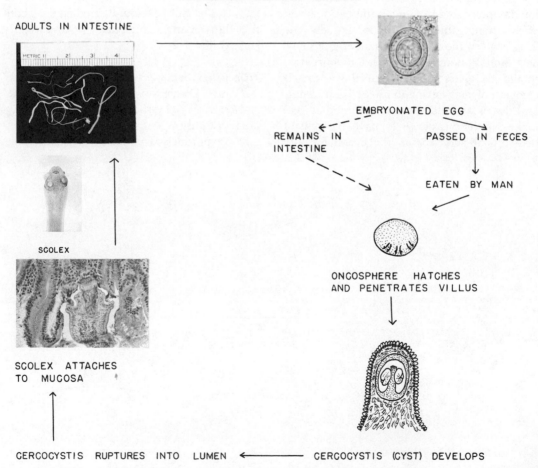

Figure 9-5. Life cycle of *Hymenolepis nana.*

breaks out of the villus into the intestinal lumen, where it attaches itself to the mucosa and becomes a strobilate worm in 10 to 12 days. In about 30 days after infection, eggs appear in the feces. Internal autoinfection results in heavy infection. The egg, instead of passing from the host in the feces, hatches in the intestinal tract; the freed oncosphere penetrates a villus and repeats its cyclic development.

Epidemiology. It is estimated that more than 20 million persons throughout the world are infected. Surveys reveal an incidence by countries of 0.2 to 3.7 percent, although in certain areas 10 percent of the children are infected. Transmission is dependent upon immediate contact, since the feebly resistant eggs, which are susceptible to heat and desiccation, cannot long survive outside the host. Infection is transmitted directly from hand to mouth and, less frequently, by contaminated food or water and possibly by insect intermediate hosts. The unhygienic habits of children favor the prevalence of the parasites in the younger age groups. Humanity is the chief source of infection, although occasional infections may arise from rodent sources. Mice and rats have been infected with *H. nana,* and children have been infected with the murine strain *H. nana* var. *fraterna,* although certain differences in the facility of development in the reciprocal hosts have been noted.

Pathogenicity. Ordinarily there is no material damage to the intestinal mucosa, but an enteritis may be produced by heavy infections, as many as 2000 worms having been reported. Light infections produce either no symptoms or vague abdominal disturbances. In fairly heavy infections, children may show lack of appetite, abdominal pain with or without diarrhea, anorexia, vomiting, and dizziness.

Diagnosis. Finding eggs in the feces is diagnostic.

Treatment. Niclosamide° (Yomesan) is given: 4 tablets (2 gm) chewed thoroughly in a single dose each day for 5 days. For children 2 to 8 years of age, the dose is half the adult daily dose, or 1 gm for 5 days. For those under 2 years, it is 0.5 gm daily for 5 days. For young children it may be necessary to crush and suspend the tablets in water or fruit juice. An alternative treatment is Paromomycin, 45 mg per kilogram daily, given in 4 doses at 4-hour intervals for a period of 5 days.

Prevention. Prevention is difficult, since transmission is direct and only a single host is involved. Control is chiefly dependent upon improving the hygienic habits of children. Treatment of infected persons, environmental sanitation, safeguarding food, and rodent control also may be undertaken.

Hymenolepis diminuta

This cosmopolitan cestode of the small intestine of rats and mice has been reported in humans more than 200 times, usually in children under 3 years of age. The adult worm, 10 to 60 cm by 3 to 5 mm, is larger than *H. nana* and has 800 to 1000 proglottides. The club-shaped scolex has a rudimentary apical unarmed rostellum and four small suckers. The mature proglottides, 0.8 by 2.5 mm, resemble those of *H. nana.* The gravid proglottid contains a saccular uterus filled with egg masses. The egg, 58 by 86 μ, differs from the egg of *H. nana* in the absence of polar filaments on the inner membrane (Figure 17-1).

The principal intermediate hosts are the larval rat and mouse fleas and the adult mealworm beetle, although other species of fleas, myriapods, cockroaches, beetles, and lepidopterans may also serve as hosts. In these insects the hatched embryo develops into a cercocystis which, when ingested by a natural definitive host, becomes a mature adult in about 18 to 20 days. Humans are infected accidentally by food or hands contaminated with infected insects. Human infections are light, and the cestode's life span in a person is short, experimental infections in an adult person lasting only 5 to 7 weeks. Diagnosis is made by finding the eggs in the stool. Treatment is the same as treatment of *H. nana,* above.

Dipylidium caninum

Disease. Dipylidiasis, dog tapeworm infection.

Life Cycle. The definitive hosts are dogs, cats, and wild carnivora. Humans are occasional hosts. The adult worm, which inhabits the small intestine, ranges from 15 to 70 cm in length and has 60 to 175 proglottides. The rhomboidal scolex has four prominent oval suckers and a retractile conical rostellum armed with 30 to 150 rose-thorn–shaped hooks arranged in transverse rows. The vase-shaped mature proglottid has a double set of reproductive organs and a genital pore midway on each lateral margin. The gravid proglottid, 12 by 2.7 mm, is packed with membranous egg capsules, containing 15 to 25 eggs. The globular egg, 35 to 60 μ in diameter, contains an oncosphere with six hooklets (Fig. 9-6).

The gravid proglottides separate from the strobila singly or in groups of two or three and are capable of moving several inches per hour. They either creep out of the anus or are passed in the feces. Their exit may cause the dog to scrape its anus along the carpet, suggesting pinworm, which it never harbors. The eggs and egg capsules (branches of the uterus containing a dozen eggs) are expelled by the contractions of the proglottid or by its disintegration outside (rarely inside) the intestine, some becoming imbedded in the host's fur, especially in the perianal region.

The intermediate hosts are larval fleas of the dog, cat, and human being, and the dog louse *Trichodectes canis*. When ingested by the larval flea, the oncosphere escapes from its covering, penetrates the wall of the gut, and develops into a pear-shaped infective cysticercoid larva in the adult flea. When the infected flea is ingested by a definitive host, the cysticercoid larva is liberated in the small intestine and in about 20 days becomes an adult worm.

Epidemiology. Several hundred human infections have been reported. Most infections oc-

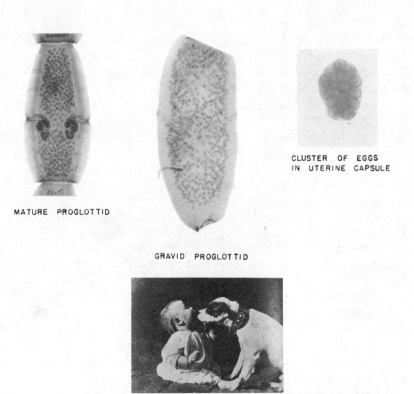

MATURE PROGLOTTID

GRAVID PROGLOTTID

CLUSTER OF EGGS
IN UTERINE CAPSULE

CHILD RECEIVES INFECTED FLEA
FROM MAN'S BEST FRIEND, THE DOG

Figure 9-6. *Dipylidium caninum.* (Dog kissing child from Riley and Johannsen: Medical Entomology, 2nd ed., 1938. Courtesy of McGraw-Hill Book Company.)

cur in children under 8 years and about one-third are in infants under 6 months of age. Transmission results from the accidental swallowing of infected fleas or lice from dogs or cats, either through the contamination of food or by hand-to-mouth contacts. A high percentage of dogs are infected.

Pathogenicity. Children, who rarely harbor more than one parasite, seldom show symptoms.

Diagnosis. Finding the characteristic proglottides or eggs in the feces is diagnostic.

Treatment. See treatment of *D. latum,* above.

Prevention. Small children should not be allowed to fondle dogs and cats infected with fleas and lice. The picturesque and touching habit of kissing a canine by adults and children should not be encouraged (Fig. 9-6). Only the dog knows what his mouth has last contacted. These household pets should be given anthelmintic and insecticidal treatments.

Taenia saginata

Disease. Taeniasis, beef tapeworm infection.

Life Cycle. The life cycle (Fig. 9-7) involves an intermediate host. Humanity is the only definitive host. The adult worm (Fig. 9-8) is 4 to 6 meters in length and is sometimes longer. It has 1000 to 2000 proglottides. Abnormalities of proglottid morphology are frequently encountered and lead to claims of new species. The pyriform scolex, 1 to 2 mm in diameter, has four prominent hemispherical suckers, but no well-developed rostellum or hooks. The mature proglottides, about 12 mm broad and somewhat shorter, have irregularly alternate lateral genital pores and differ from those of *T. solium* in having twice as many testes and a bilobed ovary. The gravid proglottides, 16 to 20 by 5 to 7 mm, are differentiated from those of *T. solium* by the more numerous lateral branches (15 to 30 on each side) of the uterus (Fig. 9-9). The gravid uterus, which has no uterine pore, contains about 100,000 eggs. The yellow-brown eggs (Fig. 9-9) cannot be distinguished from those of *T. solium.* The radially striated embryophore, 30 to 40 by 20 to 30 μ surrounds a hexacanth embryo. In the uterus the egg is covered by an outer membrane with two delicate polar filaments, which is lost soon after it leaves the proglottid.

The habitat of the adult worm is the upper jejunum. Roentgenograms reveal that the location of the worm is usually in the upper jejunum below a level of 40 to 50 cm from the duodenojejunal juncture, and that only about 6 percent of the worms are in the lower jejunum. Its life span covers up to 25 years. The proglottides, usually detached singly, may force their way through the anus by their movements or may be carried out in the stool and, when first passed, are quite active and assume various shapes. Almost immediately after passage the proglottides expel a milky fluid full of eggs from their anterior border, where the forward branches of the uterus have ruptured with the separation of the proglottid from the strobila. Thus, the liberation of the 100,000 eggs from the proglottid is not wholly dependent upon its disintegration.

Cattle are the most important intermediate hosts, but other herbivora such as camels are often infected. The eggs, infective when evacuated, are ingested from the ground or vegetation by these hosts. Hatching requires pretreatment with the gastric juices before the intestinal juices can effect the disintegration of the embryophore and the activation of the embryo. The hexacanth embryo escapes from its shell, penetrates through the intestinal wall into the lymphatics or blood vessels, and is carried to the intramuscular connective tissues, where it develops into a mature bladder worm, *Cysticercus bovis* (see Figure 8-2D), in 12 to 15 weeks. The masseters, hind limbs, and humps of cattle are the selective sites, but the cysticerci may be found in other muscles and viscera. The mature pinkish cyst, about 5 to 9 mm, has an opaque, invaginated neck and a scolex with four suckers. It undergoes degeneration and calcification in about a year, although living cysticerci have been found in cattle 3 years after experimental infections. When the living cysticercus is ingested by a person, the scolex evaginates and attaches itself to the mucosa of the jejunum, and a mature worm develops in 8 to 10 weeks. Usually

TAENIA SAGINATA

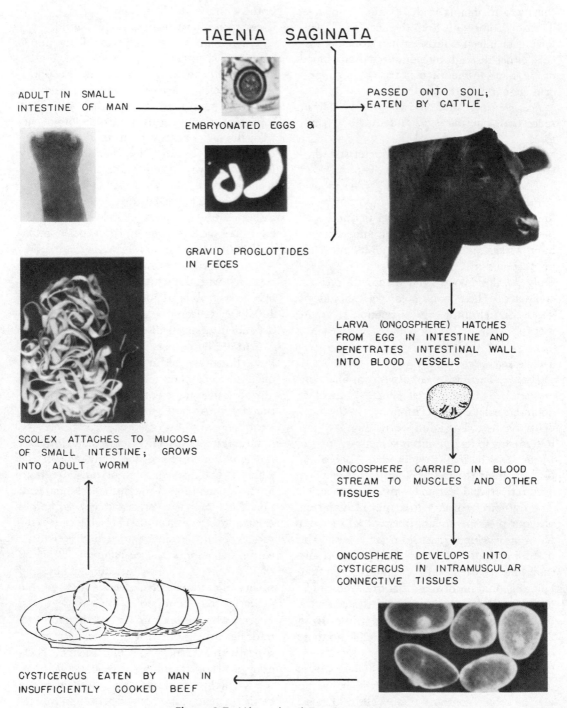

ADULT IN SMALL
INTESTINE OF MAN →

EMBRYONATED EGGS &

GRAVID PROGLOTTIDES
IN FECES

PASSED ONTO SOIL;
EATEN BY CATTLE

LARVA (ONCOSPHERE) HATCHES
FROM EGG IN INTESTINE AND
PENETRATES INTESTINAL WALL
INTO BLOOD VESSELS

ONCOSPHERE CARRIED IN BLOOD
STREAM TO MUSCLES AND OTHER
TISSUES

ONCOSPHERE DEVELOPS INTO
CYSTICERCUS IN INTRAMUSCULAR
CONNECTIVE TISSUES

SCOLEX ATTACHES TO MUCOSA
OF SMALL INTESTINE; GROWS
INTO ADULT WORM

CYSTICERCUS EATEN BY MAN IN
INSUFFICIENTLY COOKED BEEF

Figure 9-7. Life cycle of *Taenia saginata.*

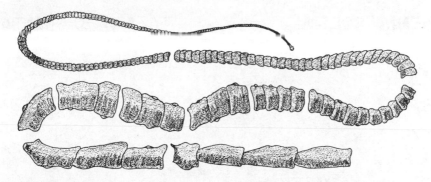

Figure 9-8. Adult *Taenia saginata.* (Redrawn from Leuckart, 1863).

only a single adult worm is present, but as many as 28 have been reported. We recovered six from a Turkish woman—a total of more than 100 feet!

Epidemiology. This parasite is cosmopolitan in beef-eating countries. Humans acquire the infection from eating raw, hemorrhaging, or imperfectly cooked beef containing the cysticerci. Cattle are infected from grazing land contaminated by human pollution, through fertilization with night soil or through sewage-laden water. Flooded pastures along the rivers are important sources of bovine cysticercosis. In these pastures the eggs may remain viable 8 or more weeks.

Symptomatology. The adult worm rarely causes symptoms of significance. Infected persons, especially those who know they harbor this large tapeworm, may complain of epigastric pain, vague abdominal discomfort, nervousness, vertigo, nausea, vomiting, diarrhea, or increased or loss of appetite. There usually is no appreciable loss of weight. There may be a moderate eosinophilia.

Gravid proglottides that lodge in the appendiceal lumen may cause slight mucosal lesions and possibly initiate a secondary appendicitis. Very rarely a mass of tangled strobila may cause acute intestinal obstruction, or the penetration of the worm into the duct of Wirsung may lead to pancreatic necrosis.

The migration out of the anus of the muscular, active, gravid proglottides give the patient the feeling of having an unsolicited stool, causing considerable consternation, depending upon where the patient is. Thus a minister preaching to his congregation cut short his sermon when 5 feet of strobila slipped down one of his trouser legs. The finding of actively moving proglottides in the underclothing, in bed, or on a freshly passed stool is also disturbing.

Prognosis is good, although it is sometimes difficult to eradicate the scolex. There is slight if any risk of cysticercosis, since only three probable instances have been reported: two in the skeletal muscles and one in the mesenteric lymph nodes.

Diagnosis. Diagnosis is based on the recovery of the gravid proglottides or the eggs from the feces or perianal region with a Scotch tape swab. Specific diagnosis is made from the 15 to 30 lateral uterine branches on each side of the main uterine stem in the gravid proglottid or from the hookless scolex recovered after therapy. Perianal swabbing with cellophane tape swabs gives a much higher recovery of eggs than examining the feces by direct smears and concentration methods, as eggs may not be present in the stool.

Treatment. See treatment of *D. latum,* above.

Prevention. Prophylactic measures include (1) removal of sources of infection by treating infected individuals and prevention of contamination of soil with human feces, (2) inspection of beef for cysticerci, (3) refrigeration of beef, and (4) the thorough cooking of beef. Cysticerci may be destroyed by freezing at −10 C for 5 days, heating above their thermal death point of 57 C, and pickling in 25 per-

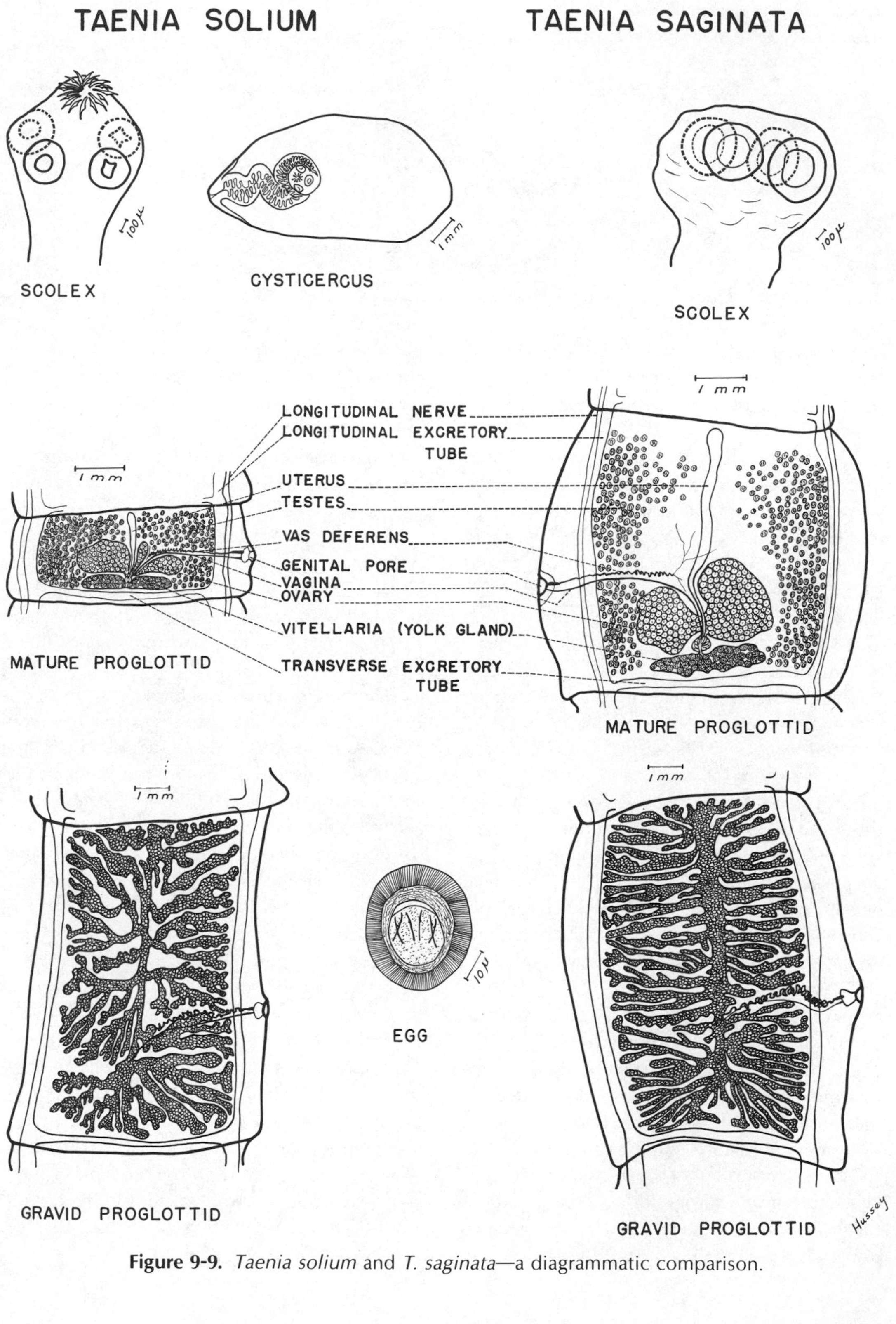
TAENIA SOLIUM
TAENIA SAGINATA
SCOLEX
100μ
CYSTICERCUS
1 mm
SCOLEX
100μ
1 mm
1 mm
LONGITUDINAL NERVE
LONGITUDINAL EXCRETORY TUBE
UTERUS
TESTES
VAS DEFERENS
GENITAL PORE
VAGINA
OVARY
VITELLARIA (YOLK GLAND)
TRANSVERSE EXCRETORY TUBE
MATURE PROGLOTTID
MATURE PROGLOTTID
1 mm
1 mm
10μ
EGG
GRAVID PROGLOTTID
GRAVID PROGLOTTID
Hussey

Figure 9-9. *Taenia solium* and *T. saginata*—a diagrammatic comparison.

cent salt solution for 5 days. The most practical safeguard is to cook beef thoroughly until it has lost its rich reddish tinge.

Taenia solium

Disease. Taeniasis; pork tapeworm infection.

Life Cycle. People are the only definitive hosts and, unfortunately, we can also be hosts of the cyst. The adult worm is 2 to 4 (occasionally 8) meters in length, and when fully developed contains 800 to 1000 segments. The globular scolex (Fig. 9-10), about 1 mm in diameter, is equipped with four cup-shaped suckers and a low, cushioned rostellum with a double crown of 25 to 30 hooks. The mature proglottid (Fig. 9-9) is roughly square, with unilateral or irregularly alternate genital pores on consecutive segments. The trilobed ovary consists of two lateral lobes and one small central lobe. *T. solium* may be distinguished from *T. saginata* by its gravid uterus with 7 to 12 thick lateral branches on each side of the main uterine stem. The mature egg, indistinguishable from that of *T. saginata,* contains a hexacanth embryo with six hooklets surrounded by a light brown, thick, striated spherical or subspherical shell, 30 to 40 μ in diameter.

The habitat of the worm is the upper part of the jejunum. Its life span is long—up to 25 years. Nourishment is obtained from the intestinal contents. The terminal, gravid, motile proglottides separate, from time to time, from the strobila in groups of five or six. The gravid proglottid liberates about 30,000 to 50,000 eggs by its rupture before or after leaving the host.

The usual intermediate hosts that harbor the cyst are hogs and wild boars. Sheep, deer, dogs, monkeys, rats and cats are less frequently infected, and humans and other primates only occasionally. The eggs, extruded by the definitive host, are ingested in food or water by a susceptible intermediate host. The hexacanth embryo escapes from its shell, penetrates the intestinal wall into lymphatics or blood vessels, and is carried to various muscles of the body. The mature cysticercus, known as *Cysticercus cellulosae,* is an ellipsoidal, translucent, thin-walled bladder, 10 by 5 mm, with an opaque invaginated scolex equipped with suckers and hooks. The lingual, masseteric, mucosal, diaphragmatic, and cardiac muscles are chiefly affected, but the liver, kidneys, lungs, brain, and eye may also be involved. When infected, measly pork is eaten by a person, the cyst is dissolved by the action of the digestive juices, and its evaginated scolex attaches to the jejunal mucosa and develops into an adult worm in several months.

Epidemiology. The incidence of *T. solium* infection in humans varies throughout the world. The adult parasite is extremely rare in humans in the United States, largely because hogs do not have access to human feces. It is common in some Central and South American countries, Africa, India, and China. Food-preparation habits and religious customs concerning meat affect the incidence of this parasite. The prevalence in hogs, in some countries 25 percent, is highest where insanitation and faulty methods of fecal disposal are prevalent, or where human feces is fed to hogs.

Symptomatology. The adult parasite, usually a single specimen, causes only slight local inflammation of the intestinal mucosa from the mechanical irritation of the strobila and the attachment of the scolex. Rare instances of intestinal perforation with secondary peritonitis and gallbladder infection have ben reported. Serious lesions result from infection with the larval cysticercus (see Figure 10-6). There may be a variable eosinophilia as high as 28 percent and a leukopenia.

The prognosis for intestinal taeniasis is good, but the infection should be terminated to reduce the risk of cysticercosis.

Diagnosis. Proglottides or eggs are often observed in the feces or perianal region. Specific diagnosis is made by the identification of the proglottides, since the eggs cannot be differentiated from those of *T. saginata.* The gravid proglottid is distinguished from that of *T. saginata* by the smaller number, 7 to 12 pairs, of the lateral branches of the uterus (Fig. 9-9). *T. solium* has hooklets on its scolex.

Treatment. See treatment of *D. latum,* above.

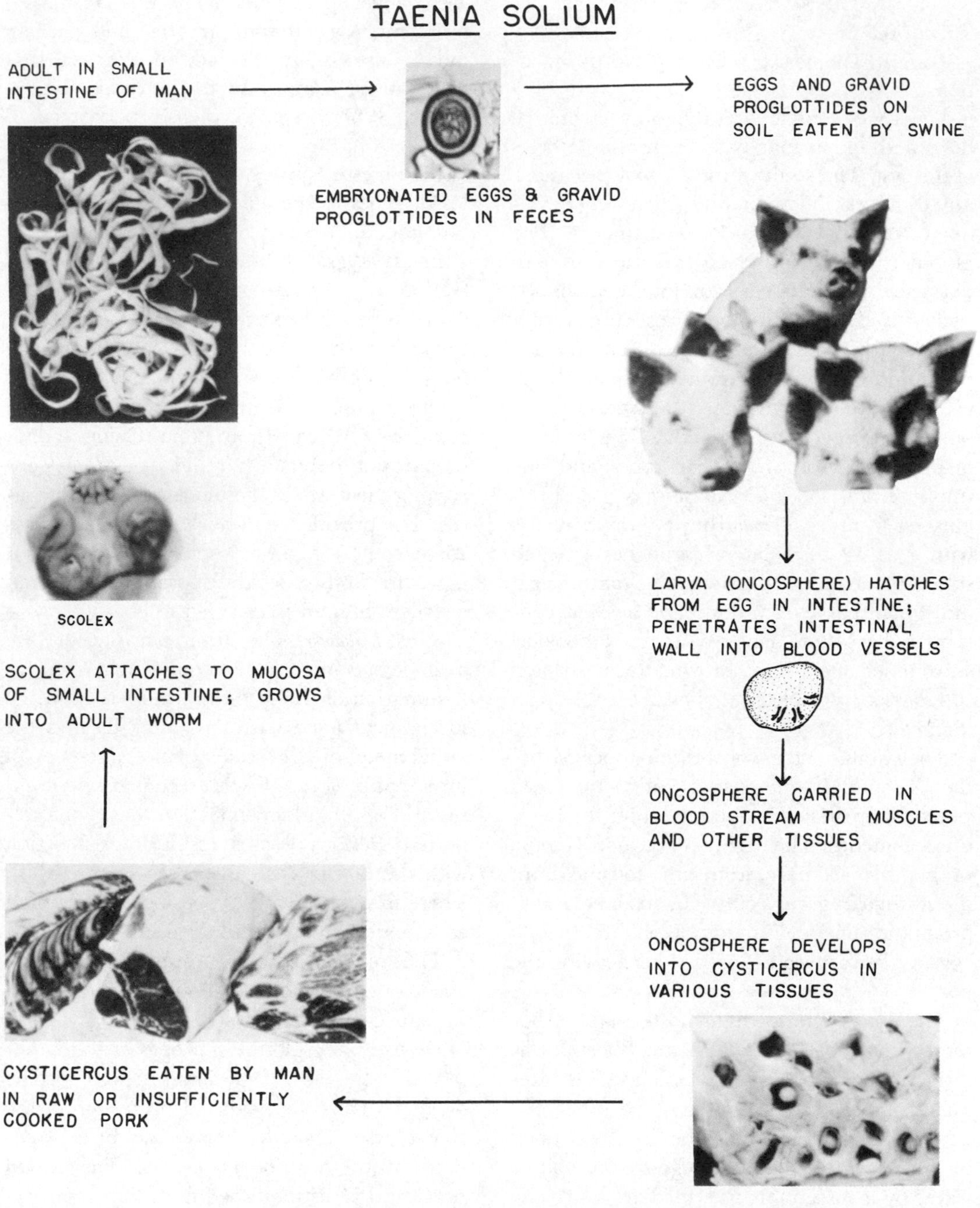

TAENIA SOLIUM

ADULT IN SMALL
INTESTINE OF MAN

EMBRYONATED EGGS & GRAVID
PROGLOTTIDES IN FECES

EGGS AND GRAVID
PROGLOTTIDES ON
SOIL EATEN BY SWINE

SCOLEX

SCOLEX ATTACHES TO MUCOSA
OF SMALL INTESTINE; GROWS
INTO ADULT WORM

LARVA (ONCOSPHERE) HATCHES
FROM EGG IN INTESTINE;
PENETRATES INTESTINAL
WALL INTO BLOOD VESSELS

ONCOSPHERE CARRIED IN
BLOOD STREAM TO MUSCLES
AND OTHER TISSUES

ONCOSPHERE DEVELOPS
INTO CYSTICERCUS IN
VARIOUS TISSUES

CYSTICERCUS EATEN BY MAN
IN RAW OR INSUFFICIENTLY
COOKED PORK

Figure 9-10. Life cycle of *Taenia solium*.

Because niclosamide and paromomycin produce disintegration of tapeworm segments, there is a theoretical risk of infection with eggs, i.e., cysticercosis. Therefore, some prefer to use quinacrine for treatment of pork tapeworm infection. However, such a complication has never been documented. Besides, there is also a risk of vomiting from quinacrine—a more likely mechanism by which autoinfection could occur.

If one wishes to be especially cautious about the theoretical danger of autoinfection complicating treatment of *T. solium* infection, the following measures can be taken. If niclosamide or paromomycin are used, a saline purge can be given a few hours after treatment. To prevent vomiting from quinicrine, prochlorperazine (Compazine) can be given an hour before treatment.

Prevention. The control of *T. solium* infection includes (1) treatment of infected persons, (2) sanitation, (3) inspection of pork, and (4) thorough cooking and processing of pork. The prompt treatment of infected persons not only reduces the sources of infection, but also eliminates the danger of autoinfection with cysticerci. In endemic areas human feces should not be deposited in areas accessible to hogs. Governmental meat inspection has lowered the incidence of human infection in countries where raw or insufficiently cooked pork is consumed, but it is impossible to guarantee freedom from infection by any system of inspection. Thorough cooking is the most effective means of prophylaxis. Cysticerci are killed by heating at 45 to 50 C, but pork should be cooked for at least a half hour for every pound or until gray. Cysticerci are killed below -2 C, but at 0 to -2 C, they survive for nearly 2 months, and at room temperature for 26 days. Freezing at -10 C for 4 days or more is an effective but expensive procedure. Pickling in brine is not always successful.

MINOR TAPEWORMS OF HUMAN BEINGS

Genus *Bertiella.* Species of the genus *Bertiella* have a large globular scolex without a definite rostellum or hooks and a relatively large strobila. The embryophore has a bicornuate process. The life cycle is not completely known, but certain species of mites are proved experimental hosts. The species that have been reported as incidental parasites of humans are natual parasites of primates. They have been found in humans several times in Africa, in Asia and neighboring islands, in the West Indies, and in Brazil.

Genus *Mesocestoides. M. variabilis,* a parasite of carnivorous animals, has been reported in three children from the United States, and another species has been reported, mainly from Japan. Niclosamide was effective in the treatment of the latest U.S. case.

Genus *Inermicapsifer.* Species of this genus have a cushion-shaped rostellum, four suckers, and grow to 4.7 cm in length. Their natural definitive hosts are probably rodents. *I. madagascariensis* has been reported in humans in the Eastern Hemisphere, several times in South America, and frequently in Cuba, in children.

Several species of adult taenial worms, other than the beef and pork tapeworms, have been occasionally reported in humans. These species are often variations or aberrant forms of *T. saginata,* characterized by the absence of external segmentation, or perforated or fenestrated proglottides. *T. confusa* has been identified in humans in the United States and has also been reported in Africa and Japan. It is probably identical with *T. bremneri,* described by Stephens in northern Nigeria. *T. africana* from an East African native, is distinguished by an unarmed scolex with a small extra apical sucker and a gravid uterus with radiating unbranched arms. Treatment is the same as for *D. latum,* above.

In veterinary practice three common taenial worms may be mentioned: (1) *T. pisiformis* of dogs, with the rabbit as an intermediate host; (2) *T. ovis* of dogs, with sheep as intermediate host; (3) *T. taeniaeformis* of cats, with mice and rats as intermediate hosts in which the cysticercus is often associated with sarcomatous growth in the liver (*T. taeniaformis* has been reported found in a child in Argentina); (4) *Dipylidium caninum* of dogs.

REFERENCES

Intestinal Tapeworms of Man
Pawlowski and Schultz: *(Taeniasis and cysticercosis*

Taenia saginata, In: Dawes (eds): Advances in Parasitology, Vol. 10. New York, Academic Press, 1972.
von Bonsdorff: Diphyllobothriasis in man, New York, Academic Press, Inc., 1977.

10

Extraintestinal Larval Tapeworms of Human Beings

The tapeworms capable of producing human infection in their larval stages include (1) the hydatid cysts of *Echinococcus,* (2) the cysticercus of *Taenia solium,* (3) the spargana or plerocercoid larvae of several species of diphyllobothriids, (4) the coenuri of species of *Multiceps,* and (5) *Hymenolepis nana* cerocystis. These larval infections, except for those of *H. nana,* produce serious symptoms and, with the exception of *Multiceps,* are not uncommon in certain areas of the world.

Hydatid Cyst of Echinococcus granulosus

Diseases. Echinococcosis, hydatid disease, hydatid cyst.

Life Cycle. The adult worm (Fig. 10-1) lives in the small intestine of dogs, wolves, jackals, coyotes, foxes, rarely in cats, and in other carnivora. These hosts acquire the adult tapeworm by devouring various organs of herbivores that contain the cyst stage with its numerous protoscolices (Fig. 10-2). It is the smallest tapeworm (2.5 to 9.0 mm) of medical importance. The globular scolex bears a prominent rostellum with a double crown of

30 to 36 hooks and four prominent suckers. The body consists of a head and neck and three proglottides, the first immature, the more elongated middle proglottid with fully developed reproductive organs, and the last or gravid proglottid has a median uterus with 12 to 15 branches distended with some 500 eggs. The egg, 30 to 38 μ, resembles those of the other taenia. Its life span is about 5 months, although it may live for more than a year. Except for inflammation of the intestine during heavy infections, it does not harm the canine host.

Hydatid Cyst. When the egg, from the feces of an infected dog or various carnivores, is ingested by an intermediate host, including a person, the liberated embryo penetrates the intestinal wall, passes into the lymphatics or mesenteric venules, and is carried by the bloodstream to various parts of the body (Fig. 10-3). If not destroyed by phagocytic cells, it loses its hooklets, undergoes central vesiculation, and becomes a cyst of about 10 mm in diameter in 5 months. The common intermediate host is the sheep, but cattle, horses, other

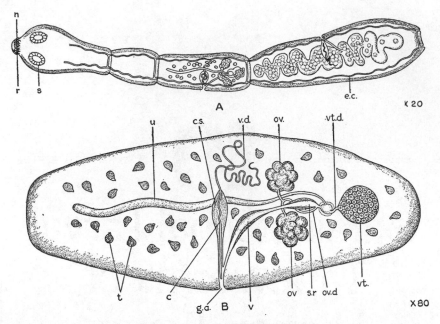

Figure 10-1. *Echinococcus granulosus.* Adult worm.

e.c., excretory canal; h, hooklets; r, rostellum; s, sucker; t, testes; u, uterus; ov, ovary; ov.d, oviduct; g.a., genital pore; v.d., vas deferens; c.s., cirral sac; s.r., seminal receptacle; vt.d., vitelline duct. (Top) Longitudinal. (Bottom) Cross-section mature segment. (Composite drawing.)

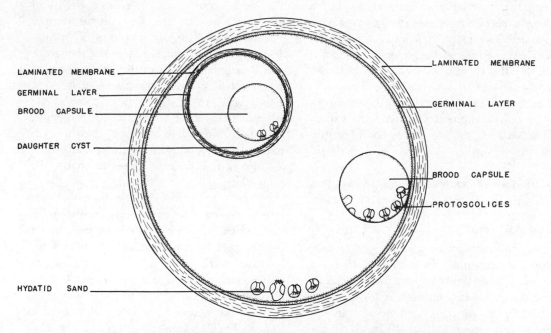

Figure 10-2. Hydatid cyst of *Echinococcus granulousus;* diagrammatic.

herbivora, and hogs may be infected. Humans also harbor the cyst stage, much to our detriment, but we do not participate in the complete cycle, since infected human organs are not eaten by dogs.

In humans hydatid cysts are of three types: (1) unilocular, (2) osseous, and (3) alveolar of *E. multilocularis*. The unilocular cyst is the most common form in humans and lower animals. It grows slowly and requires several years for development. In humans the completely de-

veloped cysts, if uninfluenced by pressure, are more or less spherical and are usually 1 to 7 cm in diameter but may reach 20 cm. The cyst has (1) an external, laminated, nonnucleated, hyaline, supporting cuticula, 1 mm thick; (2) an inner, nucleated, germinal layer, 22 to 25 μ thick; (3) colorless or light-yellow sterile fluid that causes distention of the limiting membranes; (4) brood capsules, which have only the germinal layer, containing protoscolices; and (5) daughter cysts, which

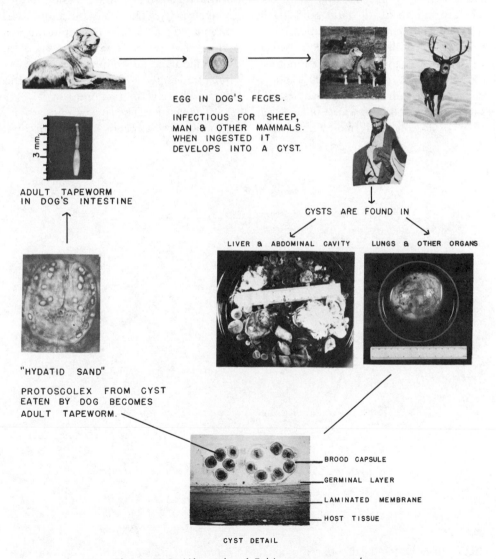

Figure 10-3. Life cycle of *Echinococcus granulosus*.

are replicas of the mother cysts. The external elastic cuticula, which is secreted by the germinal layer, permits the entry of nutritive substances but excludes substances inimical to the parasite. When ruptured it contracts, thus facilitating the dissemination of the contents of the cyst. The inner surface of the internal germinal layer is studded with small papillary brood capsules in various stages of development (Fig. 10-2). As these vesicles enlarge, small oval buds that become protoscolices develop on the inner surface. When the brood capsule ruptures, the protoscolices escape into the hydatid fluid, where they and the brood capsules are known as "hydatid sand" (Fig. 10-2). It is estimated that an average fertile cyst contains 2 million protoscolices, which when eaten by a dog would produce innumerable mature adult tapeworms in about 7 weeks. Hydatids without brood capsules and protoscolices are known as *sterile* or *acephalocysts*. The protoscolices are most remarkable,

for (1) when they are ingested by carnivores, they evaginate in the intestine and develop into adult tapeworms, and (2) if the cyst ruptures within the host, the protoscolices develop into daughter cysts (Fig. 10-4).

The endogenous daughter cyst with a thin transparent wall develops in the cystic fluid and at times may produce granddaughter cysts. Opinions differ as to its chief derivation, from protoscolices, brood capsules, or broken bits of germinative tissue. In the bones, growth of the hydatid cysts follows the line of least resistance along the bony canals, with erosion of the osseous tissues and invasion of the medullary cavity. The bony structure is slowly permeated with a gelatinous infiltration and is replaced with small semisolid cysts with little or no fluid and no scolices. Osseous cysts occur most frequently in the upper ends of the long bones, ilium, vertebrae, and ribs.

Epidemiology. The prevalence of human echinococcosis depends upon the intimate as-

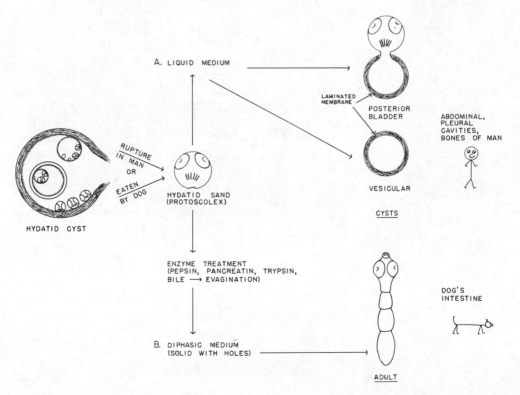

Figure 10-4. Differentiation of protoscolices of *Echinococcus granulosus*. A. Unevaginated protoscolices form hydatid cysts. B. Strobilization occurs in diphasic medium (canine intestine). (After Smyth, Hawkins, and Barton, 1966.)

sociation of humans with infected dogs. Lebanese Christians are infected with hydatid disease at about twice the rate of Lebanese Moslems, suggesting that the Moslems' belief in the uncleanliness of dogs may be responsible for their lower infection rate. The risk of infection of dog owners was 21 times that of nondog owners; 10 percent of the infected Armenians had allowed their dog to share their bed. The percentage of infected dogs in grazing countries throughout the world is 20 to 50 percent and depends upon the canine consumption of infected offal and carcasses. The prevalence of hydatid cysts in such countries is variable but runs 30 percent or more in sheep and cattle and 10 percent in hogs. In certain countries goats, camels, and water buffaloes are infected. Cattle are not a potent reservoir hazard, since their cysts are mostly sterile. The incidence of infection is high in humans in grazing countries, where association with dogs is intimate, e.g., Australia, New Zealand, the Middle East, and southern South America. In North America there have been relatively few autochthonous cases reported, but in recent years echinococcosis has been found in Mississippi, Utah, California, the upper mid-West, and among the Indians of Canada. In Canada the moose and caribou are the intermediate hosts, and the wolf the most important definitive host. Indians infect their dogs by feeding them the lungs of moose and caribou, and the dogs in turn infect their masters with their feces.

Infection often takes place in childhood, the period of unhygienic habits. Transmission is by ingestion of the eggs, chiefly a hand-to-mouth affair. A person obtains eggs on the hands from the soil or the fur of infected dogs or from uninfected dogs that have contaminated their fur by rolling on ground soiled by dog feces. Eggs are killed rapidly by direct sunlight, but they may remain alive for months in moist shady places. Thus, infection may be acquired from water and vegetables. Canine digestive juices are inimical to the oncosphere. Hence, the dog is seldom infected with the cyst.

Pathology and Symptomatology. The pathology in humans depends upon the location of the cyst. The distribution of cysts in humans is approximately as follows: liver, including secondary peritoneal invasion, 66 percent; lung, 22 percent; kidneys, 3 percent; bones, 2 percent; brain, 1 percent; other tissues (muscles, spleen, eye, heart, thyroid), 6 percent.

The unilocular cyst evokes an inflammatory reaction of the surrounding tissues that produces an encapsulating fibrous adventitia. The impairment of the organs by the common unilocular cyst is chiefly due to pressure. Erosion of blood vessels leads to hemorrhage, and torsion of the omentum to vascular constriction. The neighboring tissue cells, depending upon the density of the tissues, undergo atrophy and pressure necrosis as the cyst increases in size.

The symptoms, comparable to those of a slowly growing tumor, depend upon the location of the hydatid cyst. In the abdomen the cysts give rise to increasing discomfort, but symptoms do not appear until the cysts have obtained a considerable size. A remarkable feature is the extent of the involvement of the organs and the long existence of the cyst before symptoms may be detected. Calcified, asymptomatic cysts are found on radiograph or at autopsy—death resulting from other causes.

Hepatic cysts are essentially primary. More than three-fourths of them are found in the right lobe, mostly toward the inferior surface, so that they extend downward into the abdominal cavity. Cysts of the dome of the liver grow slowly, persisting even as long as 30 years before producing marked symptoms. Pressure on bile ducts may cause obstructive jaundice, and on the ureters, urinary problems.

The rupture of a cyst sets free protoscolices, bits of germinal membrane, brood capsules, and daughter cysts, which may reach other tissues through the blood or by direct extension and development into secondary cysts. In this respect, this infection with its metastases is like cancer. Rupture may occur from coughing, muscle strain, blows, aspiration, and operative procedures. After the rupture of a cyst, signs of secondary echinococcosis may not appear for 2 to 8 years. Hepatic cysts usually rupture into the abdominal cavity, but they may also discharge into the pleural cavity or biliary ducts. In the latter instance a characteristic triad of findings results: intermittent jaundice, fever, and eosinophilia. The peribronchial cysts that discharge into a bronchus occasionally may undergo spontaneous cure, but in the majority of cases rupture is incomplete, and a chronic pulmonary abscess results. The patient has a sudden attack of coughing usually accompanied by allergic symptoms, and the sputum contains frothy blood, mucus, hydatid fluid, and bits of membrane. Secondary infection with bacteria may occur. The first evidence of the presence of pulmonary cysts, often symptomless until complications develop, may be of an allergic character. Among the more common early symptoms are slight hemoptysis, coughing, dyspnea, transient thoracic pain, palpitation, tachycardia, and pruritus. In the brain, the cysts may be large and produce symptoms of intracranial pressure and Jacksonian epilepsy. A renal cyst may cause intermittent pain, hematuria, and kidney dysfunction, and in case of rupture, hydatid material may be present in the urine. A splenic cyst may cause a dull pain and bulging of the ribs, while spotty areas of dullness and resonance on percussion may be demonstrated with pelvic cysts. Spinal involvement may result from vertebral cysts.

The mortality rate is higher in secondary and infected cysts than in primary, uncomplicated cysts. When a cyst ruptures, the escape of fluid may give rise to allergic manifestations, usually in the form of an urticarial rash and pruritus. Rupture may be accompanied by an irregular fever, gastrointestinal disturbances, abdominal pain, cyanosis, syncope, and delirium. If considerable hydatid material suddenly enters the bloodstream, serious anaphylactic symptoms or even sudden death may result.

The osseous cyst produces a pseudotuberculous reaction with foreign-body giant cells. In the diaphysis it causes destruction of the trabeculae, necrosis, and spontaneous fracture, with thickening of cortex and distortion of the cancellous tissues. The slow, insidious growth

of osseous cysts renders diagnosis difficult, and they are often in locations where surgical removal is impossible.

Diagnosis. Clinical diagnosis is based upon the presence of a slowly growing cystic (especially hepatic) tumor, history of residence in an endemic area, and close association with dogs. Hydatid cysts require differentiation from malignancies, amebic abscesses, congenital cysts, and tuberculosis. Roentgenologic examinations are useful, especially for pulmonary cysts and calcified cysts in any location (Fig. 10-5). Various types of scanning procedures or ultrasound examination of the liver may detect an uncalcified cyst.

Laboratory diagnosis is made by finding the protoscolices, brood capsules, or daughter cysts in the cyst after surgical removal, or finding hydatid fragments from a ruptured cyst in the sputum or urine. Finding the characteristic hooklets is especially useful in diagnosis. An eosinophilia is suggestive, but many infected persons have a normal number of these cells. Serologic tests, of which there are many, are useful in diagnosis. Indirect hemagglutination (IHA) is one of the most commonly used, but low titers may be nonspecific or cross-reactions. Sera from patients with cysticercosis strongly cross-react with hydatid antigens. A higher frequency of antibodies is found in patients with liver involvement than in those with lung cysts. One antigenic fraction, "band or arc 5," has been found to be the most specific component for serologic tests. With certain tests, such as IHA, antibodies will persist in the serum of patients even after complete surgical removal of cysts. But complement-fixing (CF) and indirect fluorescent antibodies (IFA) disappear within 1 year after successful surgery. The intracutaneous test, first used by Casoni, is of value in human echinococcosis, but it may show as high as 18 percent false positive results in uninfected persons. An immediate negative reaction is good evidence of freedom from the disease, but a positive reaction may persist for years after the removal, or death and calcification, of the cysts.

Treatment. The treatment of the accessible

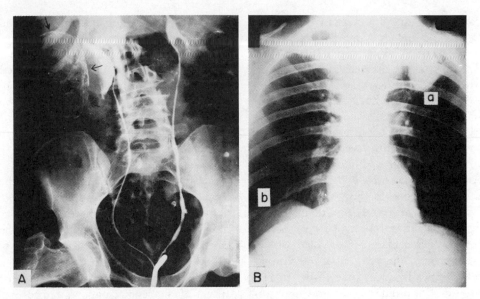

Figure 10-5. A. *Echinococcus* cyst of the kidney, undergoing calcification. B. *Echinococcus* cysts of the lungs: a, intact cyst (shown also in Fig. 10-3); b, spontaneously ruptured cyst.

unilocular hydatid cyst is surgical; the location of the cyst determines the exact surgical procedure. Chemotherapy and roentgen rays are ineffective. Whenever possible the cyst should be enucleated, but its intimate fusion with the surrounding tissues often makes enucleation difficult. Removal of cyst fluid and its replacement by 10 percent formalin to give a final concentration of 2 percent will kill the protoscolices and germinal membrane. It should be withdrawn in 5 minutes. When the cyst is large or infected, or closure is impossible, marsupialization is the operation of choice. Primary cerebral cysts require operative interference. Pulmonary cysts should be removed whenever possible. Extreme caution should be used to prevent the rupture and discharge of the cyst into the tissues. Allergic symptoms should be treated with epinephrine or antihistaminic drugs. Medical treatment with large doses of mebendazole for several months has been reported to reduce cyst size or even cure some cases of hydatid disease. A dose of at least 40 mg per kilogram per day is needed. While mebendazole is not always effective, and it may be associated with severe untoward reactions at times, use of the drug may be considered in situations where surgery is not possible.

Prevention. Preventive measures should be directed toward reducing infection with the adult parasite in dogs and with the larval worm in sheep and hogs. In endemic areas dogs should be barred from slaughterhouses and should not be fed uncooked offal; the refuse from slaughtered animals should be sterilized; and stray dogs should be destroyed. All dogs in endemic areas should be given taeniafuges once or twice a year. In Iceland this proved most effective in eliminating the infection from the country. Changes in animal husbandry, such as the slaughter of most animals at a much earlier age, will keep cyst growth to a minimum and reduce the inoculum that becomes available to dogs. The public should be informed regarding the method of transmission, warned concerning the danger of intimate contact with dogs, and instructed in personal cleanliness.

Alveolar Hydatid Cyst of Echinococcus multilocularis

The alveolar cyst is the larval stage of *E. multilocularis*. The adult tapeworm is found in foxes and cats, and the cysts in their prey, mice and voles. Dogs represent a potential source of infection for humanity if they feed on rodents. Both adult and larval stages differ from those of *E. granulosus.*

This cyst is found in humans, and occasionally in cattle, in the Bavarian-Tyrolean region, Jura, Russia, Siberia, and Alaska. The adult worm has recently been reported from foxes in North Dakota, Minnesota, Montana, and Iowa, with the cyst in rodents in these areas. The cyst, due to the very thin, laminated membrane, is not sharply defined from the surrounding tissues. It is a porous, spongy mass of small irregular cavities filled with a jellylike matrix. The cavities are separated from each other by connective tissue. In humans the cyst is usually sterile and may undergo central necrosis and even calcification while continuing growth at the periphery. Its growth is neoplastic, and metastases occur by direct extension or through the blood or lymph. It is found most frequently in the liver. Humans may be infected by eating raw plants contaminated with the feces of infected foxes, cats, or dogs, thereby ingesting eggs that develop into cysts. In Alaska, the infection is acquired from the feces of sled dogs. Humanity is apparently not a favorable host, for the cysts usually do not complete normal development and lack protoscolices.

Operation offers the only hope for treatment, but complete extirpation of the cyst tissue is difficult. Recent experience with *E. multilocularis* in Alaska using mebendazole at a dosage of up to 3 grams daily has been favorable. The drug seems more effective against this species than against *E. granulosus.*

Cysticercus cellulosae

Humanity may be both the definitive and the intermediate host of *T. solium* and thus harbor either the adult worm or the cyst. The larval stage of *T. solium* is called *Cysticercus cellulosae,* and the infection in humans is known as cysticercosis cellulosae.

Morphology. The mature cysticercus (see Figure 8-2D) is an oval, translucent cyst with an opaque invaginated scolex bearing four suckers and a circlet of hooks. It is usually enclosed in a tough host-tissue adventitious capsule, but in the vitreous humor of the eye and in the pia mater or ventricles of the brain it may be unencapsulated. It attains its full size in about 10 weeks. The cysts are oval and about 5 mm in diameter, but in the brain they may grow to a large size: several centimeters in diameter.

Life Cycle. See Figure 10-6

Epidemiology. Humans may acquire the cyst from the eggs in three ways: (1) the ingestion of food or water contaminated by infected human feces, (2) oral transmission by the unclean hands of carriers of the adult worm, and (3) internal autoinfection by the regurgitation of eggs into the stomach by reverse peristalsis. About 25 percent of patients harboring cysts give a history of having harbored the adult worm at some time. Human cysticercosis is probably more common than is indicated by its low reported incidence, since many infections escape detection. It is a disease of adult life and is more prevalent in males than in females. It is associated with insanitary porcine surroundings and poor personal hygiene.

Pathology and Symptomatology. The cysticerci, often multiple and even numbering into the thousands, may develop in any tissue or organ of the human body. The most common sites are striated muscles and the brain, but they also occur in the subcutaneous tissues, eye, heart, lung, and peritoneum. The growing cyst produces a foreign-body inflammatory reaction that results in the production of a fibrous capsule. On the death of the larva, which may survive up to 5 years, there is an increase of the cystic fluid and a pronounced tissue response to the parasitic material. The degenerating parasite usually undergoes calcification. The pathology depends upon the tissue invaded and the number of cysticerci. Invasion of the brain and eye causes serious damage.

During the stage of invasion there may be no prodromal symptoms or only slight muscular pain and a mild fever. The cysticerci are well tolerated in the muscles and subcutaneous tissues, and even in heavy infections there

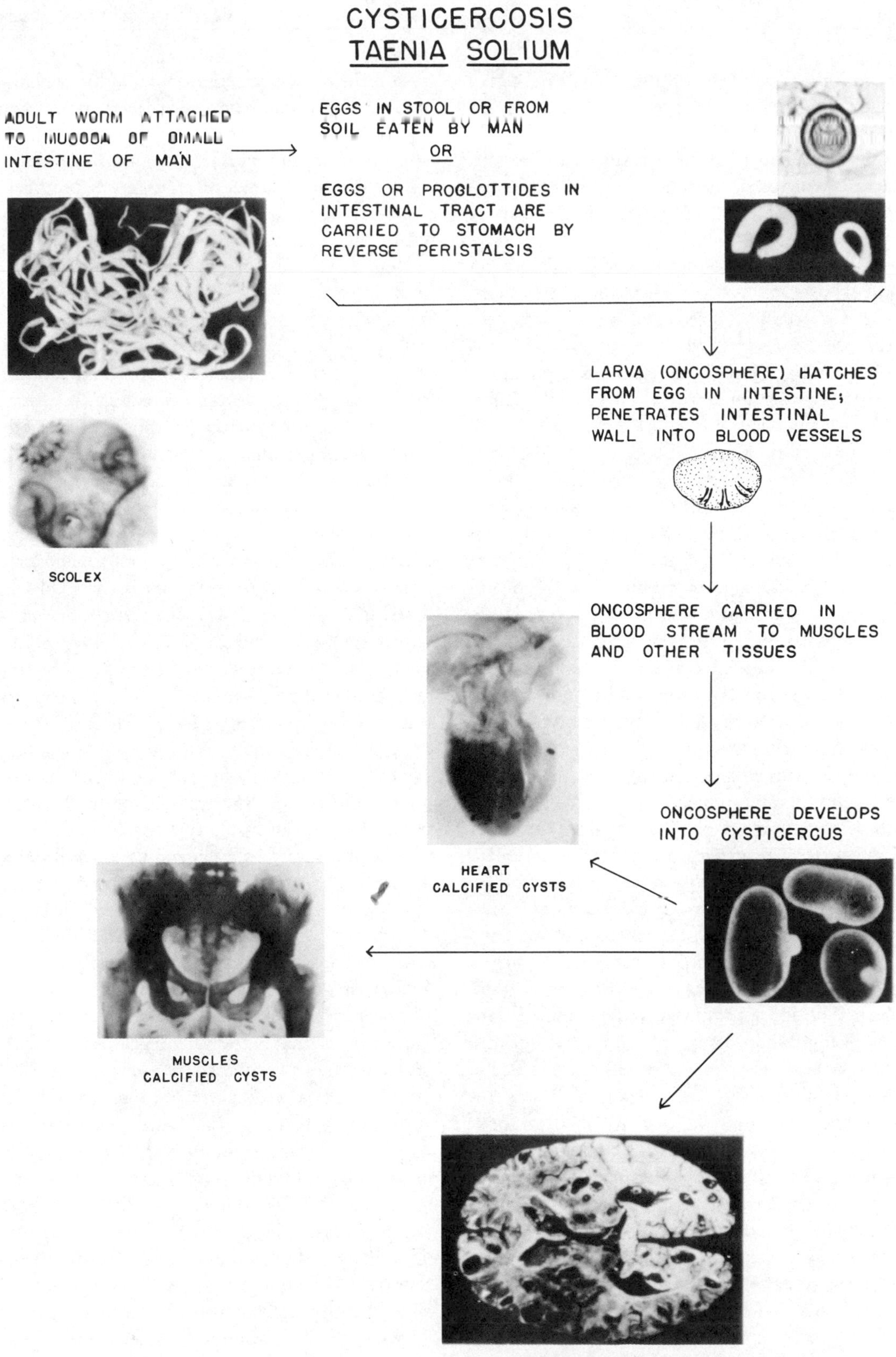

CYSTICERCOSIS
TAENIA SOLIUM

ADULT WORM ATTACHED
TO MUCOSA OF SMALL
INTESTINE OF MAN

EGGS IN STOOL OR FROM
SOIL EATEN BY MAN

OR

EGGS OR PROGLOTTIDES IN
INTESTINAL TRACT ARE
CARRIED TO STOMACH BY
REVERSE PERISTALSIS

LARVA (ONCOSPHERE) HATCHES
FROM EGG IN INTESTINE;
PENETRATES INTESTINAL
WALL INTO BLOOD VESSELS

SCOLEX

ONCOSPHERE CARRIED IN
BLOOD STREAM TO MUSCLES
AND OTHER TISSUES

ONCOSPHERE DEVELOPS
INTO CYSTICERCUS

HEART
CALCIFIED CYSTS

MUSCLES
CALCIFIED CYSTS

CYSTS IN BRAIN

Figure 10-6. Cysticercosis; *Taenia solium.*

199

may be no symptoms. Muscular pains, particularly in the back of the neck, weakness, fatigue, cramps, and loss of weight may be present. In the muscles there is degeneration and atrophy in the immediate vicinity of the parasite. Eosinophilia of varying degrees is usually present.

The serious manifestations of the disease occur in cerebral cysticercosis, usually associated with an unrecognized general cysticercosis. Cysticerci may be present in the cerebral cortex, meninges, ventricles, and, less often, in the cerebral substance. They are usually found near the surface of the brain over the frontal and parietal lobes and along the middle cerebral arteries; they are found occasionally in the occipital region and the cerebellum. Cerebral edema and pressure are produced, but there is a relative tolerance while the parasite is alive. Encapsulation results from the proliferation of neuroglia and cellular granulation tissue with inflammatory vascular changes. The neuroglia and nerve cells show pressure or toxic changes. Eventually the parasite may be absorbed and replaced by fibrous tissue that may lead to the late manifestations of epilepsy. Calcification of the parasite occurs.

Definite symptoms often do not occur for 5 to 8 years, or even for 20 years, until the death of the parasite evokes an inflammatory reaction. Symptoms may be caused earlier by pressure of the cysts and obstruction of cerebrospinal fluid. The patient, however, may show symptoms within a year if the cysticerci are located in the areas governing motor function. The most prominent late manifestations are irregularly recurrent unilateral spasms, which later may become bilateral. Early, there is no loss of consciousness, but later this may occur. These attacks range from petit mal, with or without loss of consciousness, to various stages of major epilepsy with aura. Periods of unconsciousness without convulsions may be the only manifestations. Cysticerci in various parts of the brain produce a variety of focal motor, sensory, and mental symptoms. There may be symptoms of brain tumor, meningitis, encephalitis, hydrocephalus, and disseminated sclerosis. Transitory paresis, failing vision, diplopia, sudden headaches, vomiting, and disordered mentality may be leading symptoms. The most obvious symptoms are psychic, e.g., confusion, irritability, insomnia, anxiety, changed personality, lack of concentration, hallucinations, and occasionally mental deterioration. Involvement of the spinal cord may produce hyperesthesia and altered reflexes. Increased intracranial pressure may cause papilledema and optic atrophy. A branching, unencapsulated, racemose type of larva in the subarachnoid spaces and choroid plexus may give rise to a syndrome of communicating hydrocephalus. The spinal fluid presents no consistent characteristic changes. There may be increased pressure, increased cells (mostly lymphocytes and large mononuclears), and a decrease in glucose. About 10 percent of the patients with cerebral cysticercosis show an eosinophilia of the blood.

In the eye (Fig. 10-7) the cysticercus, usually single, is subretinal or in the vitreous humor. The scolex and neck of the grayish, unencapsulated cysticercus in the vitreous is continually changing shape. Often damage other than discomfort is minimal, but sometimes the retina may be detached, the vitreous fluid clouded, the parasite surrounded by an inflammatory exudate, and the iris inflamed. The patient may experience intraorbital pain, flashes of light, grotesque shapes in the visual field, and blurring and loss of vision. Death of the parasite may lead to iridocyclitis. This parasite may be confused with retinoblastoma, which does not have movement.

Diagnosis. Clinical diagnosis of cerebral cysticercosis is made from epileptiform convulsions or other nervous manifestations in a person who has resided in an endemic area, especially if there has been a history of subcutaneous nodules. Idiopathic epilepsy usually begins in childhood; verminous epilepsy begins later in life. Differential diagnosis from other neurologic diseases is necessary. Although not always present, the finding of eosinophils in the spinal fluid can be a helpful clue. Biopsy of palpable subcutaneous cysts gives a definite diagnosis. Roentgen-ray examination of the infected muscles or brain

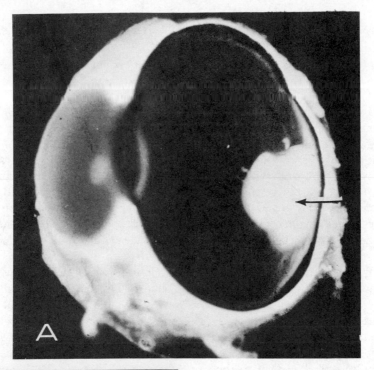

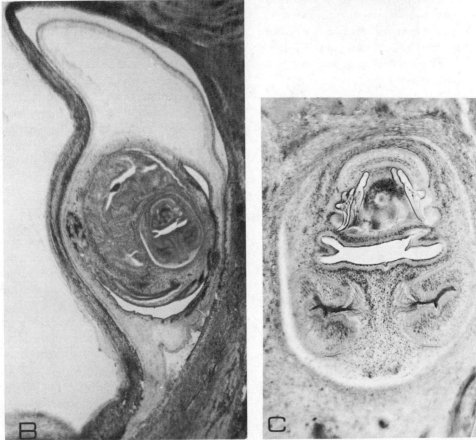

Figure 10-7. *Taenia solium* cyst in eye. A. Gross. B. Cyst embedded in retina. C. Section of scolex showing suckers and hooks. (Courtesy of Dr. J. A. C. Wadsworth, Institute of Ophthalmology, N.Y.)

may be diagnostic if the cysts have calcified. Computed axial tomography (CAT) scans are especially helpful in localizing cysticerci in the brain. In the eyes the larva may be detected with the ophthalmoscope. When tested with cysticercal antigens, hemagglutination, CF, and immunodiffusion tests are often positive with serum, and less commonly with the spinal fluid of proven cases with cerebral cysticercosis. But cross-reactions are also encountered with other helminthic infections.

Treatment. Treatment is surgical. The parasite in the eye should be removed as soon as possible. Removal of a solitary or even several cysticerci from the brain gives complete or partial recovery, but surgery is impossible when numerous cysts are present. Recent trials with praziquantel, 50 mg per kilogram daily for two weeks, plus drugs to control cerebral edema, indicate that medical treatment of cerebral cysticercosis may be possible.

Prevention. Prevention requires prompt treatment for the removal of the adult worms from patients. Personal hygiene and environmental sanitation are important.

SPARGANOSIS

The plerocercoid larvae of several species of diphyllobothriid tapeworms have been found in humans. They are known as spargana, and the disease as sparganosis. The adult worms are either found in the lower mammals or are unknown.

Nonbranching Spargana

The spargana of several species of *Spirometra* (*Diphyllobothrium*) have been described in humans.

Life Cycle. The adult worm *S. mansonoides* resembles *D. latum* but is smaller. The definitive hosts are dogs, cats, and wild carnivora. The primary intermediate hosts are species of *Cyclops,* and the secondary intermediate hosts include various small rodents, snakes, and frogs. The life cycle follows the same pattern as that of *D. latum.*

Epidemiology. This parasite is found in east and southeast Asia, Japan, Indochina, and to a lesser extent in Africa, Europe, Australia, and North and South America.

Humans may acquire sparganosis by (1) the ingestion of infected *Cyclops,* containing the procercoid, in drinking water, (2) by consuming frogs, snakes, or rodents harboring the plerocercoid, (3) by the penetration of cutaneous tissues, especially the orbit by plerocercoids from poultices made of the infected flesh of frogs or snakes. The spargana are white, up to several centimeters in length, a few millimeters wide, and exhibit considerable muscular activity.

Pathogenicity. In humans the larvae may be found in any part of the body, especially in and about the eyes, in the subcutaneous and muscular tissues of the thorax, abdomen, and thighs, in the inguinal region, and in the thoracic viscera. The spargana may migrate through the tissues. The elongating and contracting larvae within a slimy matrix cause an inflammatory and painful edema of the surrounding tissues. Degenerated larvae cause intense local inflammation and necrosis but no fibrous tissue formation. Infected persons may show local indurations, periodic giant urticaria, edema, and erythema accompanied by chills, fever, and high eosinophilia. Ocular infection, of relatively frequent occurrence in southeastern Asia, produces a painful edematous conjunctivitis with lacrimation and ptosis.

Prognosis depends upon the location of the parasite and its successful removal.

Diagnosis. The diagnosis of sparganosis is made by finding the larvae in the lesions, but the identification of species requires lengthy feeding experiments to experimental animals.

Treatment. Surgical removal of the larval plerocercoid.

Prevention. In endemic areas drinking water should be boiled or filtered and the flesh of possible intermediate hosts thoroughly cooked. The native practice of applying the flesh of frogs and other vertebrates to inflamed mucocutaneous areas should be discouraged.

Branching Spargana

A budding larval tapeworm, designated as *S. proliferum,* has been reported several times in Japan and once in the United States. The adult worm and its life cycle are unknown. The larva is characterized by irregular, lateral, supernumerary processes that may bud off as new spargana in the tissues. Diagnosis is made by finding the larvae in the chylous nodular lesions.

GENUS *MULTICEPS*

The adult tapeworm of the genus *Multiceps* is found in the intestines of dogs and wild canines. The larval worm, which is known as a coenurus (see Figure 8-2E), develops in the tissues of herbivorous or omnivorous animals. The infection is known as coenurosis, and the condition is usually serious. The identification of the particular species of *Multiceps* is extremely difficult.

Multiceps multiceps. *M. multiceps,* a common adult parasite of dogs, has a cosmopolitan distribution in sheep-raising countries. It is 40 to 60 cm in length and has a pyriform scolex with a double crown of 22 to 32 large and small hooks. The intermediate hosts are sheep and goats and, less frequently, other herbivora. The coenuri develop chiefly in the central nervous system, causing fatal "blind staggers" in sheep, although other tissues may be invaded. At least 24 cerebral infections have been reported in humans, who become infected by ingesting the tapeworm egg from the dog's stool. The larval worm is usually single, although as many as 20 have been obtained from an infant. The globular-to-sausage-shaped cysts, which range in size up to 20 mm or more, contain multiple small invaginated scolices that arise from the germinal wall. The symptoms, requiring several years to develop, depend upon the exact location of the coenurus. Usually there are symptoms of increased intracranial pressure, including loss of consciousness, convulsions, temporary anesthesia, paresis, occasional diplopia, staggering gait,

and a positive Romberg. The cellular content and protein of the spinal fluid are increased. Diagnosis can only be made by the surgical recovery of the larva. In endemic areas prevention requires the protection of food and hands from the feces of dogs.

Multiceps serialis. *M. serialis* as an adult inhabits the intestines of dogs and wild CANIDAE. The coenuri develop in the intermuscular connective tissue of rodents. Human infections have been reported.

Multiceps glomeratus. Only the larval form of *M. glomeratus* in African rodents is known. It has been reported in African natives.

REFERENCES

Cherubin: Nonspecific reactions to Casoni antigen. Am J Trop Med Hyg 18: 387–390, 1969.

Flisser, et al: Human cysticercosis: antigens, antibodies and non-responders. Clin. and Exp Immunol 39: 27–37, 1980.

Hermos, et al: Fatal human cerebral coenurosis. JAMA 213: 1461–1464, 1970.

Mueller, et al: Human sparganosis in the United States. J Parasitol 49: 294–296, 1963.

Schantz, et al: Echinococcosis in Arizona and New Mexico. Survey of hospital records, 1969–1974. Am J Trop Med Hyg 25: 312–317, 1976.

Schantz, et al: Serologic cross-reactions with sera from patients with echinococcosis and cysticercosis. Am J Trop Med Hyg 29: 609–612, 1980.

Shanley and Jordan: Clinical aspects of CNS cysticercosis. Arch Intern Med 140: 1309–1313, 1980.

Smyth: Strain differences in *E. granulosis,* with special reference to the status of equine hydatidosis in the United Kingdom. Trans R Soc Trop Med Hyg 71: 93–100, 1977.

Wilson and Rausch: Alveolar hydatid disease. A review of clinical features of 33 indigenous cases of *E. multilocularis* infection in Alaskan eskimos. Am J Trop Med Hyg 29: 1340–1355, 1980.

TREMATODA OR FLUKES

11
Trematoda

The flukes are parasitic worms of the class TREMATODA of the phylum PLATYHELMINTHES. Their parasitic existence has brought about a specialized development of the organs of reproduction and attachment, and a corresponding reduction in the organs of locomotion and digestion. The structure and life cycle vary with the type of parasitic existence, which ranges from ectoparasitism on aquatic hosts to extreme endoparasitism in the vascular system of vertebrates.

The species parasitic in humans belong to the DIGENEA, in which sexual reproduction in the adult is followed by asexual multiplication in the larval stages in snails.

Morphology. Adult digenetic trematodes are usually flat, elongated, leaf-shaped worms, but they may be ovoid, conical, or cylindrical, depending upon the state of contraction. They vary in size from less than 1 mm to several centimeters. The worm is enveloped by a noncellular tegument, which may be partially or completely covered with spines, tubercles, or ridges. The tegument is shown by electron microscopic studies to be syncytial and without nuclei, to contain many vacuoles, and many small mitochondria, and to be connected by protoplasmic tubes with an inner layer of cells. There are no microtriches or pore canals as are found in the tegument of cestodes. The tegument plays an important role in the absorption of carbohydrates. It may also serve for secretion of excess metabolites and mucus (Fig. 11-1). The worms are attached to the host by cup-shaped muscular suckers, sometimes bearing spines or hooklets. An oral sucker is situated at the anterior end of the worm, and in most species a larger, blind ventral sucker, or acetabulum, is located on the ventral surface posterior to the oral sucker. An outer circular, middle oblique, and inner longitudinal layer of muscles lie beneath the tegument, while bands of muscles traverse the body dorsoventrally. These muscles serve to alter the shape of the worm. There is no body cavity. The intervening space between the various organs is filled with fluid and a network of connective tissue cells and fibers.

A muscular, globular pharynx (Fig. 11-2) extends from the mouth in the oral sucker to a

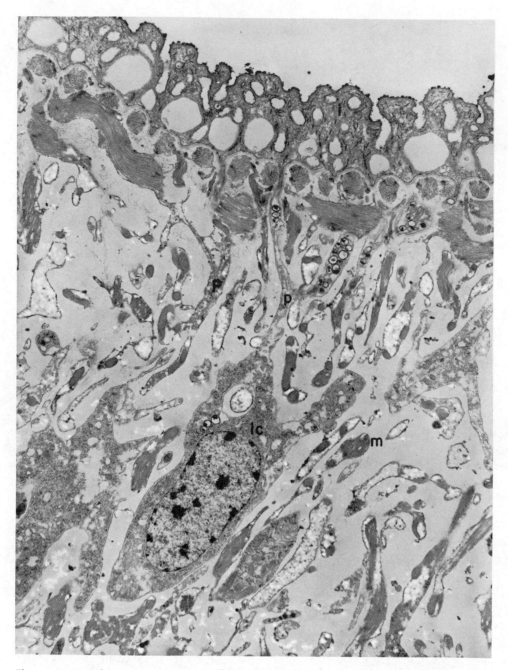

Figure 11-1. *Schistosoma mansoni.* Electron micrograph of adult male dorsal surface. P, myocytic internuncial process; p, integumental internuncial process; ic, integumental cytons; m, medullary parenchyma. (From Smith, Reynolds, von Lichtenberg: Am J Trop Med Hyg, 1969.)

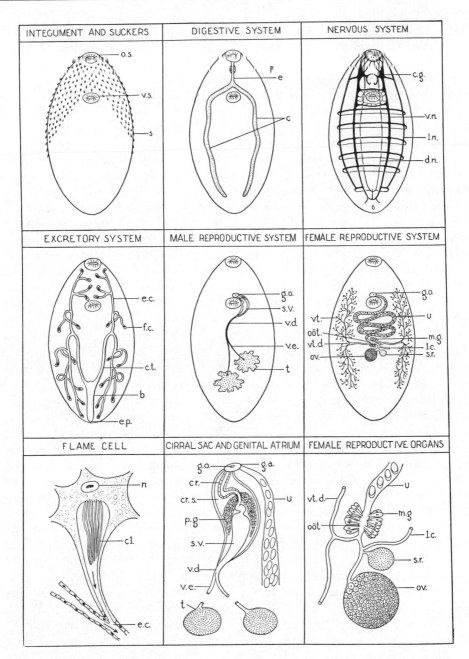

Figure 11-2. Schematic representation of morphology of a typical trematode.
b, bladder; c, ceca; c.g., cephalic ganglia; cl., cilia; cr., cirrus; cr.s., cirral sac; c.t.,
collecting tube; d.n., dorsal nerve trunk; e, esophagus; e.c., excretory capillary; e.p.,
excretory pore; f.c., flame cell; g.a., genital atrium; g.o., genital opening; l.c., Laurer's canal;
l.n., lateral nerve trunk; m.g., Mehlis' gland; n, nucleus; oöt, ootype; o.s., oral sucker; ov.,
ovary; p, pharynx; p.g., prostate gland; s, spines; s.r., seminal receptacle; s.v., seminal
vesicle; t, testis; u, uterus; v.d., vas deferens; v.e., vas efferens; v.n., ventral nerve trunk; v.s.,
ventral sucker; vt., vitellaria; vt.d., vitelline duct.

short narrow esophagus, both receiving the secretions of unicellular salivary glands. Below the esophagus the intestine bifurcates into two straight or branching ceca of variable length that usually end blindly. A system of lymph channels extend along the intestinal ceca with numerous branching canals to the various internal organs. The flow of lymph is maintained by bodily contractions.

The excretory system (Fig. 11-2) includes diffusely scattered flame cells, capillaries, collecting tubes, bladder, and an excretory pore. The terminal flame cell is a hollow cell with a tuft of cilia streaming inward toward the capillary end. Through the activity of these cilia the excreted waste products pass into the tubular excretory system and are eventually discharged from the bladder through a pore on the ventral surface at the posterior end of the worm.

The primitive nervous system (Fig. 11-2) includes two lateral ganglia in the region of the pharynx connected by dorsal commissures. From each ganglion arise anterior and posterior longitudinal nerve trunks connected by numerous commissures.

Except for the unisexual blood flukes, the parasitic trematodes of humans are hermaphroditic (Fig. 11-2). The conspicuous testes, usually two except in the schistosomes, are located most frequently in the posterior half of the body and may be globular, lobate, tubular, or dendritic, depending upon the species. The vasa efferentia, arising from the testes, unite in the vas deferens, which passes anteriorly into the cirral sac, opening into the common genital atrium.

The female reproductive organs include a single ovary, an oviduct, a seminal receptacle, vitelline glands and ducts, ootype, Mehlis' gland, and, in many species, Laurer's canal. The rounded, lobed, or dendritic ovary is usually smaller than the testes. A short oviduct leads from the ovary to the ootype, receiving Laurer's canal, the vitelline duct, and a duct from the seminal receptacle. The function of Laurer's canal, which opens on the dorsal surface in some species, is not known. The seminal receptacle is a thin-walled saccular

outpocketing of the oviduct for storing spermatozoa. The grapelike vitellaria are usually located in the midlateral part of the body, and their tubules converge to form the common vitelline duct. The ootype is a muscular dilation of the oviduct surrounded by Mehlis' gland, of uncertain function. The uterus extends forward from the ootype as a long tortuous tube, often packed with eggs, and terminates in the common genital atrium, which opens to the exterior via the genital pore.

The undeveloped egg (Fig. 11-3A) consists of the fertilized ovum, vitelline cells, vitelline membrane, and a shell. Its shape, appearance, and size are reasonably constant and diagnostic for each species. The eggshells of most species of digenetic trematodes have a caplike polar operculum, but the *Schistosoma* eggs are nonoperculated.

The adult fluke moves by contraction, elongation, and flexion. It maintains its position in the host by its suckers. The life span varies with the species, but usually covers several years—up to 30 in the schistosomes.

Nutrition is obtained from the tissues, secretion, or intestinal contents of the host, depending upon the habitat and species of the parasite. Insoluble material is regurgitated through the oral opening, while soluble material is distributed throughout the body by the lymph. Waste products are eliminated through the flame cells of the excretory system. Respiration is largely anaerobic, glycogen being split into carbon dioxide and fatty acid. The larval forms, however, require oxygen.

Self-fertilization is the common method of fecundation for the hermaphroditic species. The cirrus is the copulatory organ, and the spermatozoa traverse the uterus and are stored in the seminal receptacle. The ova are fertilized as they pass down the oviduct; yolk and shell material are added from the vitellaria. The assembled eggs in the distended uterus escape to the exterior through the common genital atrium and pore.

Life Cycle. In the definitive host, usually a vertebrate, multiplication takes place sexually with the production of eggs, and in the intermediate molluscan host by asexual genera-

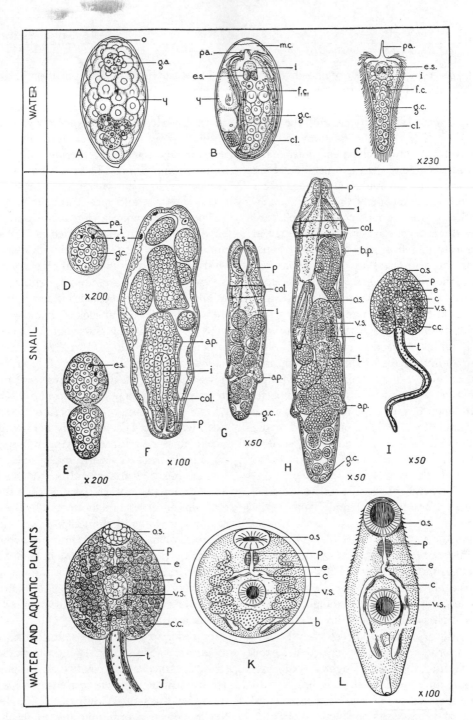

Figure 11-3. Larval forms of *Fasciola hepatica*. A. Immature egg. B. Miracidium in eggshell. C. Miracidium ready to enter snail. D. A very young sporocyst, immediately after completion of metamorphosis. E. Young sporocyst undergoing transverse fission. F. Adult sporocyst with rediae. G. Immature redia. H. Redia with developing cercariae and one daughter redia. I. Cercaria. J. Body of cercaria. K. Encysted metacercaria. L. Excysted metacercaria.

ap., appendages; b, excretory bladder; b.p., birth pore; c, ceca; c.c., cystogenous cells; cl., cilia; col., collar; e, esophagus; e.s., eye spots; f.c., flame cells; g.a., germinal area; g.c., germinal cells; i, digestive tract; m.c., mucoid cap; o, operculum; o.s., oral sucker; p, pharynx; pa., papilla; t, tail; v.s., ventral sucker; y, yolk. (A-J redrawn from Thomas, 1883. K adapted from Hegner, Root, Augustine, Huff: Parasitology, 1938. Courtesy of D. Appleton-Century Company. L redrawn from Leuckart, 1882.)

tions. In the typical life history of a digenetic trematode, the eggs escape from the definitive host via the intestinal, genitourinary, or pulmonary tracts. When discharged, the eggs may contain fully developed larvae or may require subsequent development outside the body before hatching. At the time of hatching in fresh water, the operculum pops open like a lid to permit the escape of the larval *miracidium,* whereas the nonoperculated shells are split by the energetic movement of the larva.

After escaping from the shell, the ciliated pyriform miracidium (Fig. 11-3) swims actively in the water. It has anterior secretory glands that discharge enzymes for penetrating the tissues of the snail, a paired excretory system with flame cells, a nervous system with ganglia, and a collection of germinal cells. The miracidium is attracted to an appropriate species of snail by a chemotactic stimulus, probably from the mucus or tissue juices of the snail. It penetrates the exposed portions within a few minutes by a boring motion aided by the glandular secretions, and the cilia are shed as the organism enters the snail. Unless the miracidium finds the snail within a few hours, it perishes. In some species, the unhatched eggs are ingested by the snail and hatch in its intestine.

Within the tissues of the snail the miracidium undergoes metamorphosis into an irregular saclike *sporocyst* (Fig. 11-3D–F), which serves as a brood sac for the development and production of a generation of daughter sporocysts, or *rediae,* which escape through the ruptured wall of the mother sporocyst. The mother sporocyst is usually located near the point of entry, but the daughter sporocysts and rediae migrate along the lymph spaces to the hepatic glands of the snail. The redia (Fig. 11-3G and H) is equipped with a pharynx and primitive gut, an excretory system with flame cells and collecting tubules, and germinal cells. Within the rediae and daughter sporocysts, cercariae develop and escape into the tissues of the snail and ultimately pass through the integument of the snail into the water. In certain species the rediae may produce an additional intervening generation of daughter rediae.

The mechanism of multiplication in the larval stages of digenetic trematodes involves the production of large numbers of germinal cells and is considered to be a polyembryony of the fertilized ovum. So extensive is the multiplication that thousands of cercariae may develop from one miracidium. The period of intramolluscan development varies with the temperature, snail host, and species of trematode.

The typical cercaria (Fig. 11-3I and J) has an elliptical body, an elongated tail for swimming, oral and ventral suckers, various spines or stylets, digestive tract, rudimentary reproductive system, an excretory system, and unicellular cephalic glands with ducts opening in the vicinity of the oral sucker. The lytic secretions of the cephalic glands enable the cercaria to penetrate the skin of definitive hosts *(Schistosoma)* or enter the tissues of intermediate hosts. Special cystogenous glands are present in species that encyst in secondary animal hosts or on plants. The liberated cercariae swim with their tails, the body being anterior except in those with forked appendages. The aquatic habits vary with the species, some frequenting the surface and others the lower levels. They may attach themselves to the surface film or settle to the bottom. The life of the cercaria in water is limited unless it finds a suitable plant or animal host on which to encyst or penetrates the skin of a definitive host. In the encysted cercaria, known as the *metacercaria,* the tail and cystogenous and lytic glands of the cercaria have disappeared (Fig. 11-3K and L).

In order to invade the definitive host, the metacercariae in secondary intermediate hosts (fish, crustacea, and snails) or on aquatic plants must be ingested, or the cercariae must penetrate the skin. Within the definitive host the adolescent worm migrates to its normal habitat and grows to maturity.

Snails, mostly fresh-water species, act as primary intermediate hosts for the parasitic trematodes of humans. Only certain species serve as hosts, and their identification and control play an important role in the prevention of human infection. Scarcely 70 of the 100,000 or more species of snails are known intermediate hosts of helminths of humans.

The various species and even strains of trematodes have become adapted to a single or, at most, a few species of snails. They either fail to penetrate or else do not complete their larval development in other species. Adaptation to a new host species may occur in nature, but it usually requires a concentration of infected persons and heavy deposits of eggs. Thus, while there is a potential danger, there is little chance of spreading pathogenic trematodes in new areas uninhabited by suitable snail hosts. Effective control measures for a particular species of snails, chiefly drainage and molluscacides, depend upon a knowledge of its ecology.

The designation of a species of snail as an intermediate host requires carefully controlled experimental evidence, which is difficult to obtain; it should not be based on its mere presence in a locality where the trematode is endemic. The slight differences between species, and even genera, and the great variation within species render classification confusing and subject to constant revision.

Trematodes that infect humans may also infect lower mammals and birds. In some instances, although humans may be the chief source of infection, the parasite may be of only minor importance because of limitations by climate, presence of suitable intermediate hosts, and the eating habits of the inhabitants. In other instances, humans represent an incidental host, and lower mammals are the principal hosts.

Pathology. The lesions produced by flukes depend upon their location in the host, their numbers, and the effect of their products upon the tissue in which they reside. Worms such as *Fasciolopsis* and *Metagonimus,* which inhabit the gastrointestinal tract, cause less damage than those that invade the tissues. The liver flukes that live in the biliary passages irritate the epithelium of the ducts. Adenomatous proliferation and other local changes in extremely heavy infections can result in partial biliary tract obstruction. Cystic lesions around lung flukes and their eggs coalesce into multiple pulmonary cavities. Severe pathologic changes are also associated with the eggs of schistosomes. In this case, the adult worms live in small venules of the bowel or genitourinary tract, but eggs produced by the female worm are either trapped locally or embolize to the liver, the lungs, or other tissues by shunting of the circulation. The fact that some flukes persist in the host for years is an important factor in their ability to produce tissue damage. In addition, trematodes like *Paragonimus* or the schistosomes may migrate or be shunted to aberrant sites to produce lesions in unexpected areas: the central nervous system, the skin, or any organ.

Although we cannot be sure it applies to all trematode infections, disease manifestations of schistosomiasis are largely due to immunopathology. Circulating antigen-antibody complexes are present and in large amounts in early human schistosomiasis. Developing and adult worms acquire a coating of host components over their tegument to escape immunologic attack, but they are surrounded by intense inflammatory reactions when they die. The prominent granuloma formation that is so characteristic around trematode eggs in tissue is primarily a cell-mediated reaction. But a variety of immunologic events are involved in the host response to egg antigens, which may contribute to the pathology. For example, the periportal fibrosis of the liver in severe chronic schistosomiasis is believed by some to involve some additional stimulus to fibrosis, and not simply a coalescence of granulomas around eggs. There is increasing evidence of glomerulonephritis due to immune complexes in some patients with hepatosplenic schistosomiasis. Chronic schistosomiasis of the urinary tract often leads to varying degrees of obstructive uropathy, including hydronephrosis, from the inflammatory response to eggs. Some features of the tissue response to trematodes or their products predispose to malignant change. This seems well established for squamous cancer of the bladder in urinary schistosomiasis and the relationship may also exist with biliary tract cancer and liver flukes.

Resistance and Immunity. Although our focus in thinking of resistance and immunity to trematodes is the definitive vertebrate host, and more specifically the human host, it should be noted that a high degree of host specificity is required for the snails that serve as intermediate hosts for these parasites. In general, a wide variety of animals are capable of becoming infected with liver, lung, and blood flukes. The Taiwan strain *S. japonicum* is an important exception since it matures in animals but not in humans. Yet there seems to be less specificity for definitive hosts among trematodes and fewer examples of innate resistance than with cestodes and nematodes.

Most of our information on immunity to trematode infections is based upon schistosomiasis. But extrapolation of results from experimental hosts to the situation in humans may not be warranted. For example, the rat and rhesus monkey exhibit spontaneous self-cure of *S. mansoni* infections and a high degree of resistance to reinfection. In the monkey, however, spontaneous cure requires a heavy infection; when initiated with small numbers of cercariae, infections run a chronic course.

Yet a picture of immune response is beginning to emerge from various studies that can be related to human schistosomiasis. The infected individual demonstrates a number of immunologic responses to the parasite, both humoral and cell-mediated. Some of these, including skin-test reactivity, are used in immunodiagnosis of infection. An important functional role for the eosinophil has recently been established. Schistosomula can be damaged and killed in vitro by an antibody-dependent, cell-mediated reaction with eosinophils. It is now clear that a general pattern of cell-mediated immune response to specific schistosome antigens takes place in infected patients. During the early stages, blastogenic activity is high, but after a year or two it begins to decline, and in the chronic phase lymphocytes no longer respond to the antigen. This tolerance to parasite antigens is due to suppressor activity of both cells and serum antibody.

Epidemiologic observations suggest that partial functional immunity to schistosomiasis does exist in humans. In endemic areas quantitative egg counts in a population, reflecting intensity of infection or numbers of worms, generally peak at around 10 years of age and tend to decrease thereafter. While many possible explanations can account for this, including decreased exposure to infection, the pattern is consistent enough in variable epidemiologic settings to suggest progressive resistance to infection. Passive transfer of immunity to *S. mansoni* in humans with immune globulin has been tried and was unsuccessful. In experimental animals, irradiated cercariae of schistosomes have been able to induce variable degrees of protection against subsequent challenge. Such irradiated vaccines appear promising for the control of bovine schistosomiasis.

The issue of immunity to trematodes can also be approached from the point of view of the life cycle in the definitive host. First, consideration of how the parasite gains entrance to the body and its earliest development may actually be the most vulnerable point for immunologic intervention. In the case of the schistosomes, this would be the stage of cercarial penetration and the schistosomula as it migrates through tissues. For many other trematodes the infective form is a metacercaria that is ingested and either migrates into the tissues or biliary passages or stays in the bowel. Probably only those flukes that penetrate tissue would be exposed to an effective immune response. The next phase of worm development to maturity is either in the gut, tissues, or blood vessels. In the case of schistosomes, acquisition of host antigenic determinants serves as a camouflage so the host fails to recognize the parasite as foreign. Whether a similar mechanism operates for other trematodes is not known. The final phase against which potential immunologic attack could be directed is the adult worm in its ultimate place of residence. Since schistosomes and liver and lung flukes may remain viable for 10 to 30 years or more, the adult phase of the parasite does not seem to be particularly vulnerable.

12

Intestinal, Hepatic, and Pulmonary Flukes of Human Beings

INTESTINAL FLUKES

Fasciolopsis buski

Disease. Fasciolopsiasis.

Life Cycle. Humans, hogs, and occasionally dogs are the natural definitive hosts of *F. buski*. The adult fluke (Fig. 12-1), the largest parasitic trematode of humans, is a thick, fleshy, ovate, flesh-colored worm, 2.0 to 7.5 by 0.8 to 2.0 cm. Normally, the cuticle is covered with transverse rows of small spines—these are often destroyed by the intestinal juices. The oral sucker is about one-fourth the size of the nearby ventral sucker. The intestinal tract includes a short prepharynx, a bulbous pharynx, a short esophagus, and a pair of unbranched ceca with two characteristic lateral indentations.

The two dendritic testes lie in tandem formation in the posterior half of the worm. The single branched ovary lies in the middle of the body to the right of the midline. The vitellaria lateral to the ceca extend from the ventral sucker to the posterior end of the body. From the ootype the uterus follows a convoluted course to open into the common genital atrium at the anterior border of the ventral sucker. The yellowish ellipsoidal egg, 130 to 140 by 80 to 85 μ, has a clear, thin shell with a small operculum at one end; it is undeveloped when passed in the feces (Fig. 12-2).

The fluke inhabits the small intestine, particularly the duodenum and jejunum, but sometimes it may be found in the stomach or in the large intestine. It either is attached to the mucosa by the ventral sucker or lies buried in the mucous secretions. It obtains its nourishment from the intestinal contents and secretions. Its life span is probably short in the human host. The average daily egg production per fluke is 25,000. In water at 27 to 32 C, the eggs hatch in 3 to 7 weeks. The miracidium, covered with cilia, has a spined head, pigmented eye spot, two flame cells, cephalic glands, and germinal cells; in a matter of hours it penetrates a suitable snail host or perishes.

The primary intermediate hosts are species of planorbid snails of the genera *Segmentina*, *Hippeutis*, and *Gyraulus*. In the snail the mira-

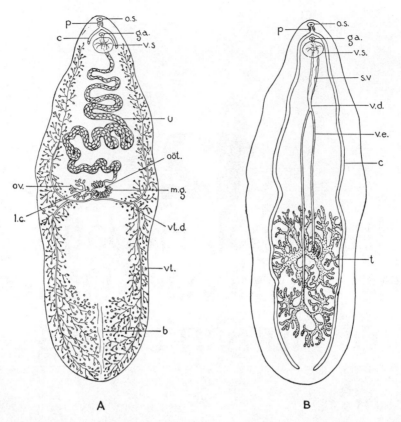

A   B

Figure 12-1. Schematic representation of morphology of *Fasciolopsis buski*♂♀(× 2). A. Female reproductive organs, ventral view. B. Male reproductive organs and digestive tract, ventral view.

   b, bladder; c, ceca; g.a., genital atrium; m.g., Mehlis' gland; l.c., Laurer's canal; oöt., ootype; o.s., oral sucker; ov., ovary; p, pharynx; s.v., seminal vesicle; t, testes; u, uterus; v.d., vas deferens; v.e., vas efferens; v.s., ventral sucker; vt., vitellaria; vt.d., vitelline duct. (Adapted from Odhner, 1902.)

cidium metamorphoses into a mother sporocyst, which migrates to the region of the heart and liver. When ripe, it ruptures to liberate mother rediae, which in turn produce daughter rediae. Cercariae, with slender muscular tails and heavy bodies 195 by 145 μ, are liberated from the daughter rediae and erupt from the snail in 4 to 7 weeks after its infection. In the water the cercaria swims by lashing the tail and crawls like a measuring worm, using its suckers. The free-swimming stage is brief, ordinarily merely of sufficient length for the cercaria to reach a suitable plant for encystment. Cercariae show little selective specificity and encyst on the surface or in the integument of all sorts of aquatic vegetation in stagnant

waters. The principal plants are the water caltrop *Trapa*, the water hyacinth *Eichhornia*, the water chestnut *Eliocharis*, and the water bamboo *Zizania*. The cercaria, casting off its tail, becomes a metacercaria by secreting an outer, friable cyst wall, 216 by 187 μ, and a firm inner wall that is soluble in the digestive juices. A single plant may harbor a large number of cysts that are resistant to cold but susceptible to desiccation at summer temperatures. When the cysts are swallowed, their inner wall is dissolved in the duodenum, and the activated larval worm attaches itself to the mucosa of the upper intestine and becomes an adult worm in 25 to 30 days (Fig. 12-2).

Epidemiology. This parasite is found in Cen-

FASCIOLOPSIS BUSKI

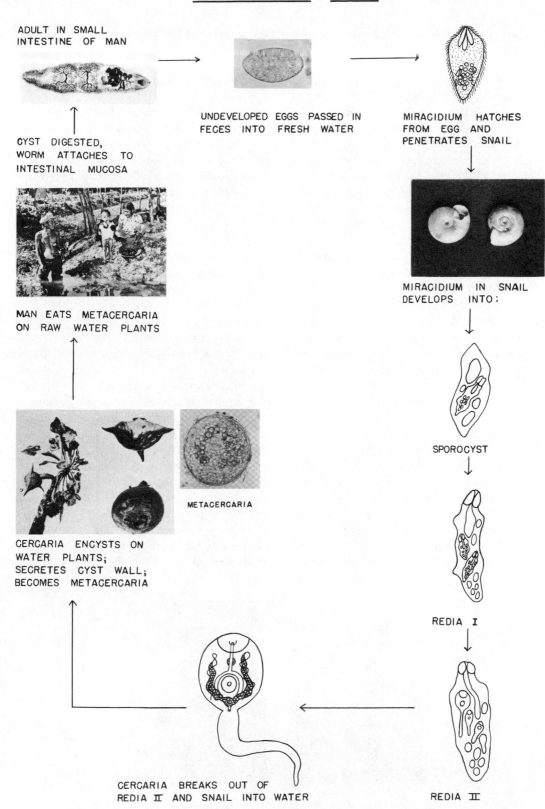

ADULT IN SMALL
INTESTINE OF MAN

UNDEVELOPED EGGS PASSED IN
FECES INTO FRESH WATER

MIRACIDIUM HATCHES
FROM EGG AND
PENETRATES SNAIL

CYST DIGESTED,
WORM ATTACHES TO
INTESTINAL MUCOSA

MIRACIDIUM IN SNAIL
DEVELOPS INTO:

MAN EATS METACERCARIA
ON RAW WATER PLANTS

SPOROCYST

METACERCARIA

CERCARIA ENCYSTS ON
WATER PLANTS;
SECRETES CYST WALL;
BECOMES METACERCARIA

REDIA I

REDIA II

CERCARIA BREAKS OUT OF
REDIA II AND SNAIL INTO WATER

Figure 12-2. Life cycle of *Fasciolopsis buski*.

tral and South China as far north as the Yangtze valley, Taiwan, Thailand, Laos, Vietnam, Cambodia, India, Korea, and Indonesia. The chief endemic area is in the Kwangtung and Chekiang provinces of China, where the incidence of human infection is high. Human infection usually results from the ingestion of metacercariae on fresh edible water plants that grow in ponds fertilized by night soil rather than in the less heavily polluted canals. When eaten raw, the pods of the water caltrop and the bulbs of the water chestnut are peeled with the teeth, thus enabling the detached metacercaria to enter the digestive tract. Dried plants are not dangerous, since desiccation kills the metacercariae.

Pathology and Symptomatology. Fasciolopsis attaches to the mucosa of the upper small intestine by means of its ventral sucker. It feeds on the intestinal contents and possibly on the superficial mucosa. Areas of inflammation, ulceration, and abscesses occur at the site of attachment. Epigastric pain, nausea, and diarrhea of varying severity occur, especially in the morning. These are relieved by food— which may be raw water nuts bringing additional infection. In heavy infections, edema, ascites, and anasarca are severe. Occasionally, intestinal stasis and obstruction are produced. The clinical manifestations are probably due to toxic products of the worm. There is slight anemia, often a leukocytosis, sometimes a leukopenia or lymphocytosis, and an eosinophilia up to 35 percent. Complete recovery follows

the removal of the worms. In advanced cases death may result from exhaustion (Fig. 12-3).

Diagnosis. The clinical symptoms are sufficiently characteristic to arouse suspicion in an endemic area. Final diagnosis is based on finding the eggs in the feces. The eggs resemble those of *Fasciola hepatica* except for the distribution of the yolk granules, those of *Gastrodiscoides hominis,* which are narrower and greenish brown, and those of *Echinochasmus perfoliatus,* which are smaller. Adult flukes are sometimes vomited or passed in the feces.

Treatment. The most effective drug is dichlorophen, given in a dose of 2 to 3 gm every 8 hours for 3 doses. For children up to 20 kilograms, each dose should be 0.5 to 1.0 gm (total 1.5 to 3.0 gm), and for children of 20 to 45 kilograms, 1.0 to 2.0 gm for each dose (total 3.0 to 6.0 gm). Abdominal pain and diarrhea are common side-effects. An alternative drug is niclosamide, in a dose of 100 mg per kilogram of body weight. In either case the treatment can be repeated after 7 to 10 days.

Prevention. While treatment will reduce the human sources of infection, it will not diminish porcine sources and will not prevent reinfection, particularly in children, in endemic areas. The infestation of water plants may be reduced by treating night soil containing the eggs by storage or unslaked lime, and by killing the eggs, miracidia, and cercariae in the water with unslaked lime (100 ppm) or copper sulfate (20 ppm). Infected hogs should be restrained from contaminating areas where wa-

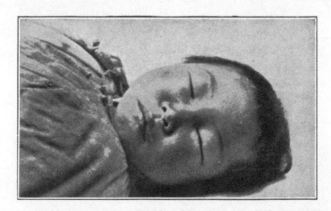

Figure 12-3. Patient with fasciolopsiasis, showing edema of cheeks and orbital area. (From Faust: Human Helminthology, 2nd ed., 1939. Courtesy of Lea & Febiger.)

ter plants are growing—a difficult task in the Far East. The intermediate snail hosts may be destroyed in various ways (see Chap. 13). The abolition of eating the raw aquatic plants would soon eliminate infection in humans, but such a measure would require education of the public and fundamental changes in eating habits. Thorough cooking or the steeping of the plants in boiling water should afford protection.

Heterophyes heterophyes

Disease. Heterophyiasis.

Life Cycle. The worm is a natural parasite of man and of domesticated and wild fish-eating mammals. The pyriform, grayish fluke (Fig. 12-4) is identified by (1) its small size, 1.3 by 0.5 mm, (2) a cuticle covered with fine scale-like spines, (3) a large central sucker in the anterior middle-third of the body, (4) a protrusible, nonadhesive genital sucker at the left posterior border of the ventral sucker, (5) two ovoid testes side by side in the posterior fifth of the body, (6) absence of cirrus and cirral sac,

the seminal vesicle opening within the genital sucker, (7) a subglobose ovary anterior to the testes, and (8) vitellaria with large polygonal follicles in the lateral posterior third of the body. The light brown, thick-shelled, operculated eggs, 29 by 16 μ, contain fully developed miracidia at oviposition. The shell has a slight shoulder at the rim of the operculum and sometimes a knob at the posterior pole. They may be differentiated from *Clonorchis* eggs by their broad ends with indistinct opercular shoulders and less developed posterior spine, and with greater difficulty from those of *Metagonimus yokogawai*, which have a light-yellow color and a thin shell.

The adult worm inhabits the middle part of the small intestine. It is usually found in the intestinal lumen, but it may be attached to the mucosa between the villi. It apparently obtains its nourishment from the intestinal secretions and contents. The life span is short.

The first intermediate hosts are brackish-water snails, *Pirenella* in Egypt and *Cerithidea* in Japan. The second intermediate hosts are

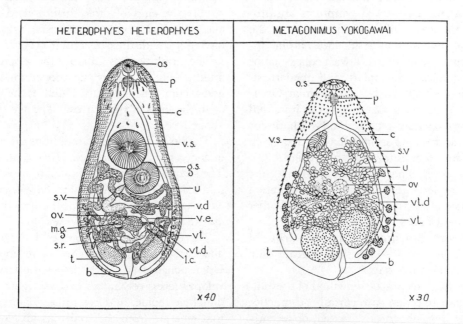

Figure 12-4. *Heterophyes heterophyes* and *Metagonimus yokogawai.*
b, excretory bladder; c, ceca; g.s., genital sucker; l.c., Laurer's canal; m.g., Mehlis' gland; o.s., oral sucker; ov., ovary; p, pharynx; s.r., seminal receptacle; s.v., seminal vesicle; t, testes; u, uterus; v.d., vas deferens; v.e., vas efferens; v.s., ventral sucker; vt., vitellaria; vt.d., vitelline duct. (*Heterophyes heterophyes* redrawn from Looss, 1894. *M. yokogawai* redrawn from Leiper, 1913.)

fish, chiefly *Mugil* (mullet) and *Tilapia* in Egypt and *Mugil* and *Acanthogobius* in Japan.

The egg is probably ingested by the snail, in which it develops successively into sporocyst, redia, and cercaria. After leaving the snail the cercaria encysts as a metacercaria in a cyst on the scales, fins, tail, gills, or, less frequently, in the muscles of susceptible fish. When raw or imperfectly cooked fish is eaten by the definitive host, the metacercaria escapes from the cyst and develops into an adult worm in about a week.

Epidemiology. This parasite is found in Egypt, particularly the lower Nile valley, Greece, Israel, Central and South China, Japan, Korea, Taiwan, and the Philippines. There is a high incidence of infection near Port Said, Egypt, where the local fishermen continually pollute the water and a high percentage of mullets are infected. Humans acquire the infection by eating raw fresh mullets or fessikh (salted mullets) pickled for less than 14 days.

Pathogenicity. Except with heavy infections there is no appreciable injury to the intestine, and as a rule no marked symptoms are produced. In heavy infections, irritation of the intestinal mucosa may result in a chronic intermittent mucous diarrhea with colicky pains and abdominal discomfort and tenderness. There is eosinophilia but no anemia. Occasionally, if the worms penetrate the intestinal wall, the eggs may get into the lymphatics or venules and set up granulomatous lesions in such distant foci as the heart and brain.

Diagnosis. Diagnosis is made by finding the eggs in the feces. They require differentiation from those of *Clonorchis*, *Opisthorchis*, and other heterophyid flukes.

Treatment. Praziquantel is the drug of choice. The dose is 20 mg per kilogram t.i.d. for two consecutive days.

Prevention. The practical method of preventing human infection is to curtail the practice of eating raw, imperfectly cooked, or recently salted fish in endemic areas. The impossibility of detecting and treating human carriers, the presence of animal reservoir hosts, and the difficulty of enforcing sanitary measures or of destroying the snail hosts render general control measures impracticable.

Metagonimus yokogawai

Disease. Metagonimiasis.

Life Cycle. The definitive hosts are humans, dogs, cats, hogs, pelicans and probably other fish-eating birds.

The adult worm (Fig. 12-4) is identified by (1) its small size, 1.4 by 0.6 mm, (2) its pyriform shape, with a rounded posterior and a tapering anterior end, (3) a cuticle covered with minute scalelike spines more numerous at the anterior end, (4) a large ventral sucker, situated to the right of the midline, with a genital opening at its anterior rim, (5) the two oval testes, obliquely side by side, in the posterior third of the body, (6) the globose ovary at the junction of the middle and lower third of the body, and (7) the coarse vitellaria in a fan-shaped distribution in the posterior lateral fields. The light yellow-brown, thin-shelled operculated eggs, 28 by 17 μ, with nodular thickening on the posterior end, contain at oviposition mature miracidia. They closely resemble the eggs of other heterophyid flukes and differ from those of *Clonorchis sinensis* by having a less distinct opercular groove.

The adult worms inhabit the upper and middle jejunum, rarely the duodenum, ileum, and cecum. They are embedded in the mucus or in the folds of the mucosa. The life span is about 1 year.

The first intermediate snail hosts are species of the genera *Semisulcospira*, *Thiara*, and *Hua*. The second intermediate hosts are fresh-water salmonoid fishes of the genera *Plecoglossus* and *Salmo*, and the cyprinoids of the genera *Richardsonium* (*Leuciscus*) and *Odontobutis*.

The egg is probably ingested by the snail, and the miracidium hatches in its intestine. Upon penetration of the tissues the larva develops successively into sporocyst, mother and daughter rediae, and cercariae. The cercaria that emerges from the snail has an elongate, spinous body attenuated anteriorly and a long tail with dorsoventral flutings. After a short swimming existence, it penetrates an appropriate species of fish, casts off its tail, and encysts in the scales, fins, tail, gills, and rarely, the muscles. When the metacercarial cyst, 140 to 225 μ, is ingested by a definitive host, the cyst wall is dissolved by the duodenal juices and ruptured by the activated larva. The excysted metacercaria becomes an adult worm in 7 to 10 days.

Epidemiology. *M. yokogawai,* the most common heterophyid fluke in the Far East, has been reported in Japan, China, Korea, the Philippines, Taiwan, Siberia, the Balkans, Greece, and Spain.

Since the infection is acquired by humans and other mammals by eating raw, infected fish, the parasite is common in people in countries where this custom prevails. The waters inhabited by susceptible snails and fish are contaminated by the fecal discharges of humans and other mammals.

Pathogenicity. Similar to that of *H. heterophyes.* Occasionally eggs may enter the lymphatics or mesenteric venules and set up granulomatous lesions in such distant foci as the heart and nervous system.

Diagnosis. Identification of eggs in feces is the method of diagnosis. They are difficult to differentiate from other heterophyid and opisthorchid eggs.

Treatment. Treatment is the same as for heterophyiasis—namely, praziquantel at a dose of 20 mg per kilogram t.i.d. for two consecutive days.

Prevention. Infection may be avoided by eating only thoroughly cooked fish.

Echinostomate Flukes of Human Beings

Species. Some 11 or more species of echinostome have been reported in humans. A few are natural, and others are incidental, human parasites. Most of these species are found in oriental countries. They are discussed here as a group, since they are of minor or only local importance as agents of human disease.

The flukes of the family ECHINOSTOMATIDAE are distinguished from other trematodes by a horseshoe-shaped collar of spines surrounding the dorsal and lateral sides of the oral sucker. They are elongated, moderate-sized trema-todes with slightly tapering, rounded extremities. The cuticle bears minute spinelike scales. The more-or-less lobate testes occupy a tandem position in the posterior half of the worm. A cirrus is present. The globular ovary is anterior to the testes. The vitellaria with small follicles usually fill the lateral borders of the posterior two-thirds of the worm. The looped uterus lies anterior to the ovary. At oviposition the large, thin-shelled egg contains an undeveloped miracidium.

Life Cycle. The ovum matures about 3 weeks after leaving the definitive host, and the miracidium enters a snail. Apparently, the sporocyst stage is abortive, and development takes place directly into mother and daughter rediae and cercariae. The cercariae escape to encyst in snails (even species that serve as first intermediate host), fish, or possibly on aquatic vegetation.

Pathogenicity. It is questionable whether the echinostomes are active pathogens, for in spite of the oral circlet of spines, they cause little damage to the intestinal mucosa other than irritation. Heavy infections may produce catarrhal inflammation and even ulceration of the mucosa. Ordinarily, no marked intestinal symptoms are produced. At times children show a clinical syndrome of diarrhea, abdominal pain, anemia, and edema.

Diagnosis. Diagnosis is made by finding the eggs in the feces. The operculated, ellipsoidal, yellow to yellowish brown, thin-shelled eggs require differentiation from the undeveloped eggs of other intestinal flukes. The various echinostome species differ in the size of the eggs, although there is some overlapping.

Treatment. Tetrachlorethylene was used in treatment but some of the newer antihelminthic drugs may be more effective.

Prevention. Snails, fish, amphibians, and plants are possible sources of infection. In endemic areas, raw or insufficiently cooked snails or fresh-water fish should not be eaten. Drinking water also should be boiled.

An example of this group is *Euparyphium ilocanum* of the Philippines, Celebes, China, and Java, a fluke 2.5 to 6.5 by 1.1 mm, with 49 to 51 spines on the circumoral disc, and eggs 83 to 116 by 53 to 82 μ. Reservoir hosts are the field rat and the dog; the first intermediate snail host is *Gyraulus*, and the second intermediate hosts are snails of the genera *Viviparus* and *Pila*, which are eaten by natives of the Philippines and Java.

Troglotrema salmincola

This is a nonpathogenic incidental parasite of humans that is associated with salmon poisoning of dogs in the northwest Pacific Coast of North America and Siberia. The adult fluke has a small, pyriform body, 0.9 by 0.4 mm. The suckers are unarmed. The uterus contains usually from 10 to 15 yellowish, broadly oval, operculate, thick-shelled eggs, 70 by 42 μ, with undeveloped miracidia.

The definitive hosts are dogs, cats, and wild fur-bearing mammals; humanity is an incidental host. The intermediate snail host on the Pacific Coast is *Goniobasis*.

The piscine hosts are species of SALMONIDAE. The eggs hatch 2 to 3 months after leaving the definitive host. The liberated miracidium penetrates a snail, where it develops into sporocyst, rediae, and cercariae, which, when liberated, encyst in the tissues of salmonoid fishes. Humans and other mammals are infected by eating raw fish; the excysted metacercaria becomes a mature worm in 5 days or more. The worms are in the small intestine.

Human beings manifest no symptoms. The presence of the flukes in dogs, foxes, and coyotes is associated with a local or generalized enteritis due to a rickettsial agent, which can be serially transmitted through the blood. The helminth acts as a reservoir host of *Neorickettsia helmintheca*. Diagnosis is made by finding the eggs in the feces. Thorough cooking of fish will prevent infection.

Gastrodiscoides hominis

G. hominis is found in Assam, Bengal, Malaya, and Vietnam. The natural definitive hosts other than humans are hogs and Napu mouse deer.

The reddish, aspinous, dorsally convex worm, 5 to 8 by 3 to 5 mm, is divided into an anterior conical portion and an enlarged posterior disc with a large ventral sucker with a thick overhanging rim. The ceca are relatively short, extending only to the middle of the discoid region. The lobate testes lie in tandem position below the bifurcation of the ceca. There is a tortuous seminal receptacle, a Laurer's canal, and a loosely coiled uterus terminating in the genital cone. The greenish-brown egg, 150 to 170 by 60 to 70 μ, is ovoid, with the anterior portion narrow and the operculum small.

The worm inhabits the cecum and ascending colon. Its life span is unknown.

The egg, unembryonated when passed in the feces, matures in 16 to 17 days at 27 to 34 C. The life cycle is unknown but probably is the same as in other species of GASTRODISCIDAE.

The definitive hosts are mammals. Redia, daughter rediae, and cercariae are produced in snails; encystment occurs on aquatic vegetation; and infection takes place by ingestion. The fluke causes mucosal inflammation of the cecum and ascending colon and may produce diarrhea. Treatment is similar to that for *Fasciolopsis* (see above).

The presence of eggs in feces is diagnostic. The eggs resemble those of *F. buski* but are narrower and greenish brown.

The only known preventive measure in endemic areas is the cooking of vegetables.

A second amphistome fluke has been reported in humans. *Watsonius watsoni*, a parasite of monkeys and baboons, has been found once in a West African black, who died of a severe diarrhea and toxic inanition. This fluke has a large, powerful ventral sucker that is the chief cause of trauma to the intestinal mucosa of primates.

LIVER FLUKES

Clonorchis sinensis

The Chinese or oriental liver fluke, *C. sinensis*, is an important parasite of humans in the Far East. The fluke is a parasite of fish-eating mammals and humans in Japan, China, South Korea, Formosa, and Vietnam.

CLONORCHIS SINENSIS

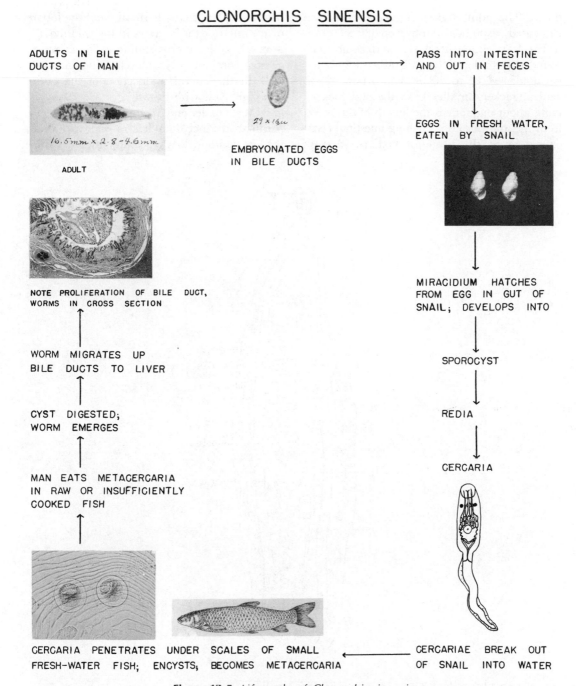

ADULTS IN BILE
DUCTS OF MAN

16.5mm x 2.8-4.6mm

ADULT

29 x 13u

EMBRYONATED EGGS
IN BILE DUCTS

PASS INTO INTESTINE
AND OUT IN FECES

EGGS IN FRESH WATER,
EATEN BY SNAIL

NOTE PROLIFERATION OF BILE DUCT,
WORMS IN CROSS SECTION

WORM MIGRATES UP
BILE DUCTS TO LIVER

CYST DIGESTED;
WORM EMERGES

MAN EATS METACERCARIA
IN RAW OR INSUFFICIENTLY
COOKED FISH

MIRACIDIUM HATCHES
FROM EGG IN GUT OF
SNAIL; DEVELOPS INTO

SPOROCYST

REDIA

CERCARIA

CERCARIA PENETRATES UNDER SCALES OF SMALL
FRESH-WATER FISH; ENCYSTS, BECOMES METACERCARIA

CERCARIAE BREAK OUT
OF SNAIL INTO WATER

Figure 12-5. Life cycle of *Clonorchis sinensis.*

Life Cycle (Fig. 12-5). The natural definitive hosts other than humans are the dog, hog, cat, wild cat, martin, badger, mink, and, rarely, ducks. The adult fluke (Fig. 12-6) is a flat, elongated, aspinous, flabby, opalescent gray worm, tapering anteriorly and somewhat rounded posteriorly. It is identified by (1) its variable size, 12 to 20 by 3 to 5 mm, (2) a ventral sucker, smaller than the oral sucker, lying about one-fourth the length of the body from the anterior end, (3) long intestinal ceca extending to the posterior end, (4) deeply lobed testes in tandem formation in the posterior part of the body, (5) a poorly developed ejaculatory duct without cirrus, cirral sac, or prostatic glands, (6) a small, slightly lobate ovary anterior to the testes in the midline, (7) a loosely coiled uterus ending in the common genital pore, and (8) minutely follicular vitellaria in the lateral midportion of the body. The light yellowish-brown eggs are 29 by 16 μ. At the smaller end, the operculum rests in a rim with distinct shoulders in such a position that its contour does not follow the curvature

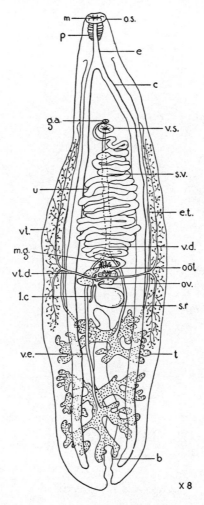

Figure 12-6. Schematic representation of morphology of *Clonorchis sinensis.*
   b, excretory bladder; c, ceca; e, esophagus; e.t., excretory tubules; g.a., genital atrium; l.c., Laurer's canal; m, mouth; m.g., Mehlis' gland; oöt, ootype; o.s., oral sucker; ov., ovary; p, pharynx; s.r., seminal receptacle; s.v., seminal vesicle; t, testes; u, uterus; v.d., vas deferens; v.e., vas efferens; v.s., ventral sucker; vt., vitellaria; vt.d., vitelline duct.

of the shell. At the thicker posterior end is a small median protuberance

The eggs, deposited in the biliary passages of the definitive host, pass from the body in the feces. Although the eggs contain fully developed miracidia, they do not hatch upon reaching water.

The first intermediate hosts are operculate snails of the genera *Alocinma, Bulimus, Parafossarulus, Hua,* and, possibly, *Semisulcospira* and *Thiara.* The miracidium, which has a blunt solid spine on the small head papilla, does not erupt from the shell until the egg is ingested by a suitable snail. In the tissues of the snail it metamorphoses into a sporocyst, rediae, and cercariae. The free-swimming cercaria perishes unless it encounters a fish within 24 to 48 hours. It penetrates beneath the scales and, losing its tail, encysts as an ovoid metacercaria, chiefly in the muscles and subcutaneous tissues, less often on the scales, fins, and gills of some 40 species of fresh-water fish belonging to 23 genera of the family CYPRINIDAE. Certain species, especially those cultivated in night-soil–fertilized ponds, are more heavily infected than others; a maximum of 2900 metacercariae per fish has been reported. The cyst, 138 by 115 μ, has an outer and an inner hyaline wall secreted by the parasite and a surrounding capsule formed by the tissues of the fish. In the human duodenum the outer wall is dissolved by trypsin, while the inner layer is ruptured by the activity of the metacercaria. The freed larva migrates to the common bile duct and thence to the distal biliary ducts, where it becomes a mature worm within a month.

The worm lies unattached in the small branches of the distal portion of the biliary tract. Occasionally in heavy infections, it may be found in the larger bile ducts, the gallbladder, and the pancreatic duct. It is not found in the duodenum, since it can only survive the action of the digestive juices for a few hours. It probably feeds on the secretions of the upper bile ducts. Its life span is 20 to 25 years. The average daily output of eggs per worm in the feces of dogs and cats, though irregular, is 1100 to 2400; in guinea pigs, 1600; in rats, 330; in humans, unknown.

Epidemiology. Humans are usually infected by eating uncooked fish containing infectious metacercariae and, less often, by the ingestion of the cysts in drinking water. The intensity of human infection is dependent upon the eating habits of the population and does not always coincide with the prevalence of the parasite in animal reservoir hosts. In North China, where little or no raw fish is consumed, antochthonous cases comprise only 0.4 percent of the population, although nearly one-third of the dogs and cats are infected. In South China—especially in the Kwangtung Province, where raw fish is served in thin slices either with vegetables and condiments or, more often, among the poorer classes by whom it is partially cooked with hot rice congee or gruel—the incidence of human infection is from 3 to 36 percent. The rearing of certain fresh-water fish in ponds fertilized by night soil is an important industry in this area, and these fish are largely used in raw-fish food dishes.

We usually associate clonorchiasis with the Oriental race. However, German-Jewish refugees of World War II who sojourned in Shanghai for several years before coming to the United States have been exhibiting *Clonorchis.* In Shanghai in 1946 some 7000 of these refugees, whose diet was low in protein, were sold small fish raised on human feces in fresh-water ponds by enterprising Chinese as "herring," a salt-water fish. During the past years clonorchiasis continues to be diagnosed in some of these people from the Shanghai epidemic in various medical centers.

Pathology and Symptomatology. The distal bile ducts inhabited by *Clonorchis* are irritated mechanically and by its toxic secretions. Early in the infection there is slight leukocytosis and eosinophilia. Depending on the severity of infection, which may run into thousands of worms, the liver may enlarge and become tender. The bile ducts gradually thicken and become dilated and tortuous, and adenomatous proliferation of the biliary epithelium develops. As the disease progresses, fibrosis and destruction of hepatic parenchyma take place, and liver function is impaired although the SGOT and SGPT are normal.

The relationship between *Clonorchis* infection and the symptoms attributed to it are not entirely clear. Light infections may produce only mild symptoms or go unrecognized. As additional worms are acquired, indigestion, epigastric discomfort unrelated to meals, weakness, and loss of weight become noticeable. In heavy infections anemia, liver enlargement, slight jaundice, edema, ascites, and diarrhea develop. Tachycardia, palpitation, vertigo, and mental depression may ensue. One of my patients, a female Chinese singer, complained of unwanted belchings during her performances. Patients seldom die of clonorchiasis, but because of lowered resistance they may succumb to superimposed diseases. With mild infections the prognosis is usually good even without treatment. With prolonged or heavy infections in highly endemic regions, the outcome is unsatisfactory and depends upon the degree of damage to the liver.

Diagnosis. Clinical diagnosis is suggestive in patients with an enlarged liver and symptoms of hepatitis in endemic areas where uncooked fish is eaten. Advanced infections require differentiation from malignancy, cirrhosis of the liver, or other causes of hepatic enlargement. Absolute diagnosis is based on finding the characteristic eggs in the feces or biliary drainage. The eggs require differentiation from those of other opisthorchid and heterophyid flukes.

Treatment. No treatment was satisfactory until recently; now praziquantel has been found effective in the treatment of this infection. The optimum dosage schedule is to give 25 mg per kilogram t.i.d. for 2 consecutive days. Headache and dizziness are common but not serious side-effects.

Prevention. The thorough cooking of fish would practically eliminate the disease in humans. This depends upon the education of the housewives and those serving raw fish in restaurants—a difficult task. Metacercariae are not killed by refrigeration, salting, or the addition of vinegar or sauce. Reduction of sources of infection is impossible because of animal reservoir hosts. Sterilization of human feces may be effected by storage or by the addition of ammonium sulfate. The curtailment of usage of night soil for fertilizing fish ponds is not economically feasible, and molluscacides capable of destroying the snails may destroy fish and other aquatic life.

Opisthorchis felineus

O. felineus is prevalent in cats, dogs, foxes, and hogs in eastern and southeastern Europe and Asiatic USSR. In the highly endemic areas of Poland and the Dnieper, Donetz, and Desna Basins, it is also found in humans.

O. felineus (Fig. 12-7), 7 to 12 by 1.5 to 3.0 mm, resembles *C. sinensis*. The eggs, 30 by 12 μ, resemble those of *C. sinensis* but are narrower and have more tapering ends, a pointed terminal knob, and a less conspicuous opercular rim. Its habitat is the distal bile ducts, occasionally the pancreatic duct. The life span is probably several years.

The first intermediate hosts are the snails *Bulimus.* The second intermediate hosts are numerous species of cyprinoid fish, of which the chub and the tench are infected most frequently. The egg, which contains a miracidium, does not hatch until ingested by a snail, in the digestive gland of which sporocysts and rediae develop. The cercariae leave the snail in about 2 months, encyst in a suitable species of fish, and become infective metacercariae. When ingested by a definitive host, they excyst in the duodenum and pass to the distal bile ducts, where they mature in 3 to 4 weeks.

The infection is acquired by eating raw or insufficiently cooked fish. Cats appear to be the most important reservoir hosts in highly endemic areas. Intermediate snail hosts are infected by feces deposited on sandy shores and washed into streams.

Pathology, prognosis, and treatment are similar to those for *Clonorchis.* The presence of characteristic eggs in feces or duodenal drainage is diagnostic. The infection may be prevented by cooking fish and by sanitary excreta disposal.

Opisthorchis viverrini

This fluke is found in Thailand and Laos in southeastern Asia. In general it is similar to *O.*

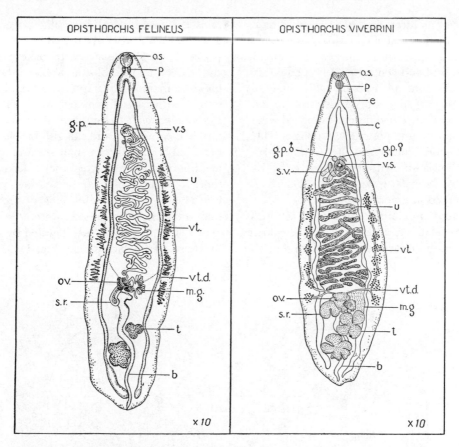

Figure 12-7. *Opisthorchis felineus* and *O. viverrini.*
  b, bladder; c, ceca; e, esophagus; g.p., genital pore; m.g., Mehlis' gland; o.s., oral sucker; ov., ovary; p, pharynx; s.r., seminal receptacle; s.v., seminal vesicle; t, testes; u, uterus; v.s., ventral sucker; vt., vitellaria; vt.d., vitelline duct. (*O. felineus* redrawn from Stiles and Hassall, 1894. *O. viverrini* redrawn from Leiper, 1915.)

felineus (Fig. 12-7). The egg is 26 by 13 μ and closely resembles that of *C. sinensis.*

The definitive hosts other than people are the civet cat, the cat, the dog, and other fish-eating mammals. Intermediate hosts are snails and several species of fish.

The disease is acquired by eating uncooked fish containing the infective metacercariae.

The hepatic lesions are similar to those of *C. sinensis.* At autopsies of patients infected with 1000 to 6000 worms, the findings included enlarged liver, marked dilatation of bile ducts, numerous worms in yellowish fluid in the lumens of ducts, thickening of walls of ducts, increase of portal connective tissue, atrophy of liver cells, and, in two cases, papillary adenomatous carcinoma. The early symptoms in these patients included loss of appetite, flatulence, epigastric discomfort and pain, and, sometimes, leukocytosis and fever. Later, there was an enlarged painful liver, transient jaundice and urticaria, watery diarrhea, weakness, and anemia. There was no marked eosinophilia.

Diagnosis is made by finding eggs in feces or duodenal drainage.

Treatment. Similar to that of *Clonorchis* (see above). The disease may be prevented by eating only cooked fish.

Fasciola hepatica

Diseases. Fascioliasis, "liver rot," sheep liver fluke.

Morphology. F. hepatica (Fig. 12-8) is identified by (1) its large size, 20 to 30 by 8 to 13 mm, (2) its flat, leaf shape with characteristic shouldered appearance due to its cephalic cone, (3) oral and ventral suckers of equal size on cephalic cone, (4) intestine with numerous diverticula, (5) highly dendritic testes in tandem formation, (6) diffusely branched vitellaria in lateral and posterior portions of body, and (7) short, convoluted uterus. The large, oval, yellowish-brown, operculated eggs, 130 to 150 by 63 to 90 μ (see Figure 11-3A), are unsegmented at oviposition.

The adult inhabits the proximal bile passages, gallbladder, and, occasionally, ectopic sites. It has an anaerobic metabolism and ob-

tains its nourishment from biliary secretions. The life span is at least 10 years.

Life Cycle. The fluke is a parasite of sheep, cattle, deer, and rabbits, as well as other herbivorous mammals. Its intermediate hosts are some 21 species of lymneid snail, of which *Lymnaea truncatula,* a snail that inhabits transitory bodies of water and sluggish brooks, is the most important. In the snail the miracidium metamorphoses into a sporocyst, rediae, at times daughter rediae, and cercariae (see Figure 11-3D-J). The latter emerge from the snail and encyst on grasses, watercress, bark, or soil (Fig. 11-3K). When ingested by definitive hosts the metacercariae (Fig. 11-3L) pass

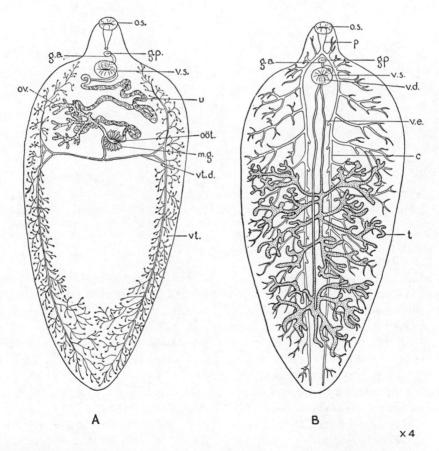

A   B

×4

Figure 12-8. Schematic representation of morphology of *Fasciola hepatica* (× 4), A. Female reproductive organs, ventral view. B. Male reproductive organs and digestive tract, ventral view.

c, ceca; g.a., genital atrium; g.p., genital pore; m.g., Mehlis' gland; oöt., ootype; o.s., oral sucker; ov., ovary; p. pharynx; t, testes; u, uterus; v.d., vas deferens; v.e., vas efferens; v.s., ventral sucker; vt., vitellaria; vt.d., vitelline duct. (Adapted from Sommer, 1880, and from Leuckart, 1863.)

through the intestinal wall, eventually penetrating the liver capsule, and migrate to the biliary tree consuming liver parenchyma en route. They mature in 12 weeks.

Epidemiology. This fluke is cosmopolitan throughout the sheep- and cattle-raising countries of the world. Human infection is frequent in Cuba, southern France, Great Britain, and Algeria. One human infection has been reported from California. An adult worm was found in an intestinal nodule in a woman who had lived in New York State all of her life, except for a visit to Hawaii, where this parasite is present (Fig. 12-9). It is common in animals in the United States.

Humans contract the disease by ingesting plants such as watercress or possibly water containing the encysted metacercariae. Herbivorous or omnivorous animals acquire the infection in low, damp pastures, where the vegetation is infested with metacercariae.

Pathology and Symptomatology. The extent of the damage and symptomatology depend upon the intensity of the infection and the duration of the disease. A single fluke can produce severe symptoms by biliary obstruction. Because of pressure, toxic metabolic products, and feeding habits, the worms provoke inflammatory, adenomatous, and fibrotic changes of the biliary tract. Parenchymal atrophy and periportal cirrhosis develop. Severe headache, chills, fever, urticaria, a stabbing substernal pain, and right upper quadrant

pains that radiate to the back and shoulders may be the first evidence of infection. As the infection progresses, an enlarged tender liver, jaundice, digestive disturbances, diarrhea, and anemia develop. Animal experiments indicate that each adult worm consumes 0.2 ml of blood per day. The erythrocyte sedimentation rate may be elevated, and there is usually marked eosinophilia early in the infection with or without leukocytosis.

Diagnosis. Clinical diagnosis is difficult because of multiplicity of symptoms, but an enlarged tender liver and a febrile eosinophilic syndrome are suggestive. Laboratory diagnosis is based on finding the characteristic eggs—operculate, 130 to 150 μ in length by 63 to 90 μ in width, and very similar to those of *Fasciolopsis*—in the feces or bile. Eggs may be found in the stools of patients eating infected liver, leading to false diagnoses. Positive complement-fixation test and intracutaneous reactions have been obtained with *Fasciola* antigens in infected and clinically cured persons, and these tests are useful in extrahepatic infections or when direct examination fails to reveal the eggs.

Treatment. Several patients infected with *Fasciola* have been treated successfully with dichlorophenol (Bithionol),° 30 to 50 mg per kilogram on alternate days for 10 to 15 doses. Dehydroemetine dihydrochloride,° 1 mg per kilogram daily intramuscularly for 10 days, or emetine dihydrochloride, 20 to 65 mg daily intramuscularly for 8 to 10 days, can be used.

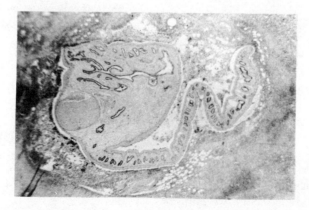

Figure 12-9. Section of intestinal nodule showing *Fasciola* adult.

Since both of these drugs are cardiotoxic, the patient should rest during therapy.

Prevention. Long-range control is dependent upon the eradication of the disease in herbivorous animals. Treatment is possible for domesticated animals, but not for wild animals. The destruction of snails and the larval parasites is difficult. Infection in humans in endemic areas may be prevented by eliminating raw watercress and other uncooked green vegetation from the diet. A safe water supply is important.

Fasciola gigantica

F. gigantica is a parasite of cattle, water buffalo, camels, wild hogs, and other herbivora in Africa, Asia, and Hawaii. The adult worm is distinguished from *F. hepatica* by its greater length, shorter cephalic cone, larger ventral sucker, more anterior position of the reproductive organs, and larger eggs (150 to 190 by 70 to 90 μ). The life cycle is similar to that of *F. hepatica,* with a snail intermediate host and encystment of the cercariae on water plants. The liver is the primary site of the adult worm, and the damage to this organ and the symptoms produced are similar to those of *F. hepatica.* In Hawaii humans are infected from eating watercress or other vegetation contaminated with metacercariae or by drinking water from streams containing floating metacercariae. In cattle of Hawaii both species of flukes are present. Raw watercress and other contaminated vegetation should not be eaten in areas where the parasite is endemic.

Dicrocoelium dendriticum

D. dendriticum has a cosmopolitan distribution in sheep and other herbivora in Asia, Africa, Europe, and North and South America. Sporadic cases of human infection have been reported.

The fluke is identified by (1) its slender, lancet-shaped, flat, aspinous body, 5 to 15 by 1.5 to 2.5 mm, (2) two large, slightly lobed testes situated obliquely to each other anterior to the small subglobose ovary, and (3) voluminous uterine coils in the posterior two-thirds of the worm. The dark-brown, thick-shelled, operculated egg, 38 to 45 by 22 to 30 μ, contains a fully developed miracidium.

The principal definitive host is the sheep. The first intermediate hosts are the land snails of the genera *Abida, Cochlicella, Helicella,* and *Zebrina,* which eat the fluke's eggs.

The egg hatches in the intestine of the snail, and the miracidium metamorphoses into two generations of sporocysts and cercariae. The latter agglomerate in groups of 200 to 300 in slime balls of secreted material in the respiratory chamber of the snail. The crawling snails shed these slime balls on vegetation, where they are ingested by the foraging ant *Formica fusca,* in whch the cercariae encyst, becoming metacercariae. When the ant is ingested by the definitive host the excysted metacercariae penetrate the intestinal wall and reach the liver and bile ducts, probably by the portal system. This complex and interesting life cycle was elucidated by W. Krull.

The pathology and symptoms are similar to those of *F. hepatica.* In animals the parasite causes enlargement of the bile ducts, hyperplasia of the biliary epithelium, formation of periductal fibrous connective tissue, atrophy of the liver cells, and finally, in heavy infections, portal cirrhosis. The hepatic changes are less pronounced in humans, in which the infection is usually light. The symptoms in humans include digestive disturbances, flatulence, vomiting, biliary colic, chronic constipation or diarrhea, and a toxemia less pronounced than in fascioliasis.

Diagnosis is made by finding the eggs consistently in the feces and eliminating spurious infections from eating livers containing the eggs. Treatment is the same as for *Clonorchis* (see above). There are no effective measures of control.

PULMONARY FLUKES

Paragonimus westermani

Diseases. Paragonimiasis, pulmonary distomiasis.

Life Cycle (Fig. 12-10). The definitive hosts, other than humans, are domesticated and wild mammals.

P. westermani is a reddish-brown fluke identified by (1) its size, 8 to 16 by 4 to 8 mm, (2) its shape, when active resembling a spoon with one end contracted and the other elongated, and when contracted or preserved an oval, flattened coffee bean, (3) spinous cuticle, (4) suckers of equal size, the ventral just anterior to the equatorial plane, (5) irregularly lobed testes, oblique to each other, in posterior third of worm, (6) lobed ovary anterior to testes on right side opposite closely coiled uterus, and (7) vitellaria in extreme lateral fields for entire length of body. The oval, yellowish brown, thick-shelled egg, 85 by 55 μ, has a thickened opercular rim and is unembryonated at oviposition.

The first intermediate hosts are operculated snails of the genera *Hua, Semisulcospira, Syncera,* and *Thiara* in the Far East, *Pomatiopsis* in North America, and possibly *Pomacea* in South America. The second intermediate hosts are the fresh-water crabs of the genera *Eriocheir, Potamon, Sesarma,* and *Parathelphusa* in the Far East, and *Pseudothelphusa* in South America, and crayfishes of the genus *Astacus* in the Far East and *Cambarus* in North America and probably elsewhere.

The eggs that escape from the ruptured pulmonary cysts leave the host via the sputum or, if swallowed, the feces. Development usually takes place in about 3 weeks at an optimal temperature of 27 C. The free-swimming miracidium cannot survive more than 24 hours unless it penetrates a suitable snail, in which it develops into a sporocyst. The first generation rediae, in the snail, migrate to the lymph sinuses near the liver and produce daughter rediae, which in turn yield cercariae that emerge from the snail about 13 weeks after infection. They perish in 24 to 48 hours unless they penetrate a fresh-water crab or crayfish, in which they encyst in the gills, legs, body muscles, and viscera as metacercariae, 250 to 500 μ in size. The crustacean also may become infected by eating the snails. One crab may harbor 3000 metacercariae. After ingestion by the mammalian host the excysted metacercariae pass through the duodenal wall into the abdominal cavity. The adolescent worms burrow through the diaphragm, enter the pleural cavity, and in about 20 days reach the lungs, where in cystic cavities near the bronchi they become adult worms in 5 to 6 weeks. During this prolonged migration, the adolescent worms may remain for long periods in the peritoneum, may enter and leave the liver, and may become lodged in organs other than the lungs—so-called ectopic lesions.

Epidemiology. *P. westermani* has a cosmopolitan distribution among mammals, but its presence in humans is chiefly confined to the Far East. The principal endemic regions are in Japan, South Korea, Thailand, Taiwan, China, and the Philippines. Human infections have also been reported in South and Southeast Asia, Indonesia, islands of the South Pacific, and northern South America. The African *Paragonimus* is possibly a different species. Only one autochthonous case in a person has been reported in North America, although *P. kellicotti* has been found in mammals in 10 or more states of the United States.

A person is infected by eating uncooked infected fresh-water crabs and crayfish. It is customary in the Orient to consume these uncooked crustaceans in brine, vinegar, or wine as "drunken crabs," in which the metacercariae may survive for several hours. Also, metacercariae, dislodged during food preparation, may contaminate eating and cooking utensils. Crushed crab juice, taken orally and used in the treatment of measles in Korea, may be a source of infection in children.

Metacercariae are killed if the crabs are roasted until the muscles turn white or if they are heated in water at 55 C for 5 minutes.

Pathology and Symptomatology. In the lungs, *Paragonimus* provokes the development by the host of a fibrous tissue capsule. Within this cyst is blood-tinged, purulent material containing eggs. Surrounding the cyst is an infiltrated area. The onset of symptoms is usually insidious: a dry cough at first and later pro-

PARAGONIMUS WESTERMANI

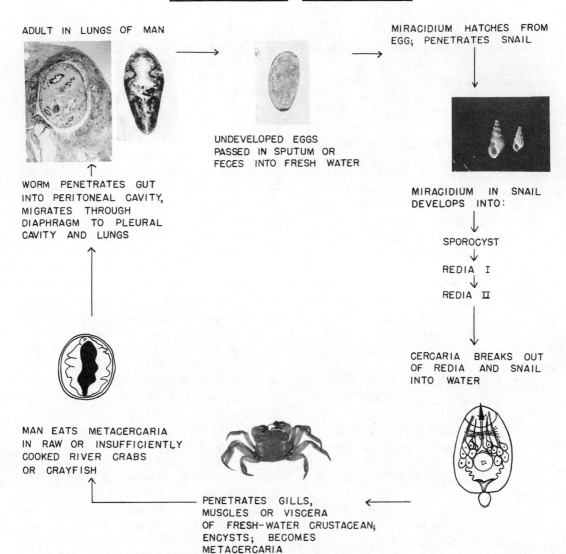

ADULT IN LUNGS OF MAN

MIRACIDIUM HATCHES FROM EGG; PENETRATES SNAIL

UNDEVELOPED EGGS PASSED IN SPUTUM OR FECES INTO FRESH WATER

WORM PENETRATES GUT INTO PERITONEAL CAVITY, MIGRATES THROUGH DIAPHRAGM TO PLEURAL CAVITY AND LUNGS

MIRACIDIUM IN SNAIL DEVELOPS INTO:

SPOROCYST

REDIA I

REDIA II

CERCARIA BREAKS OUT OF REDIA AND SNAIL INTO WATER

MAN EATS METACERCARIA IN RAW OR INSUFFICIENTLY COOKED RIVER CRABS OR CRAYFISH

PENETRATES GILLS, MUSCLES OR VISCERA OF FRESH-WATER CRUSTACEAN; ENCYSTS; BECOMES METACERCARIA

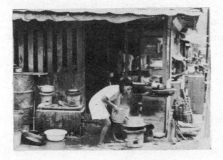

FAR EASTERN STREET RESTAURANT

Figure 12-10. Life cycle of *Paragonimus westermani*.

duction of blood-stained, rusty brown tenacious sputum most pronounced on rising in the morning. Pulmonary pain and pleurisy may be present, and hemoptysis occurs. These signs and symptoms, along with a low-grade fever and nondiagnostic radiographs, make it difficult to separate this infection from tuberculosis, pneumonia, or bronchiectasis.

Aberrant worms, with cyst formation, may localize in the abdominal wall, abdominal cavity, mesenteric lymph nodes, omentum, pericardium, myocardium, and intestinal wall. They may produce abdominal pain, rigidity, and tenderness. Eggs from the worms in the intestinal wall may be found in the stool and be accompanied by diarrhea and blood. In the brain the worms may cause Jacksonian epilepsy, hemiplegia, monoplegia, paresis of varying degrees, and visual disturbances. Worms situated in the subcutaneous tissues cause creeping tumors.

Prognosis is good with light infections, with spontaneous cure and death of the worm in 5 to 6 years. It is unfavorable in heavy pulmonary infections and in patients with cerebral involvement. Superimposed tuberculosis and pyogenic infection are especially serious.

Diagnosis. Pulmonary symptoms, blood-tinged sputum, and eosinophilia in patients in endemic regions are suggestive. At times radiographs aid in diagnosis, although it is difficult to differentiate paragonimiasis from tuberculosis, which is common in areas where *Paragonimus* is endemic. A typical roentgenographic finding is a ring-shadowed opacity, 5 to 10 cm, comprising several small contiguous cavities that give the appearance of a bunch of grapes.

Definite diagnosis is established by finding the eggs in the sputum, feces (from swallowed sputum or intestinal lesions), or less frequently in aspirated material from abscesses or pleural effusions. Although eggs are usually present in the sputum, in Taiwan the eggs were found more frequently in the stool. In Korea more than 20 sputum samples of some patients were examined before eggs were detected. At times the adult worm is found at exploratory operation. In ectopic infections, in deep foci with no eggs excreted, complement-fixation and intradermal tests with a *Paragonimus* antigen have been used.

Treatment. Bithionol,° thiobis-dichlorophenol, orally, 30 to 50 mg per kilogram of body weight every other day for 10 to 15 days, gave a cure rate of 90 percent of 1315 persons treated. Side reactions consisted of diarrhea (30 percent), rash (13 percent), and abdominal pain (11 percent). Another drug that can be used is praziquantel, at a dose of 20 mg per kilogram t.i.d. for 2 consecutive days.

Prevention. The most practical method of preventing human infection is to avoid eating raw, freshly pickled, or imperfectly cooked fresh-water crustaceans, and to refrain from drinking unfiltered or unboiled creek water in endemic districts. The best line of attack is public education, since the elimination of reservoir hosts, crustaceans, and snails is not feasible.

REFERENCES

Belamaric: Intrahepatic bile duct carcinoma and *C. sinensis* infection in Hong Kong. Cancer 31: 468, 1973.

Gutman, et al: Radiographic changes accompanying successful therapy of pulmonary paragonomiasis. Am Rev Resp Dis 99: 255–260, 1969.

Jones, et al: Massive infection with *Fasciola hepatica* in man. Am J Med 63: 836–842, 1977.

Markell: Laboratory findings in chronic clonorchiasis. Am J Trop Med Hyg 15: 510–515, 1966.

Plaut, et al: A clinical study of *Fasciolopsis buski* infection in Thailand. Trans R Soc Trop Med Hyg 63: 470–478, 1969.

Wykoff, et al: Clinical manifestations of *Opisthorchis viverrini* infections in Thailand. Am J Trop Med Hyg 15: 914–918, 1966.

Yokagawa: Paragonimus and paragonimiasis. In Dawes (eds): Advances in Parasitology, Vol 7, Academic Press, 1969, p. 375–387. New York.

13

Blood Flukes of Human Beings

The blood flukes, the most important digenetic trematodes of humans, include three important species: *Schistosoma haematobium,* an inhabitant of the vesical veins; *S. mansoni*; and *S. japonicum* of the intestinal veins.

BIOLOGY OF SCHISTOSOMES OF HUMAN BEINGS

Morphology. The schistosomes differ from the typical trematodes in their narrow, elongated shape and separate sexes. The distinctive morphologic characteristics of the three species are given in Figure 13-1. The larger, grayish male has a cylindrical anterior end, and its heavier body is folded to form a long ventral gynecophoric canal in which the darker, slender female is embraced during copulation (Fig. 13-1). The tegument is smooth or tuberculated, depending upon the species. The intestine bifurcates into two ceca, which unite in the posterior part of the body in a single blind stem. The number of testes in the male, and the length of the uterus and

number of eggs, are distinctive to the species. The excretory system consists of flame cells, collecting tubules, and two long tubules leading into a small bladder with a terminal excretory pore.

Life Cycle (Figs. 13-2 and 13-3). The delicate adult worms, which are 0.6 to 2.5 cm in length, reside in pairs, the female lying in the gynecophoric canal of the male. Depending upon the species of worm, from 300 *(S. mansoni)* to 3500 *(S. japonicum)* eggs are passed daily into the venules. A larval form, miracidium, develops within the egg; its lytic enzymes and the contraction of the venule rupture the wall of the venule, liberating the egg into the perivascular tissues of the intestine or urinary bladder. The eggs effect a passage into the lumens of these organs and are evacuated in the feces or the urine. On contact with fresh water the miracidia hatch from the eggs and swim about until they find an appropriate snail, which they penetrate. After two generations of sporocyst development and multiplication within the snail, the forked-tailed cercariae emerge. During bathing, swimming,

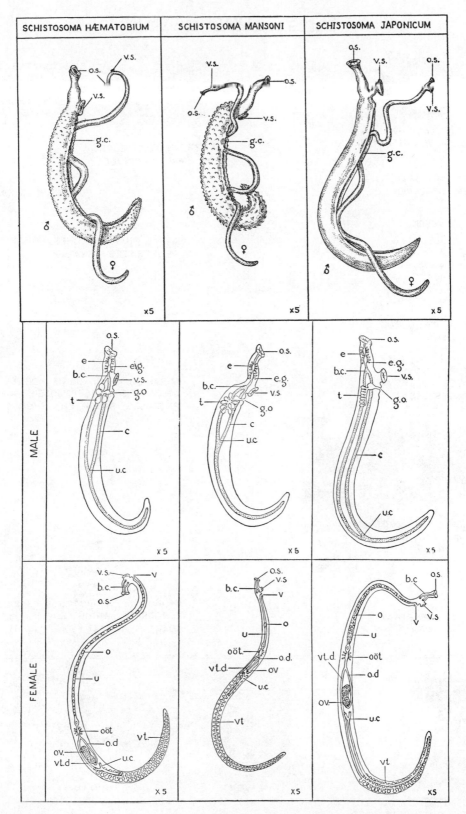

Figure 13-1. Schematic representation of important schistosomes of humans.
b.c., bifurcation of ceca; c, ceca; e, esophagus; e.g., esophageal glands; g.c., gynecophoric canal; g.o., genital orifice; o, eggs; o.d., oviduct; oöt., ootype; o.s., oral sucker; ov., ovary; t, testes; u, uterus; u.c., union of ceca; v, vulva; v.s., ventral sucker; vt., vitellaria; vt.d., vitelline duct.

SCHISTOSOMA MANSONI

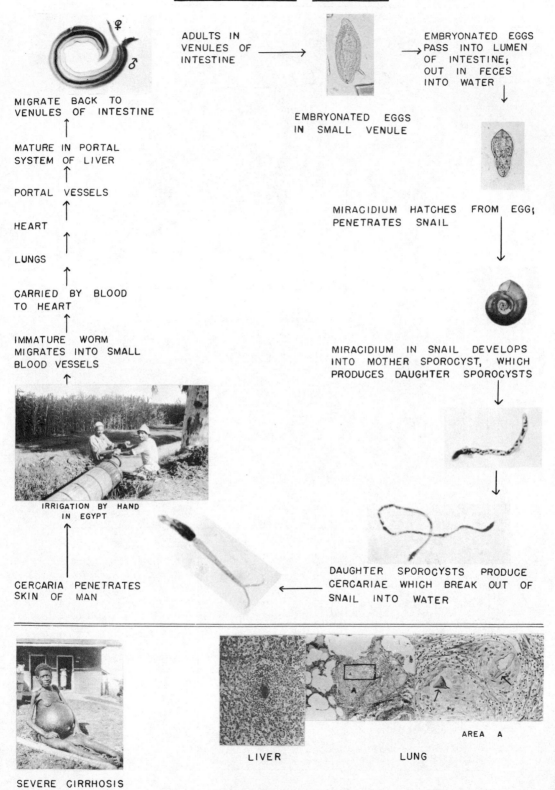

ADULTS IN
VENULES OF
INTESTINE →

EMBRYONATED EGGS
PASS INTO LUMEN
OF INTESTINE;
OUT IN FECES
INTO WATER

MIGRATE BACK TO
VENULES OF INTESTINE

EMBRYONATED EGGS
IN SMALL VENULE

MATURE IN PORTAL
SYSTEM OF LIVER

PORTAL VESSELS

HEART

LUNGS

CARRIED BY BLOOD
TO HEART

IMMATURE WORM
MIGRATES INTO SMALL
BLOOD VESSELS

MIRACIDIUM HATCHES FROM EGG;
PENETRATES SNAIL

MIRACIDIUM IN SNAIL DEVELOPS
INTO MOTHER SPOROCYST, WHICH
PRODUCES DAUGHTER SPOROCYSTS

IRRIGATION BY HAND
IN EGYPT

CERCARIA PENETRATES
SKIN OF MAN

DAUGHTER SPOROCYSTS PRODUCE
CERCARIAE WHICH BREAK OUT OF
SNAIL INTO WATER

SEVERE CIRRHOSIS
WITH ASCITES

LIVER

LUNG

AREA A

EGGS STIMULATING FORMATION OF PSEUDOTUBERCLES

Figure 13-2. Life cycle of *Schistosoma mansoni*.

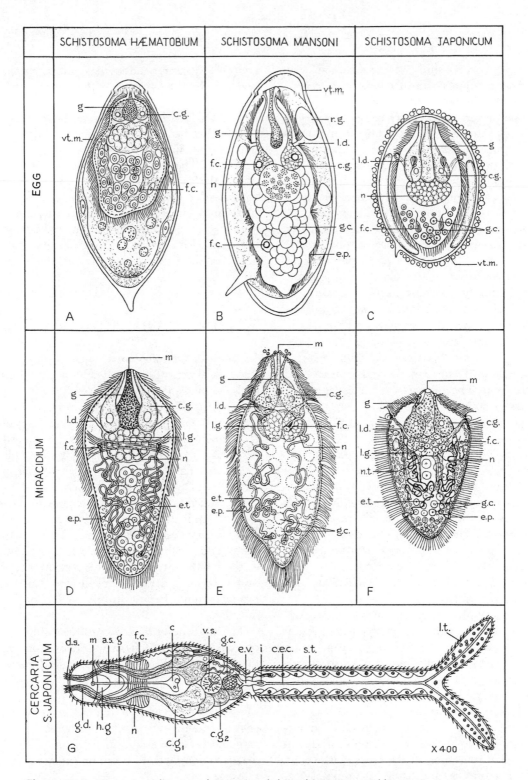

Figure 13-3. Egg, miracidium, and cercaria of the schistosomes of humans.

a.s., anterior sucker; c, cecum; c.e.c., caudal excretory canal; c.g., c.g.-1, c.g.-2, cephalic glands; d.s., duct spines; e.p., excretory pore; e.t., excretory tubule; e.v., excretory vesicle; f.c., flame cell; g, gut; g.c., germinal cells; g.d., gland ducts; h.g., head gland; i, island of Cort; l.d., lateral duct; l.g., lateral gland; l.t., lobe of tail; m, mouth; n, nervous system; n.t., nerve trunk; r.g., refractile globule; s.t., stem of tail; v.s., ventral sucker; vt.m., vitelline membrane.

working, or washing clothes, human skin comes in contact with free-swimming cercariae, which become attached and burrow down to the peripheral capillary bed as the surface film of water drains off, losing their tails as they enter the skin. If ingested with water, the cercariae penetrate the mucous membranes of the mouth and throat. The cercariae are transported through the afferent blood to the right heart and lungs. They squeeze through the pulmonary capillaries, are carried into the systemic circulation, and pass through to the portal vessels. Within the intrahepatic portion of the portal system, the blood flukes feed and grow rapidly. Approximately 3 weeks after skin exposure, the adolescent worms migrate against the portal blood flow into the mesenteric, vesical, and pelvic venules. The prepatent period for *S. mansoni* is 7 to 8 weeks; *S. haematobium*, 10 to 12 weeks; and *S. japonicum*, 5 to 6 weeks. The adult worms live as long as 30 years in humans.

Humanity is the principal host of the three species of human schistosomes.

Response of the Host. Schistosomiasis in humans may be divided into 3 stages: (1) developmental, from the penetration of the skin to the mature adult worms, (2) active oviposition and extrusion of eggs, and (3) proliferation and repair. The lesions produced by the three species are similar during the first period but, during the overlapping second and third stages, differ chiefly in tissue selectivity and site of oviposition.

The pathologic changes during the developmental period include negligible to mild cutaneous lesions at the site of cercarial entry, tissue reactions to the immature worms inside and outside of the blood vessels, and associated toxic and allergic reactions. The invasion of the tissues by the migrating larval and adolescent worms produces petechial hemorrhages and small foci of eosinophilic and neutrophilic infiltration in the lungs, with cough and hemoptysis, and acute inflammatory reactions in the liver, with fever and urticaria.

The eruption of the eggs through the vascular endothelium is brought about by collagenaselike enzymic secretions, pressure, and an endothelial or subendothelial inflammatory reaction. In the vascular endothelium, perivascular tissues, and parenchyma of the various organs, the eggs produce multiple foci of inflammatory cellular infiltration that develop into granulomas or nonnecrotizing pseudotubercles. The fundamental histopathologic unit is the pseudotubercle (Fig. 13-7), which consists of a layer of epithelioid cells, fibroblasts and giant cells surrounded by a zone of plasma cells and eosinophils. In addition to the usual selective intestinal and urinary bladder sites, the eggs are usually distributed to other organs of the body.

VESICAL SCHISTOSOMIASIS

Schistosoma haematobium

Diseases. Schistosomal hematuria, vesical schistosomiasis, urinary bilharziasis.

Epidemiology. The distribution of the schistosomes of humanity is governed by the range of their molluscan hosts (Fig. 13-4). *S. haematobium* is highly endemic in the entire Nile valley and has spread over practically all of Africa and the islands of Malagasy and Mauritius. Endemic foci are also found in Jordan, Syria, Iraq, Iran, Arabia, Yemen, and a small area on the west coast of India. In areas of Egypt and the rest of Africa, 75 to 95 percent of the inhabitants may be infected. Monkeys and baboons are naturally infected but are probably unimportant in the spread of the infection.

The snail hosts of *S. haematobium* are nonoperculate, reside in fresh water, and belong to the genera *Bulinus, Physopsis, and Biomphalaria.*

Pathology and Symptomatology. As *S. haematobium* lives primarily in the pelvic veins, its eggs are mainly deposited in the vesical plexuses and produce lesions in the urinary bladder, genitalia, and, to a minor extent, in the intestine.

The eggs of *S. haematobium* in the bladder wall are distributed in the submucosa and to a lesser extent in the mucosa, while some occlude the blood vessels (Fig. 13-3A). The resulting inflammatory condition leads to progressive changes in the bladder and neighboring tissues. The early changes are a diffuse hyperemia and minute vesicular or papular elevation of the mucosa. Papillomatous folds and polypoid excrescences develop as the disease progresses. Later inflammatory patches consisting of sloughing tissue, calcium deposits, and eggs give the mucosa a sandy or granular appearance, especially at the trigone

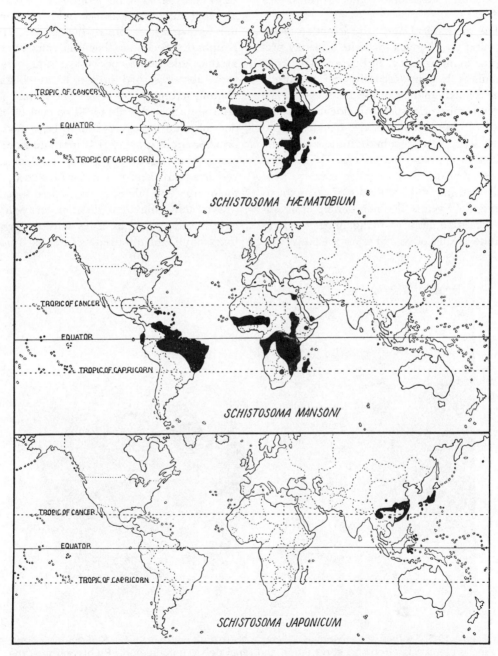

Figure 13-4. Geographic distribution of *Schistosoma haematobium, S. japonicum,* and *S. mansoni.* (From Belding: Textbook of Parasitology, 3rd ed., 1965. Courtesy of Appleton-Century-Crofts.)

of the bladder. Uric acid and oxalate crystals, phosphatic deposits, eggs, blood clots, mucus, pus, and sloughed-off papillomas may be present in the urine. The urethra may be occluded, the ureters obstructed, and the pelvis of the kidney occasionally affected (Figs. 13-5 and 13-6).

The mechanical and toxic irritation of the eggs and the chemical deposits evidently predispose to malignancy. In Egypt vesical schistosomiasis is considered the most common cause of malignancy of the bladder in male agricultural workers. The incidence of squamous cell epithelioma of the bladder in patients with vesical schistosomiasis is many times that in uninfected persons. The age incidence is below that of other cancers, most patients being under 40 years of age, some as young as 10 years. The relationship of intestinal schistosomiasis to malignancy is not as definite as that of vesical schistosomiasis.

In the male the seminal vesicles are most frequently affected, sometimes without bladder involvement, and the prostate less frequently. The changes consist of congestion, tissue proliferation, and finally adhesive fibrosis. The external male genitalia may assume an elephantoid appearance, with papillomatous growths from obstruction of the scrotal lymphatics. Secondary bacterial infection may produce ulceration, perivesical and periurethral abscesses, and fistulas of the bladder, rectum, scrotum, and penis. The female genitalia are affected in 80 to 90 percent of bladder infections: the vulva may have nodular papillomatous growths that may ulcerate; the cervix and vaginal walls may be thickened; vesicovaginal fistulas may be produced; and the ovaries and tubes may be matted together.

Symptoms may not develop for years in light infections, but in heavy infections symptoms may be first noticed as early as 1 month

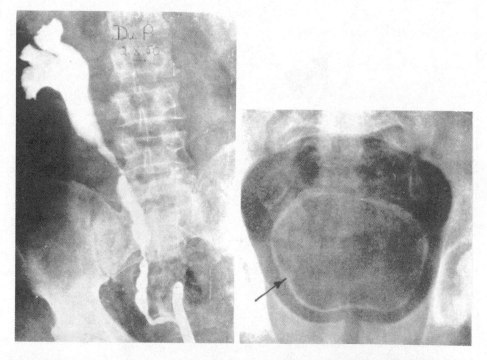

Figure 13-5. Urinary schistosomiasis. Left. *Schistosoma haematobium.* Radiograph showing ureteral dilatation and constriction and renal pelvic enlargement. Right. *Schistosoma haematobium.* Radiograph of urinary bladder showing calcification. (From Honey, Gelfand, Blair: Urological Aspects of Bharziasis in Rhodesia, 1960. Courtesy of E. & S. Livingstone, Ltd.)

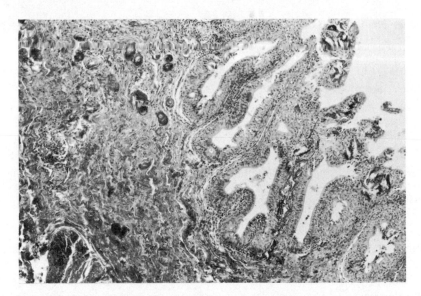

Figure 13-6. Urinary bladder heavily invaded with *Schistosoma haematobium* eggs. (× 50)

after infection. The eggs first appear in the urine in 10 to 12 weeks after infection. The most characteristic symptom is hematuria, usually with blood in the terminal drops of urine, although the whole output may be blood-tinged. As the mucosal surfaces become inflamed, painful micturition and frequency begin, and mucus and pus are found in the urine. The greatly thickened bladder wall loses its elasticity, and there is a constant urinary residual. Daily temperature elevation, sweating, malaise, weakness, and dull pain in the suprapubic region occur. The leukocyte count is increased, and there is usually eosinophilia. There is progressive cystitis with ascending secondary infection of the ureters and kidneys, and hydronephrosis. Urinary fistulas of the scrotum, perineum, and adjacent areas are common. A few patients show intestinal and rectal involvement. Liver involvement, although not less frequent, is much less severe than in *S. japonicum* and *S. mansoni* infection. Pulmonary involvement results early from the migrating immature schistosomes, and later from the embolic eggs, which produce mild parenchymatous pneumonitis around the bronchi and alveoli but at times cause more serious necrotizing and obliterative arterial lesions with hyperplasia of the endothelium,

hyaline thrombosis, and diffuse fibrous thickening of the intima. The endarteritis and periarteritis appear to be allergic responses to substances elaborated by the miracidium in the egg. The condition, known as *cor pulmonale,* results from pulmonary hypertension and leads to hypertrophy of the right ventricle and, finally, right heart failure.

Autopsy of a series of patients harboring *S. haematobium* revealed eggs in the following organs (expressed in percentages): urinary bladder, 80; ureters, 69; kidney, 46; vagina, 81; cervix, 75; uterus, 79; fallopian tubes, 12; ovaries, 67; prostate, 55; testes, 34; liver, 43; gallbladder, 38; pancreas, 35; stomach, 32; small intestine, 34; cecum, 54; appendix, 60; ascending colon, 66; transverse colon, 73; descending colon, 65; rectum, 75; suprarenal gland, 26; mesenteric lymph nodes, 32; and spleen, 34.

When large numbers of eggs are deposited in these various organs and tissues, symptoms may be produced.

Diagnosis. The eggs are identified in the urine by direct examination of the last few drops of urine passed at noon, or in the urine after exercise or prostatic massage. A simple concentration test for diagnosis is sedimentation in a conical urinalysis glass of a day's output of urine. The addition of water, previously heated to 60 C to kill any infusoria, to the sediment permits the hatched free-swimming miracidia to be detected by indirect lighting against a black background. The hatching of miracidia also furnishes an index of whether the eggs are viable.

Treatment. Correction of anemia is indicated, and the patient should be brought to a satisfactory physical state before chemotherapy. Four chemotherapeutic agents are available: Metrifonate, 7.5 mg per kilogram orally every 2 weeks for three doses; niridazole, 25 mg per kilogram orally for 5 to 7 days; praziquantel, in a single dose of 40 mg per kilogram orally; and antimony dimercaptosuccinate, in a dose of 8 mg per kilogram intramuscularly every second or third day for a total of five doses. The metrifonate and praziquantel are the least toxic. Niridazole can sometimes cause severe central nervous system symptoms, especially if liver disease is present.

Prognosis. The prognosis of vesical schistosomiasis is good, except in the late ulcerative stages, because *S. haematobium* is relatively susceptible to chemotherapy. Patients with chronic severe infections and superimposed septic infections, especially the old and debilitated, have a poor prognosis. Death usually occurs from exhaustion, pneumonia, or superimposed infections.

INTESTINAL SCHISTOSOMIASIS

Schistosoma mansoni

Diseases. Intestinal bilharziasis, schistosomal dysentery.

Epidemiology. *S. mansoni* is spread less widely in Africa than is *S. haematobium,* occurring intensely in the Nile Delta north of Cairo, and in East Africa from the Upper Nile to Southern Rhodesia, the Republic of the Congo, West Africa east and southeast of Senegal, with several foci in Natal, and on the east coast of Malagasy. Scattered foci are reported in Arabia and Yemen. The parasite, probably introduced into the Western Hemisphere by

the slave trade, is established in Brazil, Colombia, Venezuela, Surinam, Puerto Rico, Viequez, Antigua, Dominican Republic, Guadeloupe, Martinique, Montserrat, Nevis, and St. Lucia. It is not in Barbados, Cuba, Haiti, Jamaica, Trinidad, or the Virgin Islands.

The fresh-water snail intermediate hosts are *Biomphalaria* in Africa and *Biomphalaria (Australorbis)* and *Tropicorbis* in South America and the West Indies.

Rodents, monkeys, and baboons have been found infected in nature.

Schistosoma japonicum

Diseases. Oriental schistosomiasis, Katayama disease.

S. japonicum is confined to the Far East. It is highly endemic in the Yangtze River valley of Central China and it is present in less abundance on the east coast, south to Hong Kong. There are five endemic areas in the coastal river valleys of Japan, numerous foci in the islands of Mindanao, Mindoro, Luzon, Samar, and Leyte in the Philippines, a small focus in the Celebes, and a focus in Thailand. An animal focus is present in Taiwan, but no human infections have been found. *Oncomelania* which inhabit canals, ditches, and marshes serve as intermediate hosts. The numerous reservoir hosts include rats, mice, cats, dogs, horses, cows, water buffalo, and swine. A focus of human schistosomiasis similar to *S. japonicum,* but belonging to a distinct species called *S. mekongi,* has been discovered in Laos, along the Mekong River. The eggs are similar to those of *S. japonicum,* as are the disease and the treatment for it.

S. mansoni and S. japonicum

Pathology and Symptomatology. The incubation period is initiated by the penetration of the skin by cercariae, which may produce a transient pruritus and rash. During the invasion of the liver and other organs by the immature worms, petechial hemorrhages and foci of eosinophilic and leukocytic infiltration are produced. Toxic and allergic reactions may cause urticaria, subcutaneous edema, asthmatic attacks, leukocytosis, and eosinophilia. Toward the end of the incubation period the liver becomes enlarged and tender, and there are abdominal discomfort, fever, sweating, chilliness, and sometimes diarrhea. The young worms now migrate against the bloodstream—*S. japonicum* mainly to the superior mesenteric and *S. mansoni* mainly to the mesenteric veins—and their eggs invade the walls of the small and large intestines, respectively.

With the initiation of egg laying, the acute stage begins. In the normal cycle the eggs work their way through the intestinal wall and escape in the feces. When numerous, they are accompanied by blood and necrotic tissue cells. Many eggs are swept back into the bloodstream to the liver and spleen.

Autopsies of 110 persons infected with *S. mansoni* revealed eggs in the following organs (expressed in percentages): liver, 20; gallbladder, 4; lungs, 24; pancreas, 5; stomach, 11; small intestine, 16; cecum, 23; appendix, 8; ascending colon, 29; transverse colon, 36; descending colon, 38; rectum, 44; suprarenal gland, 2; mesenteric lymph nodes, 2; spleen, 2; urinary bladder, 14; vagina, 19; cervix, 6; uterus, 21; kidney, 2; ureters, 6; prostate, 7; and testes, 6.

The stage of acute symptoms marks the onset of invasion of the intestines, liver, and lungs by the eggs. It is characterized by fever, malaise, urticaria, eosinophilia, abdominal discomfort, diarrhea, weight loss, cough, a slightly enlarged liver, and sometimes an enlarged spleen. In the chronic disease, which begins after 1.5 years in heavy infection and in 4 to 5 years in light infection, there is loss of weight, anemia, symptoms referable to the intestinal tract, and, often, splenomegaly, periportal fibrosis (Symmer's) of the liver, and ascites.

The eggs of *S. mansoni* and *S. japonicum* are deposited in the mesenteric lymph nodes and the intestinal wall. The most severe lesions are caused by *S. japonicum,* which produces about 10 times as many eggs as *S. mansoni.* The invading eggs evoke an intense cellular infiltration in the intestinal wall with extensive fibrous tissue proliferation, formation of papillomas, and thrombosis of the small blood vessels (Fig. 13-7). The early changes are congestion, granular or hypertrophic mucosa, yellowish papillae (diagnostic), and ulcerations, and in the late disease, polyps and strictures. The entire intestinal wall, including the peritoneal surface, may be included in the process and may be bound down by mesenteric and omental adhesions. Fibrous constrictions of the irregularly thickened wall may cause the tearing off of papillomas and polyps, and secondary bacterial infections may produce the discharge of blood, pus, and eggs into the intestinal lumen. In advanced cases, relaxation of the anal sphincter may permit the prolapse of pedunculated papillomatous masses. Fistulas may extend to the ischiorectal fossa, perineum, buttocks, or bladder. Eggs are found in the appendix in 75 percent of intestinal infections, at times accompanied by

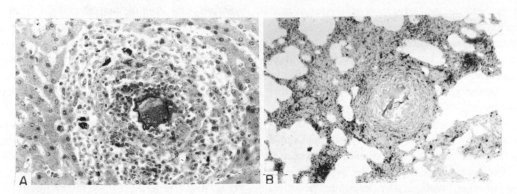

Figure 13-7. Pseudotubercle formation around eggs of *Schistosoma mansoni.* A. Liver. ($\times$ 200) B. Lung. ($\times$ 50)

secondary bacterial invasion, but they rarely are responsible for an appendicitis syndrome.

The embolic eggs are chiefly responsible for the progressive fibroblastic proliferation and periductal fibrosis with rising portal hypertension (Fig. 13-2). Toxins from the adult worms, pigment, and hypoproteinemia from malnutrition may also play a part in the production of the hepatic lesions. Hepatic fibrosis, which leads to cirrhosis, is common in *S. mansoni* and *S. japonicum* infections but is infrequent in *S. haematobium* disease. It is difficult to separate the contribution of schistosomiasis from other causes of liver disease, such as viral hepatitis, alcoholism, and nutritional factors. Ultrasound examination appears to be useful in demonstrating schistosomal periportal fibrosis. In late cases, ascites and its attendant complications may develop. The condition of the portal system may be ascertained by roentgenography and venography.

In early stages of the initial infection, the spleen may show congestion, medullary hyperplasia, and slight enlargement. In the late stages, splenomegaly is caused chiefly by portal obstruction and, to a lesser extent, by the invasion of the eggs and the reticuloendothelial reaction to the toxic products of the worms. Splenomegaly occurs less frequently with *S. haematobium* than with the other two species. Splenectomy may be indicated when there are esophageal varicosities, progressive cirrhosis of the liver with portal hypertension, ascites, and leukopenia.

Abdominal tenderness, hepatitis, anorexia, fever, headache, myalgia, dysentery, and weight loss are characteristic of intestinal schistosomiasis. The acute stage lasts 3 to 4 months, and it is more severe in heavy infections and in *S. japonicum* infections because of the larger number of eggs produced by this species.

The chronic stage of the disease may develop in 18 months with heavy infections and as late as 25 years in light *S. mansoni* infections.

The liver is enlarged in the acute stage of the disease, but as the infection becomes chronic the liver recedes in size and, although usually slightly enlarged, may become subnormal in size. A firm, palpable left lobe under the xiphoid is a characteristic finding in Symmer's fibrosis. The liver cells are atrophied, and there is a periportal fibrosis. Although the fibrosis of the liver may be extreme, especially in *S. japonicum* infections, interference with bile flow rarely occurs. Severe ascites may develop, and dilated abdominal, thoracic, and esophageal veins are often present. The SGOT and SGPT may be normal or slightly elevated.

Depending upon the intensity and duration of the chronic infection, the patient may have a colitis of varying degree, with the formation of polyps. Headache, malaise, irregular slight fever, diarrhea, and abdominal pain are common. The appetite becomes poor, and the patient loses weight. As the disease progresses the red blood cells gradually decrease to below 3 million with a corresponding reduction in hemoglobin, producing hypochromic anemia. There is leukocytosis of above 10,000 in 75 percent of patients in the early stages of the disease, and leukopenia in the late stages. Eosinophilia, which occurs early in the infection, often disappears in chronic infections. The blood serum shows an increase in gamma globulin and a decrease in albumin. The sedimentation rate is increased. Eggs that pass into the systemic circulation and are filtered out in the lungs, brain, or spinal cord produce various pulmonary and nervous disorders.

The uncommon cerebral infections, chiefly caused by *S. japonicum,* are due to embolic eggs, which act mechanically, as foreign proteins, and as toxic agents, to set up an intense reaction with edema, neural cellular infiltration, foreign body cells, phlebotic changes, and degeneration of the surrounding tissues.

The symptoms encountered are headache, disorientation, coma, aphasia, amnesia, confusion, paraplegia, spasticity, altered reflexes, incontinence, cranial nerve involvement, and Jacksonian epilepsy. Eggs carried to the lungs produce an arteriolitis and fibrosis resulting in cor pulmonale and a right ventricular failure.

The chronic stage may be prolonged for years, and the patient may die of pneumonia or other infections or of rupture of esophageal varices.

Diagnosis. As schistosome eggs may be few in number, large quantities of stool must be sedimented. This is one product that the patient can supply abundantly and free. The examination of a small specimen may give negative results. Eggs may be few in number owing to a light infection, the intermittency of their discharge, or a chronic infection; hence, concentration by sedimentation should be employed. A whole stool should be thoroughly broken up in 0.5 percent glycerol water and, after sedimentation in a conical glass, the supernatant fluid poured off. Mixing and decanting should be repeated until only a small residue remains, which should be examined microscopically for eggs.

Biopsies by sigmoidoscopic method often yield eggs when the fecal examinations are negative. These mucosal snips, unfixed and unstained, should be pressed between two glass microscope slides and examined for eggs under the low power of the microscope. Occasionally, when eggs cannot be found in the feces or rectal mucosa, a liver biopsy may reveal their presence.

All eggs from the feces, urine, or tissues should be examined under high power to determine their viability by the activity of the cilia of the excretory flame cell of the enclosed miracidium. Dead eggs may persist for a long time after successful therapy or natural death of the worms, and their presence should not lead to therapy.

Various serologic and intradermal tests are useful and, when positive, should stimulate a thorough search for eggs. Various animal schistosomes which temporarily invade man may cause falsely positive results. The complement-fixation test remains positive at least 4 years after chemotherapeutic cure.

Treatment. The most effective drug for treatment of *S. mansoni* infection is an oral drug, oxamniquine. It is used in a single dose of 15 mg per kilogram for infections of New World origin, but infections of Old World origin generally require two to four doses of oxamniquine. Niridazole° and praziquantel can also be used, in similar doses as used for *S. haematobium* infections. Antimony dimercapto-succinate can also be used, but it is generally more toxic than the drugs suggested above; in addition, it must be given parenterally.

S. japonicum is the most resistant form of human schistosomiasis to drug treatment. While some of the oral drugs used for treatment of other species, such as niridazole and oxamniquine, show some effect against *S. japonicum,* they are clearly suboptimal. Fortunately, the new oral drug, praziquantel, is quite effective against *S. japonicum.* The dose is 20 mg per kilogram every 4 hours for three doses.

Prevention. Prevention of schistosomiasis includes (1) reduction of sources of infection, (2) protection of snail-bearing waters from contamination with infectious urine or feces, (3) control of snail hosts, and (4) protection of persons from cercaria-infested waters.

Theoretically, the sources of infection of *S. mansoni* and *S. haematobium* may be reduced by the detection and treatment of infected persons, but difficulties in diagnosis, the unsuitability of chemotherapeutic agents to mass therapy, and constant reinfection reduce the effectiveness of this method unless combined with vector control. The presence of animal reservoir hosts renders chemotherapy of less value for the control of *S. japonicum.* Until a cheap, nontoxic, effective, preferably oral, chemotherapeutic agent is developed, mass treatment cannot be attempted with any expectation of success.

The protection of waters from contamination involves excreta disposal. The sanitary disposal of human feces and urine should eradicate the disease, but its practice runs counter to economic, racial, and religious customs, and to the primitive habit of promiscuous defecation and urination in or near snail-infested waters. The economic need for night soil for fertilizer in the Orient is a complicating factor, although composting of night soil prior to use will kill the eggs. Populations must be educated to use sanitary toilet facilities and to avoid contact with infected water. Safe facilities for bathing and washing of clothes must be provided.

The eradication of snails may be attempted

by removal of vegetation, desiccation by drainage, reduction in number by capture with hand nets or palm-leaf traps, introduction of natural enemies, and molluscacides. Control of snails is accomplished with copper sulfate, sodium pentachlorphenate, dinitro-o-cyclohexylphenol, Bayluscide, and zinc dimethyldithiocarbamate. The cercariae are killed by chlorine, 1 ppm, in 10 to 20 minutes. Aquatic migration of snails from nontreated areas into treated areas complicates this method of control.

The avoidance of contact with waters infested with cercariae affords complete protection, but, unfortunately, prohibition of bathing, wading, or working in and the drinking of infested waters cannot be enforced and is nullified by agricultural and other practices. Agricultural workers may be partially protected by clothing, boots, or repellents, but economic considerations, conveniences of working, and ignorance tend to make such measures impracticable.

SCHISTOSOME DERMATITIS

Diseases. Swimmer's itch, clam digger's itch.

Schistosome cercariae of several avain and mammalian hosts penetrate the skin but can progress no further and are destroyed in the skin, producing a dermatitis. A number of migratory birds, including several species of ducks, harbor the adult worms and, wherever in their travels the suitable snail host is present, the dermatitis may be found in humans. Recognition of this clinical entity is gradually expanding the known geographic distribution of the disease (Fig. 13-8).

Geographic Distribution. Distribution is probably cosmopolitan. At least 25 species of cercariae from fresh-water snail hosts and at least 4 from marine snails have been reported, and probably many other species exist. The disease was first recognized in Michigan in 1928 by Cort and has been reported from the United States, Canada, Europe, Mexico, Central America, Japan, Malaya, Australia, India, Af-

rica, Alaska, South America, Cuba, and New Zealand. Marine forms cause a dermatitis among clam diggers and sea bathers on the east and west coasts of the United States and in Hawaii. The cercariae from the snails either swarm in shallow water or are swept toward the shore by wave action. Their free-swimming existence lasts about 24 hours. The distribution and habits of the snail hosts determine the infestation of bathing beaches.

Pathology and Symptomatology. The cercariae, "strangers in a strange land," are walled off and destroyed in the epithelial layers of the skin, although occasionally some may escape to the lungs. They evoke an acute inflammatory response with edema, early infiltration of neutrophils and lymphocytes, and later invasion of eosinophils. Penetration may take place in the water, but usually it occurs as the film of water evaporates on the skin. A prickling sensation is followed by the rapid development of urticarial wheals, which subside in about half an hour, leaving a few minute macules. After some hours of severe itching, edema, and the transformation of the macules into papules, occasionally pustules occur, reaching maximal intensity in 2 to 3 days. The papular and sometimes hemorrhagic rash heals in a week or more, but may be complicated by scratching and secondary infection. In cases of heavy infection there may be a general reaction with prostration. There is marked individual variation in the reaction to infection.

The reaction is essentially a sensitization phenomenon. The local skin lesions produced by the schistosomes of humans are slight, but with continuous reinfection, sensitized persons may show a definite dermatitis. The dermatitis produced by the animal schistosomes ranges from mild to severe, depending upon the immune response of the individual. Repeated infections tend to become more and more severe.

Diagnosis. History of contact with water and a cutaneous rash. Serologic and skin tests may be positive, leading to a mistaken diagnosis of human schistosomiasis. Patients should not be

SCHISTOSOME DERMATITIS

FRESH-WATER   **"SWIMMER'S ITCH"**   **"WATER ITCH"**

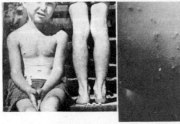 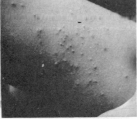

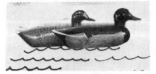

ADULTS IN MESENTERIC VENULES OF
DUCKS, SHORE BIRDS, MICE, MUSKRATS

LESIONS PRODUCED
BY CERCARIAE IN
SKIN OF MAN

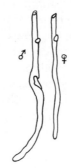 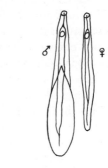

♂   ♀   ♂   ♀

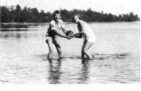

TRICHOBILHARZIA SPP.   SCHISTOSOMATIUM SP.

NORMAL CYCLE

  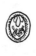

EGG   PASSED   IN   FECES   INTO   WATER

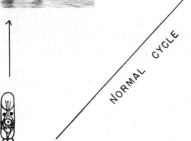

MIRACIDIUM   HATCHES   FROM
EGG, PENETRATES   SNAIL

CERCARIA   BREAKS   OUT
OF   SNAIL   INTO   WATER,
PENETRATES   SKIN   OF
WARM-BLOODED   ANIMALS

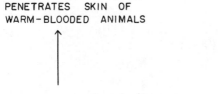

DAUGHTER SPOROCYST ← MOTHER SPOROCYST
IN   SNAIL   SNAIL   HOSTS

MARINE   "CLAM-DIGGER'S ITCH"   "SEA-BATHER'S ERUPTION"

ADULTS, MICROBILHARZIA SP.,
IN DUCKS AND SHORE BIRDS

SNAIL

HOST

Figure 13-8. Schistosome dermatitis.

245

treated for schistosomiasis until live eggs are found.

Treatment. Antipruritic and antihistaminic lotions are of palliative value. Antimicrobial drugs should be used for secondary bacterial infection.

Prevention. The removal of snails from the neighborhood of bathing beaches is the most practical method of combating "swimmer's itch." The snails may be destroyed by removal of vegetation, and by molluscacides. A mixture of two parts copper sulfate and one part copper carbonate at 3 pounds per 1000 square feet has proved effective. Sodium pentachlorphenate should also be of value. Vigorous rubbing of the body with a towel immediately after the bather leaves the water tends to prevent the penetration of the skin by cercariae.

REFERENCES

Blood Flukes of Man
Hiatt, et al: Factors in the pathogenesis of acute schistosomiasis mansoni. J Infect Dis 139: 659–666, 1979.

Lo Verde, et al: Parasite-parasite interaction of *Salmonella typhimurium* and *Schistosoma*. J Infect Dis 141: 177–185, 1980.

Nash, et al: Schistosome infections in man. Perspectives and recent findings. Ann Intern Med. In press, 1982.

Warren: Regulation of the prevalence and intensity of schistosomiasis in man. Immunology or ecology? J Infect Dis 127: 595–609, 1973.

ARTHROPODA

14

Arthropods Injurious to Human Beings

The widely distributed and diversified phylum ARTHROPODA contains more species than all the other phyla of the animal kingdom and is humanity's principal competitor for this earth.

Adult and larval arthropods may injure humans by venenation, vesication, blood sucking, and tissue invasion, and they transmit bacterial, rickettsial, spirochetal, viral, and animal parasitic diseases.

Arthropods are characterized by bilateral symmetry, metameric segmentation, jointed appendages, and a hard exoskeleton. The body comprises head, thorax, and abdomen. The paired appendages are modified into walking legs in the terrestrial species and swimming organs in the aquatic. The appendages of the head are variously adapted as sensory, masticating, or piercing organs. The eyes are compound or simple. Digestive, vascular, excretory, and nervous systems are present. Respiration usually is accomplished in the aquatic forms by gills and in the terrestrial by tracheae, tubular extensions of the outer covering. Usually the sexes are separate, and re-

production is sexual, although parthenogenesis may occur.

The ARTHROPODA are divided into five classes. The ONYCHOPHORA are not injurious; the MYRIAPODA have only the poisonous millipedes and centipedes; and the CRUSTACEA contain a few species that serve as intermediate hosts for animal parasites. The INSECTA and ARACHNIDA include most of the parasitic species or vectors of disease.

CLASS MYRIAPODA

The elongated, terrestrial myriapods have numerous segments bearing legs and tracheal stigmata. The two principal orders are the DIPLOPODA (millipedes) and the CHILOPODA (centipedes). The herbivorous millipedes have been incriminated as hosts of the cestode *Hymenolepis diminuta,* and some produce vesicating agents, i.e., material that can irritate the skin.

Order Chilopoda. The poisonous, carnivorous centipedes, 5 to 25 cm in length, have flattened bodies and a single pair of legs on most segments. They live in damp localities under bark, rubbish, or stones, and feed on insects and small animals. The first body segment bears a pair of claws with openings at the tips for the expulsion of a paralyzing venom that is contained in a gland at the base of the claw. The small centipedes of the temperate zones are often incapable of penetrating the skin, and their mild bites seldom produce little more than a sharp pain, erythema, and, sometimes, induration. The larger tropical and subtropical genus *Scolopendra* (Fig. 14-1) inflicts painful bites and even causes necrotic local lesions. No authenticated deaths from uncomplicated centipede bites have been reported.

The puncture wounds caused by the ven-omous claws of centipedes may be treated locally with ammonia, alcoholic iodine, or soothing lotions. The painful systemic symptoms produced by the larger centipedes may require analgesics.

CLASS CRUSTACEA

The aquatic CRUSTACEA contain the species that are intermediate hosts of animal parasites of human beings.

Order Copepoda. Copepods are small, graceful, symmetrical animals with the head and first two thoracic segments fused into a cephalothorax, and a slender abdomen of 3 to 5 segments. *Cyclops* are intermediate hosts of the Guinea worm *Dracunculus medinensis*, the ces-

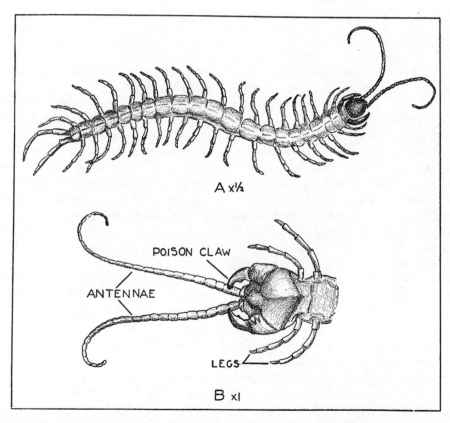

Figure 14-1. Schematic representation of centipede *(Scolopendra)*. A. Dorsal view of centipede. B. Ventral view of head.

tode *Diphyllobothrium latum,* and the nematode *Gnathostoma spinigerum.* Species of *Diaptomus* are hosts of *D. latum.*

Order Decapoda. The DECAPODA include the large crustaceans, such as shrimps, crayfish, lobsters, and crabs. Species of fresh-water crabs and crayfish are second intermediate hosts of the lung fluke *Paragonimus westermani.* Land crabs *(Cardisoma, Birgus,)* and the fresh-water prawn harbor the infective rat lung-worm larvae *(Angiostrongylus)* that infect the human brain.

15

Class Insecta

The numerous species of insects play an important role in the economic life of human beings. Relatively few species are parasites of humans or act as vectors of human diseases, but these few are intimately concerned with our welfare and have been responsible for the spread of the worst scourges of humanity: malaria, typhus, and plague, among many others.

Morphology. The primitive insect (Fig. 15-1) has a head of six fused segments, a three-segmented thorax bearing three pairs of legs and two pairs of wings, and an eleven-segmented abdomen. The segmentation of the ancestral form is evident only in the abdomen of present-day insects. The body is encased in a more-or-less rigid integument consisting of hard plates, or *sclerites,* connected by a flexible, slightly chitinous membrane.

The cephalic appendages of the primitive arthropod have been converted into sensory organs, such as multijointed antennae, compound and simple eyes, and masticatory organs of varying structures, depending upon feeding habits. The simplest form of the latter is the chewing or biting mouth (cockroach), but in the highly specialized insects the mouth parts have been modified for piercing-sucking (mosquito) and sponging-lapping (housefly). The thorax is composed of the prothorax, mesothorax, and metathorax, each of which bears a pair of legs. Winged insects theoretically have a pair of wings each on the meso- and metathorax, but there are modifications, such as the degeneration of the posterior wings in the flies to structures called *halteres.* The number of abdominal segments is reduced in the more specialized insects.

The abdomen of the adult insect is devoid of appendages. The last segments may be modified for sexual purposes into the *hypopygium* of the male and the *ovipositor* of the female.

In the typical insect (Fig. 15-2), the nervous system is represented by a chain of ventral ganglia, from which nerves pass to the tissues and sensory organs. The respiratory system comprises branching tracheal tubes communicating with the exterior by *spiracles.* The poorly developed circulatory system consists of a dorsal pulsating organ and aorta, and an

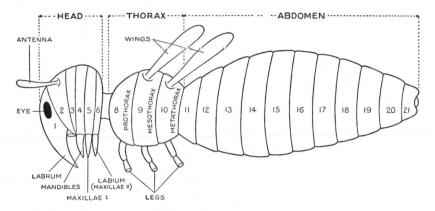

Figure 15-1. Diagram of primitive insect, showing segmentation of head, thorax, and abdomen. The numbering includes 20 segments and the neck piece. (Adapted from Patton and Cragg, 1913, after Berlese.)

open body cavity (hemocele). The digestive system comprises a pharynx, a slender esophagus, proventriculus, distensible stomach or midgut, intestine or hindgut, rectum, and anus. In bloodsucking insects the muscular pharynx acts as a suction pump. Paired salivary glands open into the mouth parts. The excretory system includes several slender malpighian tubules that empty into the intestinal canal just above the juncture of the mid- and hindgut. The male reproductive organs consist of two testes, a seminal vesicle, accessory glands, and hypopygium. The female reproductive organs include ovaries, oviducts, seminal receptacle (spermatheca), shell and cement glands, and ovipositor.

Life Cycle. Insects are oviparous, viviparous, and ovoviviparous. The types of life cycle,

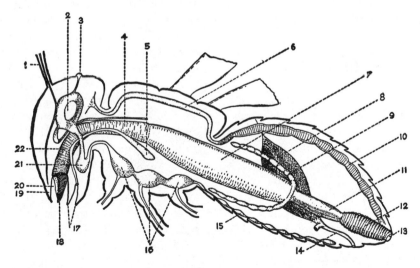

Figure 15-2. Internal structure of a typical insect.
1, antennae; 2, supraesophageal ganglion; 3, ocellus; 4, esophagus; 5, salivary gland; 6, aorta; 7, midgut; 8, gonad; 9, malpighian tubule; 10, dorsal pulsating vessel; 11, intestine; 12, rectum; 13, anus; 14, gonaduct; 15, abdominal nerve ganglion; 16, thoracic nerve ganglia; 17, maxillae; 18, mandible; 19, labrum; 20, mouth; 21, subesophageal ganglion; 22, pharynx. (From Hegner, Root, Augustine, Huff: Parasitology, 1938, as redrawn from Berlese, "Gli Insetti." Courtesy of D. Appleton-Century Company.)

which afford a basis for classification, are direct development, incomplete metamorphosis, and complete metamorphosis. In the uncommon first type, the newly hatched insect is a small replica of the adult. Incomplete metamorphosis, in which the nymphs differ from the adult only in size, proportion, and absence of wings and external genitalia, occurs in the more primitive insects. Complete metamorphosis is found in the highly specialized insects; the wormlike larva differs from the adult in feeding habits and after several molts passes through a pupal stage, during which the larval structures are transformed into those of the adult. The larva and pupa possess characteristic hairs, bristles, and appendages that aid in the differentiation of species. The duration of life in both the adult and larval stages varies with the species and with the environment.

The insects of special interest as parasites of human beings belong to four orders: SIPHONAPTERA (fleas), ANOPLURA (sucking lice), HEMIPTERA (bugs), and DIPTERA (flies, including mosquitoes).

Of less importance are the COLEOPTERA (beetles), HYMENOPTERA (bees, wasps, hornets, ants), LEPIDOPTERA (butterflies and moths), and ORTHOPTERA (cockroaches).

ANOPLURA (SUCKING LICE)

Lice are small, dorsoventrally flattened, wingless insects that have incomplete metamorphosis. The order includes only the sucking lice, which have mouth parts modified for piercing and sucking, and are ectoparasites of humans.

Species. The parasitic lice of humans include three species or varieties: (1) *Pediculus humanus* var. *capitis* (head louse), (2) *Pediculus humanus* var. *humanus* (body louse), and (3) *Phthirus pubis* (crab louse). The body and head lice interbreed; their descendants are fertile; and their morphologic differences overlap.

Diseases. Pediculosis, crabs. Vectors of epidemic typhus, trench fever, and relapsing fever.

Morphology. The flattened, elongated, grayish white body has an angular ovoid head, a fused chitinous thorax, and a nine-segmented abdomen (Fig. 15-3). The head bears a pair of simple lateral eyes, a pair of short five-jointed antennae, and extensile piercing stylets. Each of the three fused segments of the thorax bears a pair of strong, five-segmented legs that terminate in a single hooklike claw and an opposing tibial process for gripping hairs or fibers. The last abdominal segment in the female bears a median dorsal genital opening and two lateral blunt gonopods, which clasp the hairs during oviposition. The body louse is more robust than the head louse; both are 2 to 3 mm in length. The crab house is distinguished by its small size, 0.8 to 1.2 mm, oblong turtle shape, rectangular head, short indistinctly segmented abdomen, and large, heavy claws (Fig. 15-4).

Life Cycle. The operculated, white eggs, 0.6 to 0.8 mm, called "nits," are deposited on and firmly attached to the hairs or to the fibers of clothing. They may remain viable on clothing for a month. The eggs hatch in 5 to 11 days at 21 to 36 C. Metamorphosis is incomplete. The nymph develops within the egg case and emerges through the opened operculum. It undergoes three molts within 2 weeks. The average life cycle of the body or head louse covers 18 days, and that of the crab louse 15 days. The life span of the adult is approximately 1 month.

The total number of eggs deposited during the lifetime has been estimated at 300 for the body louse, 140 for the head louse, and 50 for the crab louse.

Epidemiology. These lice are exclusively human parasites and have worldwide distribution. The favorite locations are the hairs on the back of the head for the head louse, the fibers of clothing for the body louse, and the pubic hairs for the crab louse. The body and head lice readily pass from host to host, but the crab louse changes its position infrequently. The body and head lice survive for a week without food, but the crab louse dies in 2 days. They suck blood for long periods. They exist between 15 and 38 C but die at over 40 C. Moist heat at 60 C destroys the eggs in 15 to 30 minutes.

Pediculosis is most common in persons of unclean habits in cold climates where heavy clothing is required and bathing is infrequent; in occupants of flophouses, jails, or crowded tenements; and in soldiers, as "cooties" or "motorized dandruff," during wartime. The head louse, which is easily transmitted by brushes, combs, and hats, is most prevalent in school children. The body louse is transmitted by contact or by clothing or personal effects infested with nits. The crab louse is usually transmitted during coitus by the transfer of adults or nits on broken hairs and less frequently through toilet seats, clothing, or bedding (Fig. 15-4). Recent sexual promiscuity has led to an increase in the prevalence of this louse.

Pathogenicity. The irritating saliva, injected

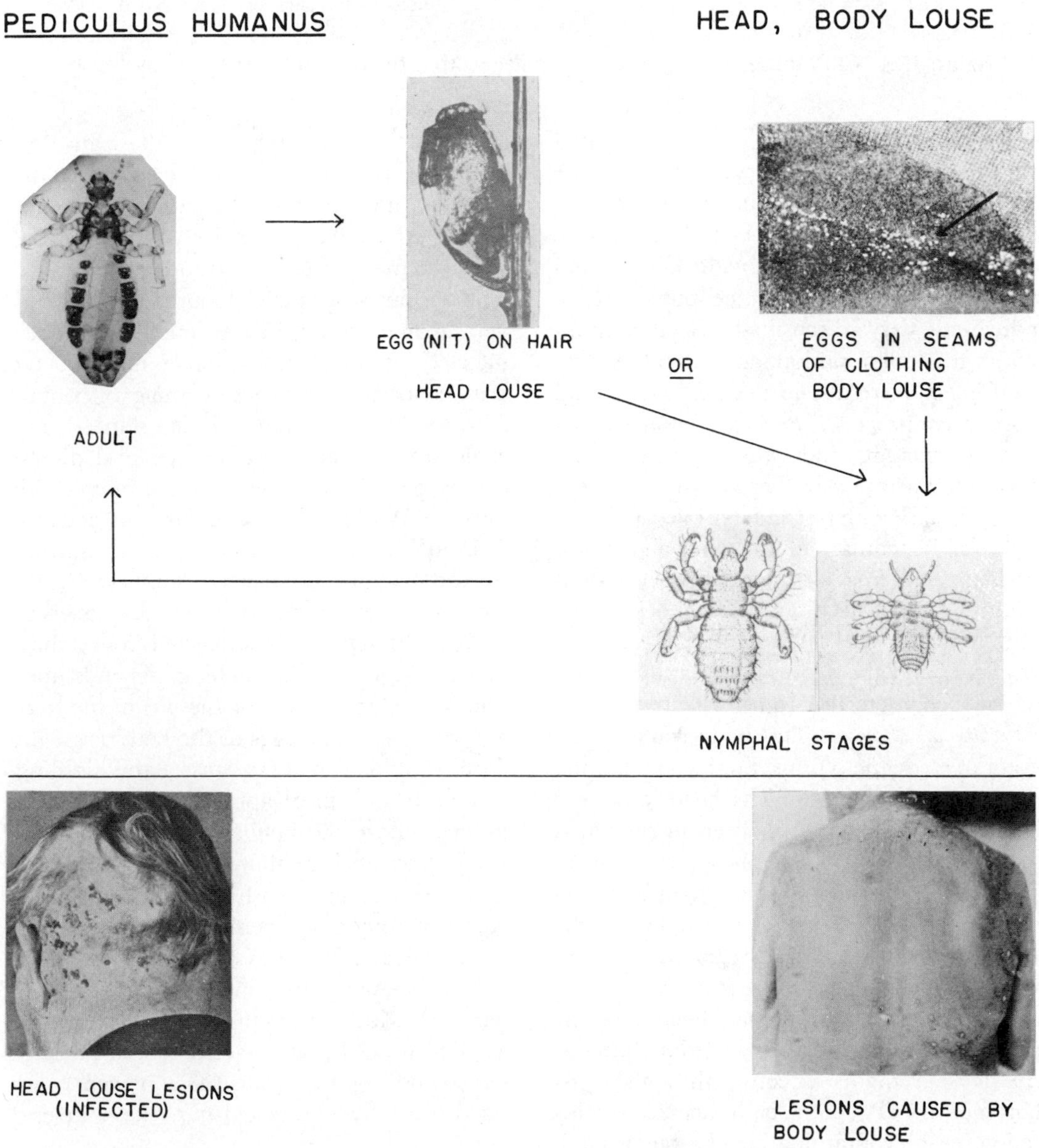

PEDICULUS HUMANUS

HEAD, BODY LOUSE

ADULT

EGG (NIT) ON HAIR

HEAD LOUSE

OR

EGGS IN SEAMS
OF CLOTHING
BODY LOUSE

NYMPHAL STAGES

HEAD LOUSE LESIONS
(INFECTED)

LESIONS CAUSED BY
BODY LOUSE

Figure 15-3. Life cycle of head and body louse.

PHTHIRUS PUBIS   CRAB LOUSE

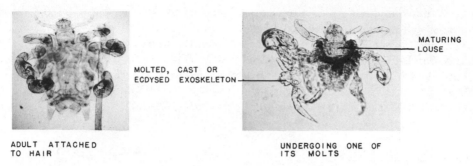

Figure 15-4. Crab louse. The life cycle is similar to that of the head and the body louse.

during feeding, produces a roseate elevated papule accompanied by severe itching. The head louse sucks most frequently on the back of the head and neck; the body louse, on the parts of the body in contact with clothing; and the crab louse, chiefly in the pubic region. Individuals vary in sensitivity. Scratching increases the inflammation, and secondary bacterial infection results in pustules, crusts, and suppurative processes. Severe infestations may produce scarring, induration, pigmentation, and even ulceration of the skin. Infestation of the eyelashes with secondary infection may lead to phlyctenular conjunctivitis and keratitis. The symptoms are the result of cutaneous irritation, loss of sleep, and mental depression. Itching is the earliest and most prominent symptom, and the sequelae of scratching are the most characteristic signs.

Vectors of Diseases. The body louse is the vector of epidemic typhus, European relapsing fever, and trench fever. The head louse and the crab louse have never been incriminated in disease transmission. Typhus fever occurs in epidemics in crowded jails, in armies, and during famines. Lice become infected with the causative organism, *Rickettsia prowazeki,* by ingesting the blood of a diseased person. The parasites multiply in the epithelium of the midgut of the louse and are passed in the feces. The louse remains infective throughout its shortened life. People usually acquire the infection by the contamination of a bite wound, abraded skin, or mucous membranes with the infected feces or crushed bodies of the lice. The

spirochete *Borrelia recurrentis,* the causative agent of epidemic relapsing fever, when ingested with the blood of the patient, multiplies rapidly throughout the body of the louse, which remains infective throughout its life. The various strains of tick-borne relapsing fever do not survive in the louse. People are infected by the contaminative method, the crushed body of the louse coming in contact with the bite wound or abraded skin. Trench fever, an incapacitating but nonfatal disease caused by *R. quintana,* was present in epidemic form in World War I and later in endemic form in Europe and Mexico. It is transmitted by the bite of the infected louse or by the contamination of abraded skin by its feces.

Diagnosis. Diagnosis, suspected from itching and the sequelae of scratching, depends upon finding the adult louse or the nits of the head and crab lice. The eggs of the body louse are usually hidden in the seams of the clothing.

Treatment. Topical applications of soothing lotions relieve the itching and thus, by preventing scratching, allow the lesions to heal.

HEAD LICE. First wash the hair and dry it. Apply shampoo of 1 percent gamma benzene hexachloride (Kwell) as directed in the package insert. Alternatives include pyrethrins (0.2 percent) with 2 percent piperonyl butoxide applied topically as directed in the package insert and copper oleate (0.03 percent), applied topically as directed in package insert.*

---

*Recent experience indicates this to be equally effective and potentially less toxic than benzene hexachloride.

BODY LICE. Treat as for head lice. An alternative is 1 percent gamma benzene hexachloride or 1 percent malathion dusts containing 0.2 percent pyrethrin or 0.3 percent allethrin synergized with piperonyl butoxide (1:10). Some lice recently have become resistant to malathion.

CRAB LICE. On pubic area, treat as for head lice. For infestation on the eyelashes, nits and lice may be removed with forceps. Ophthalmic ointments of Eserine (0.25 percent physostigmine) or of yellow oxide of mercury are both effective.

Control. Mass delousing methods are designed not only to exterminate the lice but also to control the epidemic diseases that are transmitted by lice. Various types of delousing plants for handling large numbers of persons have been devised for military personnel and civilian populations. For the mass delousing of civilians, it is much simpler to administer insecticidal powders such as 10 percent gamma benzene hexachloride or 10 percent DDT simultaneously to the body and clothing. Persons coming in contact with lice-infested individuals in typhus epidemics may be protected by wearing silk or rubber outer garments fastened tightly at the wrist, ankles, and neck, and by impregnating their clothing with repellents. Strains of lice resistant to DDT have been reported in Korea, Egypt, Japan, and North China. Strains resistant to gamma benzene hexachloride (Lindane) and malathion have been noted outside of the U.S.

Availability of some residual insecticides for vector control has been made difficult by legislation in the U.S. banning their widespread use in the environment. But they are still used for public health purposes in many countries.

ORDER SIPHONAPTERA (FLEAS)

Fleas are bloodsucking ectoparasites that, for feeding purposes, temporarily infest mammals and birds.

Morphology. Fleas are small, brown, wingless insects, 2.0 to 2.5 mm, with laterally compressed bodies. The small head may bear eyes and combs; all have antennae and suctorial mouth parts. Each segment of the three-segmented thorax bears a pair of powerful legs terminating in two curved claws (Fig. 15-5).

Life Cycle. The hosts of fleas are domesticated and wild animals, especially wild rodents. The various species tend to be host specific, but their activities permit the infestation of animals other than their preferred hosts. The life span is about a year under favorable conditions of cool, moist temperature, but the maximal survival period apart from the host is 38 to 125 days, depending upon the species. The larvae die at 36 C, but the adults can withstand 38 C for 24 hours.

The adult fleas feed on their hosts, while the larvae live on any nutritive debris, particularly dried blood and the feces of the adults. Both sexes are able to suck blood. Fleas have unusual leaping powers, which enable them to transfer readily from host to host.

In order to produce a large number of eggs, the female must copulate more than once and take frequent blood meals. The small, ovoid, white or cream-colored eggs (Fig. 15-6), about 0.5 mm in length, are laid in the hairs or in the habitat of the host. In houses they are deposited in small batches under rugs, in floor cracks, or on the ground near and under buildings. Those deposited on the host usually drop off before hatching.

Fleas develop by complete metamorphosis, passing through a larval and a pupal stage in the host's environment (Fig. 15-6). In 2 to 12 days the larva emerges from the egg as an active wormlike, white, eyeless, legless, bristled creature of 14 segments, approximately 4.5 mm in length. It has a chewing mouth. It avoids light and seeks crevices. The larval period usually lasts 7 to 30 days, during which time it undergoes two or three molts, the last being within the silky pupal cocoon. The pupal stage lasts 14 to 21 days but at low temperatures may extend over a year. When the development of the pupa is completed, the adult flea breaks out of the cocoon.

Epidemiology. The incidence of human infestation varies with hygienic standards and the

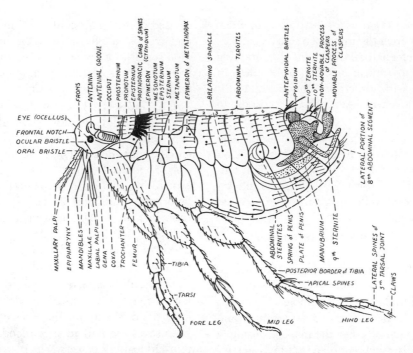

Figure 15-5. External anatomy of a male flea *(Nosopsyllus fasciatus)*. (Adapted from Stitt, Clough, Clough: Practical Bacteriology, Hematology and Animal Parasitology, 1938. Courtesy of The Blakiston Company.)

association of man with animals. Some of the differential morphologic characteristics of the more common species associated with the diseases of man are shown in Figure 15-7. Classification is based chiefly on the presence, size, and position of the eyes; the location of the ocular bristles; presence, arrangement, and spines of combs; structure and appendages of the head; and the genitalia. Humanity is an important host of *Pulex irritans, Ctenocephalides canis, Ct. felis,* and *Tunga penetrans,* and an incidental host of several species parasitic on other animals.

Vectors of Disease. Fleas are of medical interest chiefly in connection with the transmission of plague and endemic typhus. They also may act as intermediate hosts of animal parasites.

PLAGUE. Humans acquire plague caused by the gram-negative bacillus, *Yersinia pestis,* from the fleas that transmit the infection from rat to rat. However, human infection can also occur from direct contact with tissues of infected wild rodents. On the death of the rat near human habitations, the infected fleas seek new

hosts, either humans or other rats. *Xenopsylla cheopis* is the most important and efficient vector. It is readily infected, remains infectious for a long time, and has a wide distribution. Other species of fleas are prominent locally in various parts of the world. *Pulex irritans* has been found infected on persons dying of plague and is a plague vector in the Chilean Andes, above the "rat line." *Y. pestis* may be transferred from flea to person by infected mouth parts, by the regurgitation of organisms that have multiplied in the gut, particularly if the proventriculus has been blocked, and, infrequently, by the contamination of the wound by the feces. Most successful transmissions are from blocked fleas, which are persistent in their efforts to feed. Sylvatic plague in Asia, Africa, and North America is spread by the fleas of wild rodents. *Diamanus montanus* is an important vector among ground squirrels in the United States for both plague and tularemia.

TYPHUS. Endemic or murine typhus is transmitted from rat to rat and from rat to

XENOPSYLLA CHEOPIS

RAT FLEA

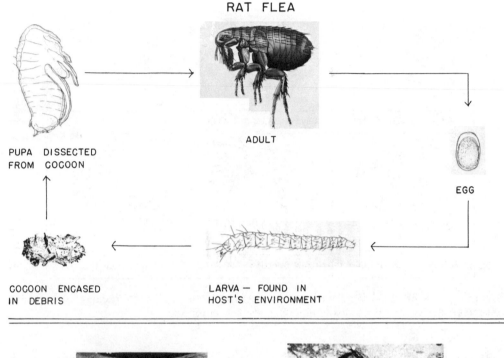

PUPA DISSECTED
FROM COCOON

ADULT

EGG

COCOON ENCASED
IN DEBRIS

LARVA — FOUND IN
HOST'S ENVIRONMENT

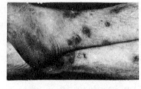

FLEA BITES ON ANKLE

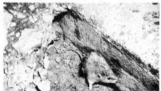

RAT FLEAS ARE
VECTORS OF DISEASE

Figure 15-6. Life cycle of *Xenopsylla cheopis.*

human being by fleas. *X. cheopis* and *Nosopsyllus fasciatus* are considered the common vectors, but any species frequenting rats may be incriminated. A single feeding renders the flea infectious for life. The causative agent, *Rickettsia typhi,* is excreted in the feces. Infection is transmitted by the contamination of the bite wound or abraded skin with the infectious feces or the crushed bodies of the fleas.

MISCELLANEOUS DISEASES. Fleas may act as mechanical vectors of a number of bacterial and viral diseases, chiefly through contaminated feces wind-borne onto mucous membranes. *Ct. canis, Ct. felis,* and *P. irritans* act as intermediate hosts of the dog tapeworm, *Di-*

pylidium caninum and, together with *N. fasciatus, X. cheopsis,* and *Leptopsylla segnis,* of the rat tapeworm *Hymenolepis diminuta.* Both of these tapeworms are incidental parasites of man, acquired by accidental ingestion of infected fleas.

Pathogenicity. The cutaneous irritation caused by the salivary secretions of the flea in different persons varies from no reaction to a raised, roseate, slightly edematous lesion, and in sensitive individuals to a more extensive inflammation or papular rash.

TUNGA PENETRANS. The chigoe, jigger, nigua, sand flea, or burrowing flea is a parasite of humans, hogs, and dogs in tropical America

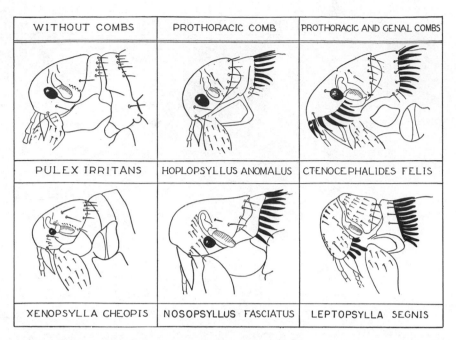

WITHOUT COMBS	PROTHORACIC COMB	PROTHORACIC AND GENAL COMBS
PULEX IRRITANS	HOPLOPSYLLUS ANOMALUS	CTENOCEPHALIDES FELIS
XENOPSYLLA CHEOPIS	NOSOPSYLLUS FASCIATUS	LEPTOPSYLLA SEGNIS

Figure 15-7. Schematic representation of heads of various fleas, showing differential characteristics of shape, combs (ctenidia), eyes, and antennae.

and parts of Africa, the near East, and India. The flea is differentiated from the other fleas by its small size (1 mm) and its shortened thorax. In addition to sucking blood, the fertilized female flea burrows into the skin of mammals and humans for oviposition. Humans are infected by contact with soil infested with immature fleas. The burrow is usually located about the toes, soles of the feet, fingernails, or interdigital spaces. The lesion, at first characterized by a central black spot in a tense, pale area, becomes a festering, painful sore. Secondary bacterial infection may produce an extensive, painful ulcer, sometimes crippling and even causing the death of the host (Fig. 15-8) because of bacterial infection of the lesions. The burrowing *Tunga penetrans* may be removed surgically. A 10 percent DDT powder dusted into shoes will prevent infestation.

PULEX IRRITANS. The human flea is the most common flea found on humans in Europe and the western United States. It also

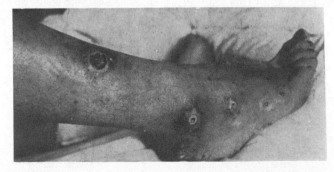

Figure 15-8. Lesions caused by *Tunga penetrans*. (From Manson-Bahr: In Andrews, Domonkos (eds): Diseases of the Skin, 5th ed., 1963. Courtesy of W. B. Saunders Co.)

infests hogs, calves, dogs, rats, mice, cats, and small wild rodents.

FLEAS OF LOWER ANIMALS. The Indian rat flea, *X. cheopis,* is the most abundant rat flea in tropical and subtropical regions. It is the most important flea associated with the transmission of plague. It attacks people and other mammals, as well as its natural host, and has cosmopolitan distribution. *Hoplopsyllus anomalus* and *D. montanus* are common fleas of ground squirrels and other rodents in the western United States. *Ct. canis* and *Ct. felis* infest dogs and cats, but may attack humans and other animals. These cosmopolitan fleas are the most common species in house infestations in the eastern and southern parts of the United States. The mouse flea, *L. segnis,* is a common parasite of the house mouse, rat, and other small rodents. The stick-tight or southern chicken flea, *Echidnophaga gallinacea,* infests birds, dogs, cats, rats, and humans.

The bites of fleas cause an itching dermatitis in some persons, most often at the garter or belt line. The local irritation may be relieved by calamine lotion or menthol-phenol paste.

Control. Environmental control of fleas consists of spraying rat runways, harborage areas, floors, and other areas with one of the following solutions in kerosene, fuel oil, or in emulsion concentrates: chlordane (2 percent); DDT (5 percent); Diazinon (1 percent); Lindane (1 percent); Malathion (3 percent); Methoxychlor (5 percent); Ronnel (1 percent); Trichlorfon (1 percent). The oil sprays are applied at a rate of 1 gallon per 1000 square feet. Powders in inert dust of 10 percent DDT, 1 percent Ronnel, and 1 percent Trichlorfon may be used. Before an antirat campaign is initiated, their environment should be thoroughly sprayed to kill all fleas. Otherwise, as the rats die and the fleas seek new hosts, humanity may be the only one available to receive their attentions. Dogs and cats may be dusted with 4 percent malathion powder, 1 percent Rotenone dust, 10 percent Methoxychlor, or a 10 percent DDT powder or pyrethrum. Cats groom themselves with their tongue, hence care must be exercised in applying these potentially toxic products to them.

Their sleeping areas should also be dusted or sprayed. Collars impregnated with various flea-killing agents are available for dogs and cats.

ORDER HEMIPTERA (TRUE BUGS)

Cimex Bedbugs

The genus *Cimex* contains important blood-sucking species, of which *C. lectularius,* the common bedbug, and *C. hemipterus,* the tropical bedbug, are human parasites.

Morphology. The bedbugs have oval, dorsoventrally flattened, chestnut-brown bodies covered with short, stout, simple or serrated hairs (Fig. 15-9). The female, slightly larger than the male, has a length of 5.5 mm. Its flattened, pyramidal head bears prominent compound eyes, slender antennae, and specialized mouth parts in a long proboscis flexed backward beneath the head and thorax when not in use. The large, conspicuous prothorax has a concave border and rounded lateral horns that give the head a shrunken appearance. Each of the three thoracic segments bears a pair of legs that terminate in a pair of simple claws. The hind wings are absent, and the forewings are reduced to small pads.

Habits. Bedbugs feed at night on humans and small mammals. They conceal themselves during the day in the crevices of wooden bedsteads, in wainscoting, or under loose wallpaper. They pass readily from house to house and are easily transported in clothing and baggage. In cold weather they remain inactive in their hiding places. They can survive starvation for over a year. They emit a characteristic odor from stink glands. A blood meal seems essential to the production of a normal quota of eggs.

Life Cycle. The common bedbug may deposit as many as 200 eggs at the rate of about 2 per day. The white ovoid eggs, about 1 mm in length, have an oblique, projecting, collar-like ring with an operculum at the anterior end and are coated with an adhesive gelatinous substance (Fig. 15-9). Hatching takes place in 4 to 10 days. Development is by incomplete metamorphosis. The yellowish white to brown larval bedbug passes through five or six molts at intervals of about a week to become a sexually mature adult. The life span of the adult is 6 to 12 months.

Pathogenicity. The bite of the bedbug produces red itching wheals and bullae. Some persons show little or no reaction. Others, particularly children, have local urticaria, and still others may manifest allergic symptoms with generalized urticaria and even asthma.

The role of the bedbug in the transmission of human disease is minimal. It may act as a mechanical carrier, but it is not a proved biologic vector of human diseases. Hence, at present, this detested bug must be given an approved bill of health. Although capable of harboring pathogenic organisms in the digestive tract, there is no regurgitation of infected

CIMEX LECTULARIUS

BEDBUG

ADULT

INFESTED WOODWORK OF
BACK OF PICTURE FRAME
I- EGGS; 2 - BUGS;
3 - EXCREMENT

PROGRESSIVE NYMPHAL STAGES ← EGGS

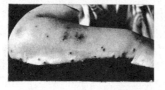

BITES IN TYPICAL GROUPS OF 2

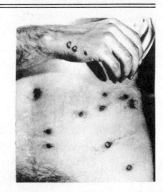

HEMORRHAGIC BULLAE

Figure 15-9. Life cycle of *Cimex lectularius* (bedbug).

blood on biting a second host, and the feces rarely contaminate the bite wound. However, there is evidence to indicate that hepatitis B surface antigen may be transmitted.

Treatment. The irritation and itching of the bites of bedbugs may be relieved by ammonia, spirits of camphor, menthol-phenol paste, or calamine lotion.

Control. In infested houses the repair of cracked plaster and wallpaper and the substitution of iron for wooden bedsteads are recommended. A 5 percent DDT solution in kerosene, a 0.1 percent Lindane oil solution, or a 1 percent malathion solution is applied to floors, walls, furniture, and mattresses. It may be supplemented by the dusting of DDT or malathion powder into the crevices of the floors and walls. Dichlorvos at 0.5 percent, 0.5 percent diazinon, or 1.0 percent Ronnel can also be used. Care must be exercised in using these compounds on bedding used by infants.

Reduviid, Triatomine, or Cone-Nosed Bugs

The reduviid bugs are called "cone-nosed" bugs because of the pointed head, "barbers" or "kissing bugs" because they bite the face, "assassin" bugs, and "flying bedbugs." They are found as disease vectors in North and South America.

Morphology. The triatomid bugs (Fig. 15-10) have long, narrow heads with prominent compound eyes, usually two ocelli, four-jointed antennae, a three-segmented, ventrally folded, slender proboscis, and an obvious neck. The long, rather narrow, flattened body has functional wings and elongated legs with three-jointed tarsi. The color is dark brown with red and yellow markings on the thorax, wings, and sides of the abdomen.

Life Cycle. The female lays white or yellowish pink, smooth, barrel-shaped eggs, in batches of 8 to 12, which hatch in 10 to 30 days. Development is by incomplete metamorphosis. The young bug must obtain its first blood meal within days, and undergoes a lengthy metamorphosis during 6 to more than 12 months to the adult stage, with blood meals between each molt.

Pathogenicity. Both sexes require blood meals, for which they have well-adapted mouth parts for entering a capillary with ease and without disturbing the victim. Reactions in humans to this "mainlining" insect are variable: Some have no reactions initially but are capable of becoming sensitized; others

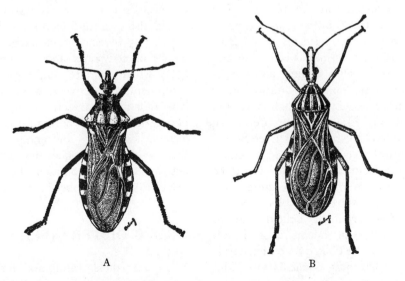

A   B

Figure 15-10. A. Adult male *Panstrongylus megistus.* B. Adult male *Rhodnius prolixus.* (After Brumpt: In Hegner, Root, Augustine, Huff: Parasitology, 1938. Courtesy of D. Appleton-Century Company.)

have prominent, pruritic local skin reactions that develop within 30 minutes after the first exposure. The likelihood of local reactions at the bite site may be partly dependent upon the species of bug.

Vectors of Disease. Several species of reduviid bugs are important vectors of *Trypanosoma cruzi,* the causative agent of Chagas' disease, and of *T. rangeli,* which appears to be non-pathogenic for humans. Most reduviid bugs are capable of transmitting this pathogenic organism, but only certain species are efficient vectors. The most important vectors are *Triatoma infestans, Panstrongylus megistas,* and *Rhodnius prolixus.*

The domiciliary species that readily adapt to living in houses, especially native huts made of mud and sticks, are the most important for human transmission of *T. cruzi.* They hide and breed in crevices and recesses, avoiding bright light and venturing out for a blood meal in subdued light or at night. Only adult bugs can fly, and not for very long distances, but they move rapidly on foot. Species that infest rodent burrows and oppossum nests are referred to as *sylvatic* vectors. Depending upon the frequency of *T. cruzi* infection in the animal or human reservoir, up to 50 percent or more of the bugs in houses or in sylvatic habitats may be infected with the parasite. The trypanosome multiplies in the mid- and hind-gut of the bug and transforms to infective stages. Infection is transmitted when the bug defecates during or after feeding, and the infective stages contaminate the bite wound or mucous membranes. Even though bugs and wild animals infected with *T. cruzi* are known to occur in most of the southern United States, only two naturally acquired human infections have been documented. This is believed to be due partly to the prolonged "defecation time" (time from onset of starting the blood meal to defecation) of vectors in the United States as compared to vectors in endemic areas. In addition, the bugs in the United States have little propensity for becoming domiciliary, i.e., invading houses.

Treatment. The irritation and itching of the bites of reduviid bugs can usually be relieved by calamine lotion or a menthol-phenol paste. If the reaction is severe and lasts for days, it may be necessary to use topical steroids, such as 1 or 2 percent hydrocortisone cream, or orally administered antihistamines.

Control. The control of reduviid bugs is difficult because sylvatic habitats are too dispersed and inaccessible to get at, and because houses that have been sprayed can later be reinvaded by sylvatic vectors. Benzene hexachloride (BHC), and the more active pure gamma isomer of this compound, Lindane, are the most effective insecticides. Lindane can be applied as a 5 percent emulsion in kerosene with 0.3 percent Triton X-45 as an emulsifier to walls, roofs and other surfaces. It may also be applied as a dusting powder on beds, cracks and holes in the walls, and other possible hiding places of the bugs. An application on inside surfaces retains activity for 3 to 6 months. But it, and many other insecticides, has no effect on the egg, requiring repeated applications. Dieldrin is another effective insecticide against triatomine bugs, but it has greater toxicity for humans than BHC. No serious insecticide resistance of reduviid bugs has been observed as yet, except for Dieldrin resistance in one area of Venezuela. Of course, improved housing that would not provide habitats for domiciliary vectors in mud cracks and thatched roofs would also prevent infestation of houses.

Current investigations suggest that analogues of ecdysones and juvenile hormones (JH), which regulate moulting and insect development, respectively, offer promise of a new biologic approach to control of insect populations. These hormones exert their effects at extremely low concentrations, and their synthetic analogues may retain biologic activity when incorporated into solid organic vehicles, such as rubber-base paints.

ORDER DIPTERA (FLIES)

From a medical standpoint, DIPTERA is the most important order of arthropods. It embraces many species of bloodsucking and non-bloodsucking flies, some of which are intermediate hosts or mechanical vectors of bacterial, viral, protozoan, and helminthic agents of disease.

Morphology. The general morphology is that of insects. The relatively large head bears two large compound eyes. The boxlike thorax is chiefly a base of attachment for the powerful muscles of flight. The enlarged mesothorax (second segment) comprises most of the thorax and bears the large membranous wings, the prothorax (first segment) and the metathorax (third segment) being reduced to small rings that unite the thorax with the head and abdomen, respectively. Each thoracic segment carries a pair of variously colored legs adorned with spines and hairs.

The jointed legs may terminate in a pair of toothed claws and elongated hairy pads, the pulvilli. These hollow hairs associated with a gland secrete a sticky substance. The first two segments of the abdomen are atrophied, and the remaining segments are not always distinguishable.

The antennae, equipped with sensory organs, are composed of a series of similar and dissimilar joints, the number, shape, and hirsute adornment of which are characteristic for the various genera (Fig. 15-11). The more primitive flies have long antennae with numerous joints, while the more highly developed species have short antennae with fewer and heavier joints.

Various adaptations of the mouth parts en-

able flies to feed upon the blood and tissue juices of animals, the nectar of flowers, liquids, or food that may be liquefied by their digestive secretions. The various modifications of the mouth parts are important in distinguishing genera and species (Fig. 15-12). The penetration of the skin is accomplished by the maxillae and the mandibles. The food channel is formed by the labrum-epipharynx and hypopharynx (Fig. 15-12A and B). In the bloodsucking muscid flies, the cutting organs are highly developed, consisting of two stylets, the labrum-epipharynx, the hypopharynx, and teeth at the tip of the labium (Fig. 15-2D). In the nonbloodsucking species, the fly absorbs its food in liquid state through its labellum (Fig. 15-12C).

Flies have paired true wings arising from the mesothorax and small clublike halters, considered homologous with the metathoracic wings of other insects. The true wings are thin, membranous extensions of the tergal integument, supported by longitudinal, chitinous, tracheal tubes or veins that radiate from the base of the wing and are connected at intervals by cross veins. They may be transparent or covered with spines, scales, or hairs that give an iridescent or mottled appearance. The spaces between the veins are called *cells.* The number and position of the veins and enclosed cells, and the distribution of hairs and scales, are of value in identifying genera and species (Fig. 15-13).

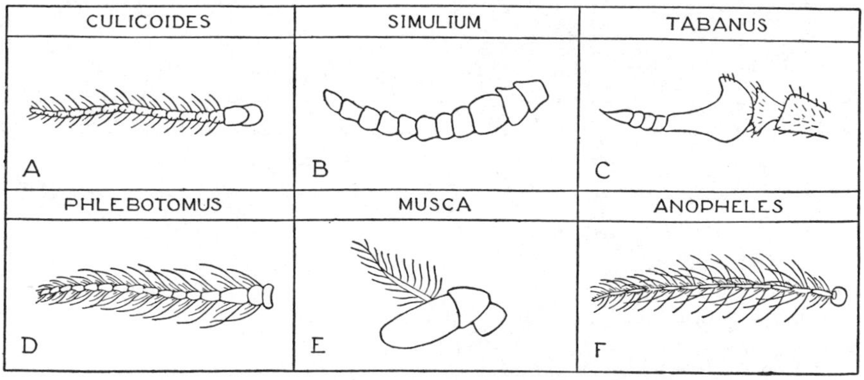

Figure 15-11. Antennae of various genera of Diptera. (A, B, C, and E redrawn from Hegner, Root, Augustine, Huff: Parasitology, 1938. Courtesy of D. Appleton-Century Company.)

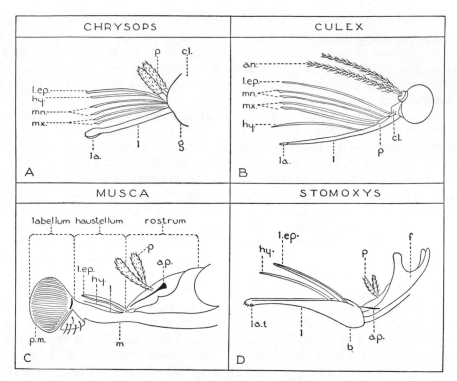

Figure 15-12. Schematic representation of mouth parts of various genera of Diptera. Orthorrhaphous flies. A. *Chrysops* (bloodsucking). B. *Culex* (bloodsucking). Cyclorrhaphous flies. C. *Musca* (nonbloodsucking). D. *Stomoxys* (bloodsucking).

an., antennae; ap., apodeme of labrum; b, bulb; cl., clypeus; f, fulcrum; g, gena; hy., hypopharynx; l, labium; la., labella; la.t., labellar teeth; l.ep., labrum-epipharynx; m, mentum; mn., mandibles; mx., maxillae; p, palps; p.m., pseudotracheal membrane.

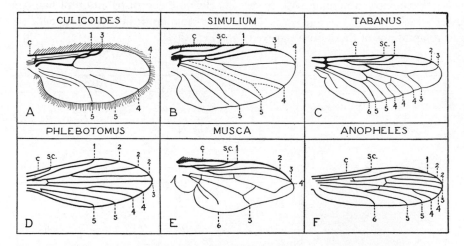

Figure 15-13. Wing venation of certain genera of Diptera of medical importance.

c, costal vein; sc., subcostal vein; 1-6, longitudinal veins. (A, B, C, and E redrawn with modifications and D and F redrawn from Hegner, Root, Augustine, Huff: Parasitology, 1938. Courtesy of D. Appleton-Century Company.)

Life Cycle. Most species of flies are oviparous, but a few deposit larvae in various stages of development. The eggs or larvae are deposited in water, on the ground, in decomposing organic matter, in excreta, or in the bodies of animals. Metamorphosis is complete. The elongated, legless, wormlike larva (see Figure 15-21) leads an aquatic or terrestrial existence. It feeds voraciously with its chewing mouth parts on organic material or becomes adapted to a parasitic existence. After three to four molts, it becomes a nonfeeding pupa that eventually develops into an adult fly.

Mosquitoes

Mosquitoes are slender, delicate flies of evil reputation. The bloodsucking mosquitoes of the family CULICIDAE include important vectors of viral, protozoan, and helminthic diseases of humans and lower animals. Some species feed only on plant juices.

Morphology. Mosquitoes (Fig. 15-14) are distinguished from other flies by (1) the elongated mouth parts, adapted in the females for piercing and sucking blood, (2) the long 15-jointed antennae, plumose in the males and pilose in the females, and (3) the characteristic wing venation, with scales. The roughly spherical head is almost covered by a pair of compound eyes that nearly meet. The rigid thorax, covered by a dorsal scutum, bears three pairs of long, slender legs. The coloration and pattern of the thoracic scales and bristles are useful in differentiating genera and species.

The mouth parts of the bloodsucking female

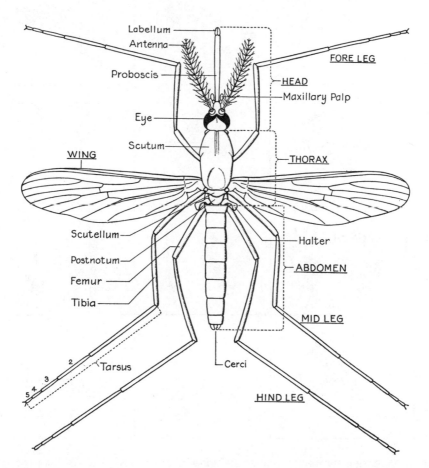

Figure 15-14. Diagram of mosquito (female). Dorsal view, showing nomenclature of parts. (Adapted from MacGregor, 1927, and Marshall, 1938.)

consist of the grooved lower labium, the upper labrum-epipharynx, the hypopharynx, the styletlike paired mandibles, and the serrated maxillae (Fig. 15-12B). The maxillary palps of the female are slender and hairy, while those of the male are long and ornamented like the antennae with tufts of hair, giving a plumed appearance (Fig. 15-15). The salivary glands are located in the prothorax. The male mosquito with its weak mouth parts is unable to penetrate human skin and is therefore relegated to a vegetarian diet—plant juices.

A pair of strong wings is attached to the mesothorax and a pair of vestigial wings to the

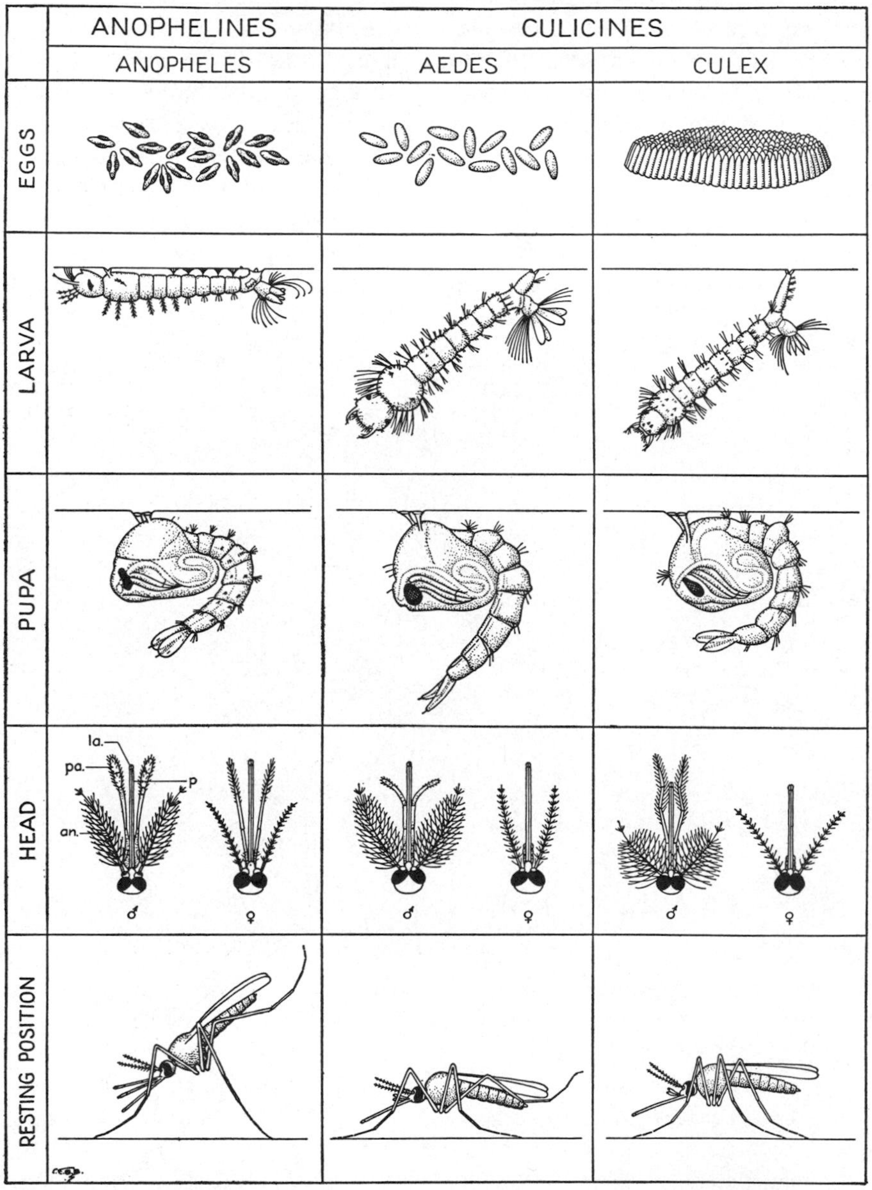

Figure 15-15. Schematic representation of differential characteristics of anopheline and culicine mosquitoes.
  an., antennae; la., labella; p, proboscis; pa., palp.

metathorax. The venation, especially the anterior and posterior forked cells, and the structure, size, and distribution of the flat squamous and long plume scales distinguish the mosquito from other flies and help to differentiate genera and species.

Habits. Each species has an effective flight range between the breeding grounds and the sources of the blood meal, as well as a maximal range—from 1 to 3 miles for *Anopheles,* up to 10 miles for *Culex,* and 50 to 100 miles for some *Aëdes,* often windblown.

Mosquitoes are attracted by bright light, dark-colored clothing, and the presence of humans and animals. Long-distance attraction is due to the olfactory stimulus of animal emanations, especially CO_2 and certain amino acids, and immediate localization to warmth and moisture. Certain species are preeminently anthropophilic (human) in their blood-sucking preferences, and others are essentially zoophilic (animals). Host preferences of the different species may be determined by precipitin tests on the blood meals. Predilection for humans determines the importance of an anopheline species as a vector of malaria. The females are the bloodsuckers; as a rule, females cannot produce fertile eggs without ingesting blood. The biting activities of the different species vary with age, time of day, and environment. Likewise, the daily rhythm of attack varies with the season and temperature. Certain species frequent houses for feeding and resting, while other species enter houses only for feeding and spend their resting periods elsewhere. The former are readily destroyed by residual spraying of the interior of the houses with insecticides.

Mating is preceded by the prenuptial swarming of the males in some species. The anopheline and culicine mosquitoes deposit their eggs in water, but many *Aëdes* mosquitoes select shaded ground subject to intermittent flooding. The maximal number of eggs deposited at one time is from 100 to 400. Many anopheline species lay more than 1000 eggs in a lifetime. The average life span of the adult female mosquito is about 14 to 30 days. The females of species frequenting houses may

hibernate as adults during winter, and a few species pass the winter in the egg or larval stage. Species vary in their natural susceptibility to environmental conditions and, possibly, in their ability to develop resistance against insecticides. Birds, bats, toads, frogs, and dragonflies are natural enemies of the adults, and waterfowl, fish, and aquatic insects prey on the larvae and pupae.

Life Cycle. The larval development of the diverse species occurs under extremely varied environmental conditions, moisture being the chief essential. Most species use fresh water for their aquatic stages, but some, chiefly culicines, breed in brackish or salt water. Domesticated mosquitoes, such as *C. quinquefasciatus* and *A. aegypti,* breed in small amounts of water present in various artificial containers in the vicinity of human habitations.

The egg, about 0.7 mm in length, is encased in a three-layered shell that has a funnel-shaped passage for the entry of the spermatozoa. The eggs of *Anopheles* resemble boats with lateral, ribbed, exchorionic floats. The tapering eggs of *Culex,* with cup-shaped corona, are cemented in raftlike masses. The elliptical eggs of *Aëdes* are polygonally sculptured. The eggs that are laid in water hatch in 1 to 3 days at 30 C but may require 7 days at 16 C, while those of *Aëdes* do not hatch until the ground is flooded with water. The eggs of different species vary in their resistance to desiccation and to high and low temperatures. Anopheline eggs usually perish above 40 C and below 0 C and do not develop below 12 C.

The elongate, limbless larva (Fig. 15-15), with simple or transversely branched tufted hairs symmetrically arranged along its body, passes through four instars to attain a length of about 10 mm. The head bears eyes, hirsute antennae, and chewing mouth parts. The eighth abdominal segment bears two spiracles. The anal aperture is surrounded by four flexible papillary processes, the anal gills. Their function is probably the absorption of water rather than respiration. The resting anopheline larvae are suspended horizontally at the surface of the water and the culicine hang at an angle (Fig. 15-15). The larvae feed on algae, bacteria, and forms of particulate matter. The anopheline larvae obtain their food at the surface, and the culicine larvae beneath the surface by sweeping particles with their mouth brushes or by nibbling decaying matter at the bottom. They swim with a jerky motion, rising to the surface to breathe. They are able to withstand moderately cold temperatures. The length of the larval cycle, under optimal conditions, averages a little over 3 weeks.

The fourth instar larva becomes a megalocephalic curved pupa that resembles a comma (Fig. 15-15). The pupa has respiratory trumpets on the thorax, an air vesicle situated between the future wings of the adult, and a pair of overlapping paddles with terminal hairs on the last abdominal segment. These paddles enable the pupa to dive rapidly in a succession of jerky somersaults in response to stimuli. Pupae are readily destroyed by freezing or drying. The nonfeeding pupal stage lasts 2 to 5 days. In hatching, the pupal skin is ruptured by the air vesicle and the activity of the escaping adult insect.

Classification. The family CULICIDAE is divided into three subfamilies, of which only the ANOPHELINAE (the large genus *Anopheles*) and the CULICINAE (containing the *Theobaldia-Mansonia*, the *Aëdes*, and the *Culex* groups) have species that are vectors of human diseases. The principal genera thus associated are *Anopheles*, *Culex*, *Aëdes*, and *Mansonia*, and to a lesser extent *Haemagogus*, *Psorophora*, and *Culiseta*.

Species are differentiated by the coloration and pattern of scales and bristles, wing venation and scales, male hypopygium, and the type of distribution of hairs, bristles, and appendages of the fourth-instar larva. The main differences between anopheline and culicine mosquitoes are given in Figure 15-15.

The numerous species of *Anopheles* vary greatly as to habitat, being found in open country and in wooded areas, in both urban and rural communities, and at various altitudes. The different species have a wide range of preferential breeding grounds, from shaded to sunny places, from fresh to strongly brackish water, and from puddles of water to moderately swift streams, with a wide range in free-oxygen content. Anopheline mosquitoes are the only vectors of human malaria, and certain species transmit Bancroft's and Malayan filariasis.

The genus *Aëdes* includes many species of mosquitoes of cosmopolitan distribution. They breed in tree holes and in temporary pools of fresh or tidal waters. Many North American species are troublesome biters. Certain species may act as vectors of yellow fever, dengue, filariasis, and the viral encephalitides.

A large number of species of the genus *Culex* with its many subgenera are distributed throughout the world, mostly in warm regions. These small- to medium-sized mosquitoes breed for the most part in permanent bodies of water and have both an urban and a rural distribution. Certain species transmit filariasis and the viral encephalitides.

Adults of the genus *Mansonia* have white-banded legs and usually a mixture of black and white scales on the wings. Their distribution is cosmopolitan but largely tropical. The eggs are deposited in clumps on aquatic plants *(Pistia)* from which the larvae obtain oxygen. Certain species are vectors of Malayan filariasis.

Pathogenicity. In biting, the piercing apparatus probes beneath the skin until a blood supply is tapped, at which time feeding may take place from the blood vessel or from the extravasated blood. The intermittently injected saliva may contain substances that stimulate capillary dilation or slow coagulation. Some bites cause little irritation, and others a considerable amount. The ordinary bite is followed by erythema, swelling, and itching. Vesicular bullae may appear, and secondary infections may result from scratching. Salivary antigens elicit immediate allergic, as well as delayed-type, skin reactions.

Vectors of Disease. Mosquitoes serve as biologic or mechanical vectors of bacterial, helminthic, protozoan, and viral diseases of humans and lower animals. In addition, day-flying and day-biting mosquitoes of the genera *Psorophora* and *Janthinosoma* carry the eggs of the myiasis-producing warble fly, *Dermatobia hominis,* to the skin of humans and other mammals. The species that are important vectors are listed under the respective diseases.

MALARIA. The only vectors of human and simian malaria are anopheline mosquitoes, while both anopheline and culicine mosquitoes carry avian malaria.

Many species of *Anopheles* may be infected experimentally, but relatively few are important natural vectors. Some 110 species have been associated with the transmission of malaria, of which 50 are of general or local importance. The aptitude of a species for transmitting malaria is determined by (1) its presence in or near human habitations, (2) its preference for human rather than animal blood, although when animals are scarce, zoophilic species may feed on humans, (3) an environment that favors its propagation and provides a life span sufficiently long for the plasmodia to complete their life cycles, and (4) physiologic susceptibility to infection.

The suitability of a species as a potential vector may be determined by recording the percentage of infected mosquitoes after feeding on a malarial patient, but its importance as a vector is ascertained by obtaining the index of natural infections, usually from 1 to 5 percent, in female mosquitoes collected in houses in a malarial district. The following species are among the more important vectors of malaria:

Americas

A. albimanus	Central and South America, West Indies, Mexico
A. albitarsis	South America
A. aquasalis	South America, West Indies
A. bellator	Caribbean and South America
A. cruzii	South America
A. darlingi	South and Central America
A. freeborni	Western U.S.A., Mexico
A. nuneztovari	South America
A. pseudo-punctipennis	Central and South America, Mexico, Southwestern U.S.A.
A. punctimacula	Central and South America
A. quadrimaculatus	East, Central and South U.S.A.

Europe and Mediterranean area

A. atroparvus	Europe
A. claviger	Eastern Mediterranean, Near East
A. labranchiae	Southern Europe, North Africa
A. maculipennis	Southeastern Europe
A. sacharovi	Southeastern Europe, Near East, Asia
A. sergenti	Egypt, Near East
A. superpictus	Eastern Mediterranean, Near East

Asia

A. annularis	
A. balabacensis	
A. culicifacies	Southern Asia
A. hyrcanus sinensis	Southeast Asia, Pacific Islands
A. fluviatilis	India
A. maculatus	Southeast and East Asia, Taiwan
A. minimus	Southeast and East Asia, Taiwan
A. stephensi	South Asia
A. sundaicus	South and Southeast Asia, Indonesia
A. umbrosus	Southeast Asia, Indonesia

Africa

A. funestus	East, West, Central, and South Africa; Malagasy; Mauritius
A. gambiae	East, West, Central, and South Africa; Malagasy; Mauritius, Reunion, and Cape Verde Islands
A. melas	West African coast, Mauritius
A. pharoensis	North Africa

Pacific Islands

A. farauti	Solomons, Hebrides, New Guinea, from New Britain to

	eastern Celebes, Australia
A. punctulatus	New Guinea, Solomons, other islands
A. subpictus	Pacific Islands

FILARIASIS. Mosquitoes are vectors of *Wuchereria bancrofti* and *Brugia malayi*. Numerous species of *Anopheles, Aëdes, Culex,* and *Mansonia* have shown complete development of *W. bancrofti,* but most of these species are unimportant as natural vectors. In the tropics and subtropics *C. quinquefasciatus* (= *fatigans*), a night-biting mosquito of domesticated and urban habits that breeds in partially polluted water near human habitations, is the common vector of the nocturnal periodic form of Bancroftian filariasis. In Africa, *A. gambiae* and *A. funestus* are important vectors, while in Southeast Asia species of *Anopheles* and of *Mansonia* are involved in the transmission of periodic and subperiodic *Brugia. A. polynesiensis* is the common vector of the nonperiodic type of Bancroftian filariasis in certain South Pacific islands. This rural mosquito, rests in bushes (never in houses), breeds in coconut shells and cavities of trees, and feeds on domesticated mammals and chickens but prefers humans.

Yellow Fever and Dengue. Yellow fever, a viral disease of high mortality, exists as an endemic zoonosis in forests of Central and West Africa, as well as in the jungles of South America. Jungle yellow fever is transmitted by species of *Aëdes* mosquitoes in Africa and by *Haemogogus* mosquitoes in the Americas. Various types of monkeys and possibly other forest animals are the reservoirs of the jungle form, with humans occasionally becoming infected when they invade the forest. Recent evidence indicates that the yellow fever virus can be transmitted transovarially in the laboratory, although the frequency of this event is very low. Nevertheless, vertical transmission may be a mechanism for maintenance of the virus in nature, since animal reservoirs are often scanty in numbers.

The main threat of yellow fever is the periodic invasion of the virus to densely populated urban areas where it can be transmitted by the almost ubiquitous, human-biting species, *A. aegypti.* Urban yellow fever can spread in epidemic fashion. *A. aegypti* breeds in all manner of domestic water receptacles, in clean or foul water containing organic material. While the breeding of *A. aegypti* can be controlled, it is an expensive and laborious task in refuse-ridden, overpopulated, tropical urban slums. In fact, the job was undertaken by our Public Health Service but was soon given up for reasons that are still debated. People can be protected against both epidemiologic forms of the disease by a very effective live virus vaccine.

Dengue is another virus disease of the tropics that is transmitted by *A. aegypti.* The disease is world-wide in distribution, and can occur in epidemic fashion. A clinical form of the disease characterized by hemorrhagic skin lesions and gastrointestinal bleeding can have substantial mortality.

Viral Encephalitides. A variety of viral encephalitides are transmitted mainly by species of *Culex* and *Aëdes,* and occasionally by *Anopheles* and *Mansonia.* Japanese B encephalitis, which has its natural reservoir in domestic mammals, such as pigs, and occurs in epidemics at times with high mortality, is transmitted by *Culex* mosquitoes, especially *C. tritaeniorhynchus.* In the central and western United States, St. Louis encephalitis, which has its reservoir mostly in domesticated birds, is transmitted chiefly by *C. tarsalis, C. pipiens,* and *C. nigripalpus,* but other genera have been found infected in nature. Equine encephalomyelitis, a highly fatal disease of horses and at times of humans, the virus of which is found in wild and domesticated birds, is capable of being transmitted by *Aëdes, Culex, Anopheles,* and *Mansonia* mosquitoes. *C. tarsalis* is probably the most important vector of the western type, and *Culiseta melanura* of the eastern type. The Venezuelan type is carried mainly by *Culex* mosquitoes of the subgenus *Melanoconium,* by some species of *Aëdes,* and by *Psoropohora confinnis.* The virus of West Nile fever, which can occasionally cause encephalitis, is transmitted by several species of *Culex.* The California group viruses, which include a virus called LaCrosse, cause sporadic but severe encephalitis in California, Wisconsin, and a few other midwestern states; they are transmitted by species of *Aëdes* and *Culex*. Numerous other viruses have been isolated from mosquitoes.

Control. Mosquito control requires a knowledge of the habits of the particular species, the climate of the country, the habits and socioeconomic status of the population. Mosquitoes may be controlled by (1) elimination or reduction of their breeding grounds, (2) destruction of the larvae, and (3) destruction of adult mosquitoes. More than one method may be required. The effectiveness of control measures may be evaluated by the reduction in mosquito population and decline in incidence of the transmitted diseases.

The destruction of breeding grounds, essentially an engineering problem, gives permanent results but involves high initial and maintenance costs. Drainage is applicable to species of limited flight range that breed in quiet bodies of water, but it must be supplemented by the filling of depressions. Extensive drainage operations are seldom practicable, but they are of value at selected sites. Water-level management and the removal of vegetation from the banks and surfaces of streams and ponds reduce the breeding grounds of many species. Changing the water level by intermittent flushing has proved useful for controlling species that breed in impounded waters and flowing streams. Tide gates have been installed for the control of brackish-water-breeding mosquitoes.

Various measures, including the use of both chemical and biologic agents, are used for the control of mosquitoes, as well as other medically important arthropods. Aquatic, surface-inhabiting larvae can be killed by application of oils or other organic surface films that interfere with the gas exchange of larvae or affect the emergence of adults. Many insecticides of four different chemical classes may be used against larval or adult stages of mosquitoes. These include (1) the chlorinated hydrocarbons, such as DDT, BHC, and Dieldrin, (2) the organic phosphates, such as malathion and parathion, (3) the carbamates, such as landrin and bendiocarb, and (4) the pyrethroids, such as permathrin and decamethrin. These insecticides can be used in different ways, in aerosols for rapid knock-down of adult mosquitoes or incorporated into liquid or solid materials for slow-release residual action after being sprayed or dusted on surfaces.

The residual spraying of the interior walls of houses or outbuildings with DDT was the main instrument of malaria control and eradication programs throughout the world for many years. This practice was based upon the knowledge that many anopheline vectors entered buildings for their human blood meals and rested on the walls before or after feeding, thereby coming into contact with the insecticide. But almost as fast as new insecticides have been introduced, resistant strains of mosquitoes have been selected out and emerged. Thus, the effort of human beings to control insect vectors goes on—a never-ending battle. Another complicating factor has been the increasing awareness of nature lovers and environmentalists of the actual and potential damage to other elements of the biologic chain of life by the indiscriminate and widespread use of insecticides. In view of these developments, the manufacture and use of many insecticides has been banned in the United States. This is not a problem for U.S. citizens, for whom malaria, onchocerciasis, and sleeping sickness are exotic, far-away diseases. But unavailability of these insecticides creates great problems for much of the rest of the world, for whom these diseases are a living, current reality, while environmentalism is a luxury for tomorrow. Ironically, the contamination of the environment and the development of insecticide resistance has resulted mainly from the agricultural use of pesticides rather than from their use for vector control in public health programs.

The problems associated with insecticide use have also stimulated new approaches to vector control. These involve biologic methods and include such measures as introduction of larva-eating fish (*Gambusia* spp.) in lakes and ponds, use of hormones that inhibit insect growth and development, other hormones that attract insects (pheromones), and toxins produced by bacteria *(Bacillus thuringiensis)*. These biologic methods of control are still in their early development.

The protection of humans against mosquitoes comprises mosquito-proofing of buildings with 18-mesh wire screening; mosquito nets over beds; protective clothing, such as head nets, gloves, and high boots; and repellents applied to skin and clothing. Effective repellents, such as indalone, dimethyl phthalate, Rutgers 612, and diethyltoluamide (Off), are effective for several hours.

Culicoides (Midges)

The genus *Culicoides* includes several hundred species of aggressive biters and contains species that are vectors of human parasites. They are cosmopolitan, except in Patagonia and New Zealand.

Common Names. Midges, gnats, punkies, and no-see-ums.

Morphology. These delicate brown or black flies (Fig. 15-16) are chiefly identified by their small size, 1.0 to 1.5 mm, slightly humped thorax that projects over the head, and the venation of, and spots on, the wings.

Habits. The midges swarm during the day near ponds and swamps. They breed in forest, jungle, and swampland, in fresh and brackish water, but may be found far from these breeding places: Some species breed in moist decomposing organic matter, not requiring standing water. Only the bloodsucking female has bladelike cutting mouth parts.

Life Cycle. The small oval eggs are deposited on plants or vegetable material in such shallow water as the margins of ponds, puddles, and tree holes. In about 3 days the smooth, elongated, 12-segmented larvae wriggle into the bottom mud, where they feed on vegetable debris with their toothed mandibles. In 1 to 12 months they become elongated pupae with terminal spines and respiratory trumpets. The adult fly emerges from the pupa in 3 to 5 days.

Pathogenicity. The bite of the fly causes considerable irritation, and sensitive persons may experience severe local pruritus and fever.

Vectors of Disease. Certain species are hosts of filarial parasites that infect humans: in Africa, *C. austeni* and *C. grahami* of *Dipetalonema perstans* and *C. grahami* of *D. streptocerca;* in the Western Hemisphere, *C. furens* and *C. paraensis* of *Mansonella ozzardi,* and *Dipetalonema.* Other species are intermediate hosts of filarial and various blood protozoa parasites of lower animals and birds. A number of viruses have been isolated from *Culicoides.*

Control. Control measures are unsatisfactory. Local breeding grounds may be reduced

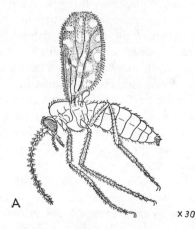
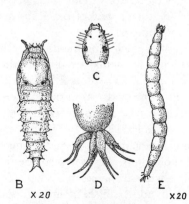

Figure 15-16. The genus *Culicoides*. A. *C. austeni,* adult female. B. Pupa of *C. kiefferi.* C. Head of larva of *C. kiefferi.* D. Last segment of larva of *C. kiefferi* showing tracheal gills extruded. E. Larva of *C. kiefferi.* (A redrawn from Sharp, 1928. B-E redrawn from Patton, 1913.)

by drainage and filling operations. Ordinary screens do not exclude these small flies. The residual spraying of the door and window screens and interiors of houses with DDT or other insecticides may prevent their entrance. Individuals may be protected by repellents.

Phlebotomus and Lutzomyia (Sandflies)

Common Names. Members of the genera *Phlebotomus* and *Lutzomyia* are called sandflies, humpbacked sandflies, moth flies, and owl midges.

Geographic Distribution. *Phlebotomus* is cosmopolitan in tropical and subtropical countries of the Old World, and the genus *Lutzomyia* in the New World.

Morphology. The slender, humpbacked, yellowish or buff-colored sandflies (Fig. 15-17) are characterized by their small size (3 mm), extreme hairiness of bodies and wings, and the erect V-shaped position of the wings at rest. The hairy, oval, or lanceolate wings are devoid of scales, and the second longitudinal vein forks near its middle with a second fork in the anterior branch before reaching the margin. The 16-jointed antennae are long and hairy. The mouth parts have bladelike cutting organs.

Habits. Most species feed on mammals, a few on reptiles. As a rule, the females are the bloodsuckers, but in some species the males have piercing mouth parts. Most species are active nocturnal feeders, especially on warm, humid nights. During the daytime the flies rest in crevices in stone, concrete, or earth constructions, or in rodent burrows. Inability to fly against slight winds limits their flight range to less than a mile from their breeding places. They enter houses in a series of short, intermittent flights and rest on the walls before biting humans.

Life Cycle. In 30 to 36 hours after the blood meal, the female fly deposits, in dark, moist crevices near nitrogenous waste, 30 to 50 elongated eggs (Fig. 15-17). After 6 to 12 days the egg develops into a sluggish, segmented, caterpillarlike larva with long caudal bristles, which feeds on dead leaves and nitrogenous wastes. The larva undergoes four molts in 25 to 35 days before it becomes a buff-colored pupa with a triangular head and curved abdomen. The adult fly, which emerges from the pupa in 6 to 14 days, has a life span of about 14 days. The entire period from egg to adult is 5 to 9 weeks.

Pathogenicity. The bite of the fly produces a rose-colored papule surrounded by an erythematous area 10 to 20 mm in diameter.

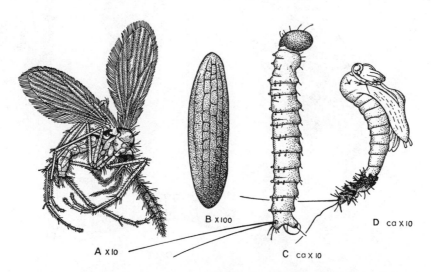

Figure 15-17. The genus *Phlebotomus.* A. Adult fly. B. Egg of *P. papatasii.* C. Larva of *P. papatasii.* D. Pupa of *P. papatasii.* (A redrawn from Hegner, Root, Augustine, Huff: Parasitology, 1938. Courtesy of D. Appleton-Century Company. B-D redrawn from Newstead, 1911.)

There is a stinging pain and an itching that persists for some time. In sensitive persons the local lesions are more pronounced and may be accompanied by nausea, fever, and malaise.

Vectors of Disease. Sandflies are the vectors of leishmaniasis, sandfly fever, and bartonellosis. *Leishmania donovani,* the cause of kala-azar, *L. tropica,* the agent of oriental sore, and *L. braziliensis* and *L. mexicana,* the etiologic agents of American leishmaniasis, are transmitted by sandflies.

Sandfly fever is a nonfatal, febrile viral disease caused by a group of antigenically related viruses of the *Phlebotomus* fever group. It is most prevalent in the Mediterranean region and southern Asia, but occurs sporadically in the Americas. Transovarial transmission of the virus helps in its survival, hence it can be recovered from male sandflies that do not take a blood meal.

Bartonellosis occurs in northwestern South America as the acute febrile Carrión's disease and as a chronic granulomatous verrucous condition. The causative bacillus, *Bartonella bacilliformis,* is transmitted by the Andean sandflies.

Control. Residual spraying of the interiors of houses with DDT and other insecticides has proved highly successful in freeing dwelling houses of sandflies and reducing leishmaniasis, although the flies remain abundant outdoors. Persons may be protected by repellents such as diethyltoluamide (Off).

Simulium (Black Fly)

Common Names. Black flies, buffalo gnats, turkey gnats, and Kolumbtz flies.

Geographic Distribution. Cosmopolitan.

Morphology. Black flies (Fig. 15-18) are identified by their small size (2 to 3 mm), stout hump-backed forms, short legs, conspicuous compound eyes, short smooth antennae, and venation of the unspotted wings. The short proboscis has bladelike cutting organs. The body is covered with short golden or silver hairs that give it a longitudinally striped appearance.

Habits. Black flies breed in moderately swift woodland streams in upland regions. They remain near, or move along, these shaded watercourses. Their migratory range is usually 2 to 3 miles, but this distance is sometimes

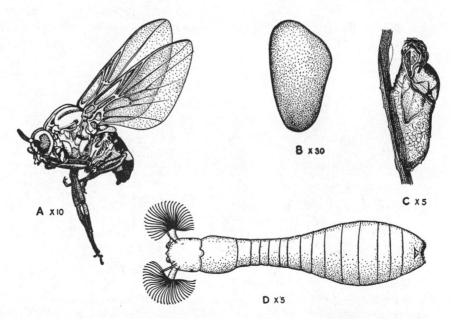

Figure 15-18. The genus *Simulium.* A. Adult fly. B. Egg. C. Cocoon and pupa of *S. mexicanum,* lateral view. D. Larva, dorsal view. (A and D redrawn from Hegner, Root, Augustine, Huff: Parasitology, 1938. Courtesy of D. Appleton-Century Company. C redrawn from Bequaert, 1934.)

greatly extended by movement with winds. The females bite during the daytime, particularly in the morning and toward evening, in open places at the edge of thick vegetation. They may enter houses, and they bite humans in the vicinity of buildings. They are a scourge to fishermen at certain seasons.

Life Cycle. The triangular eggs are laid in batches of 300 to 500 and are attached by a gelatinous secretion to stones, leaves, submerged plants, stakes, and branches. In 3 to 5 days a yellowish green, cylindrical larva with hairy mouth parts and fingerlike anal gills emerges and attaches itself in an upright position to rocks, aquatic vegetation, and other debris. In Africa the larva and pupa of *Simulium neavei* are found on the surface of freshwater crabs *(Potamon)*. It molts seven times in 13 days before spinning a cocoon with an open pocket, in which the dark brown pupa with posterior hooklets and long respiratory filaments is attached. The adult emerges in about 3 days; the females live only a few weeks.

Pathogenicity. The bite, painless at first, often bleeds profusely. Later, swelling, pruritus, and pain develop, which may continue for some days. In susceptible individuals even a few bites may cause marked local inflammation and general incapacity.

Vectors of Disease. In Africa *S. damnosum* and *S. neavei,* and in the Americas *S. metallicum, S. ochraceum,* and *S. callidum,* are vectors of onchocerciasis. Other species are probably minor vectors, and still others transmit onchocerciasis of cattle and protozoan diseases of birds. Species of *Simulium* have recently been found to be vectors of *Mansonella ozzardi* in the Brazilian Amazon and in Colombia. This human filarial parasite is usually transmitted by *Culicoides.*

Treatment. The painful, itching, slow-healing bites of black flies may be partially relieved by antiseptic and soothing lotions.

Control. Black flies are difficult to control. The adult flies may be reduced in number by spraying their bushy resting places with DDT or BHC. Better results are obtained by using DDT as a larvicide in the form of a wettable powder or in solution for streams, usually by the drip method. An initial concentration of 0.1 ppm applied for 3 minutes for streams with a flow of less than 5000 gallons per minute and 2 ppm for streams with more than 5000 gallons is effective for 2 miles. A large-scale vector-control program against onchocerciasis has been under way in West Africa for several years. An organophosphate, temephos (Abate), applied in emulsion form via helicopter, has been used extensively. The reduction of onchocerciasis has been promising. Mechanical destruction of breeding places is effective but expensive. Travelers in black fly districts may be protected by fine head nets, tight sleeves and trouser bottoms, and repellents.

Chrysops (Deer Fly)

Of the 60 genera of the family TABANIDAE, only the genus *Chrysops* contains vectors of human diseases, although other species are vicious biters.

Common Names. Species of *Chrysops* are known as deer flies. Other tabanids are known as horse flies, mangrove flies, breeze flies, green-headed flies, clegs, and seroots.

Geographic Distribution. Chrysops flies ae cosmopolitan and are more abundant in the Americas.

Morphology. The tabanid flies are recognized by their robust shape and brilliant color. *Chrysops* flies are small tabanids with conspicuous markings, slender antennae, brilliantly colored eyes, yellow-banded abdomens with dark stripes, and clear wings with one dark band along the anterior margin and a broad crossband at the level of the discal cell. The bloodsucking female has an awl-shaped epipharynx, bladelike mandibles, and serrated maxillae (Fig. 15-12A).

Habits. Chrysops flies are found in shady woodlands. In Africa their main habitats are the woodlands and the savanna grasslands, and the rain-forest species have probably been derived from this source. The bloodsucking females attack humans most actively in the early morning and late afternoon. This midday diminution probably is associated with light intensity, since at ground and canopy level there is no marked bimodal activity.

Life Cycle. The female deposits from 200 to

800 elongated, spindle-shaped eggs in adhesive masses on aquatic plants, grasses, or rocks overhanging water. The carnivorous larvae, which hatch in 4 to 5 days, pass through six molts in mud and water before they pupate in dry ground. The adult emerges from the pupa in 10 to 18 days. The life cycle may be completed in the tropics in 4 or more months, but in the temperate zones it may extend over 2 years.

Pathogenicity. The fly usually makes several thrusts of the cutting mouth parts before it starts drawing about 30 mm³ of blood from the hemorrhagic pool. The ugly puncture wound is not immediately painful. Within a few hours there is considerable irritation and often swelling that may persist for days. In Japan the aquatic larvae of several species puncture the hands and feet of workers in the paddy fields.

Vectors of Disease. Species of *Chrysops* are associated with the transmission of the filarial parasite *Loa loa.* The chief cyclic vectors of human loasis are the numerous *C. silacea* and *C. dimidiata,* both of which have close contact with people.

Treatment. Soothing lotions.

Control. Control measures are unsatisfactory. The adult flies may be killed by DDT. Larvicidal measures are effective only for certain species. Domestic animals may be given some protection by smudges, sprays, and repellent dips. People may be protected by nets and repellents.

BLOODSUCKING FLIES OF THE FAMILY MUSCIDAE

The bloodsucking flies of the family MUSCIDAE include relatively few genera: *Stomoxys* (stable flies) and *Glossina* (tsetse flies), which attack humans and animals, and *Haematobia* and *Philaematomyia,* which prey on domesticated animals.

Stomoxys (Stable Flies)

The cosmopolitan stable fly, *S. calcitrans,* is a typical representative of the genus *Stomoxys,* which includes 10 or more similar species. It is an annoying pest of humans and animals and a mechanical vector of animal diseases.

Common Names. Stable fly, storm fly, stinging fly, and dog fly.

Morphology. The oval, grayish fly resembles, but is slightly larger than, the house fly. It may be distinguished by its bayonet-shaped proboscis, robust appearance, dark color, thorax with four dark longitudinal stripes, and banded abdomen. The labium, which in other flies usually forms a sheath for the mouth parts, is itself a piercing organ (Fig. 15-12D).

Life Cycle. The flies usually frequent stables and farmyards, attracted by animals and decaying vegetation. They also breed in the fermenting tidal deposits of bay grasses and in seaweed on beaches. Both males and females attack domesticated animals and humans during the day. They invade houses during or after rain storms. The life span of the adult is about 17 days. The female deposits up to 275 eggs during her lifetime, in batches of 20 to 50, on moist, decaying vegetation in barnyards, marshy ground, or on the banks of streams. The elongated, creamy-white, banana-shaped egg produces in 1 to 3 days, a creamy-white, translucent, footless larva that becomes a pupa in 1 to 3 weeks. Under favorable conditions, the life cycle is completed in 3 to 4 weeks.

Pathogenicity. The bite causes a sharp initial, and subsequent prickling, pains, but after the extraction of blood there is little discomfort. A drop of blood collects at the site of the puncture and a small roseola with a scarlet center persists for some time. Cattle and horses, subjected to frequent and heavy attacks, lose flesh and are unable to work.

Vectors of Disease. The habit stable flies have of leaving one animal to feed on another makes them ideal mechanical vectors of disease. *S. calcitrans* is the natural mechanical vector of *Trypanosoma evansi* (surra) in cattle and horses.

Several human diseases have been experimentally transmitted by the stable fly, such as African sleeping sickness, oriental sore, and poliomyelitis. Stable flies have also been accused of spreading anthrax and the infectious anemia of horses among animals.

Treatment. Soothing lotions.

Control. Control is best achieved by destroying the breeding places through the removal of decaying vegetable material. Chemical treatment of manure, without impairing its value as fertilizer, will kill the larvae. Stables may be screened and their walls sprayed with DDT, organophosphates, or pyrethroids to destroy the adult flies.

Glossina (Tsetse Flies)

The genus *Glossina* includes some 20 or more African species of tsetse flies, several of which

are vectors of the trypanosomes of humans and animals.

Geographic Distribution. Equatorial Africa from 18 N to 31 S latitude. *G. tachinoides* is also found in southern Arabia.

Morphology. The yellow, brown, or black flies (Fig. 15-19), 6 to 13 mm, are distinguished by (1) the resting position of the wings, which fold over each other like the blades of scissors, (2) the slender, horizontal proboscis with its bulbous base, (3) the branched, curved bristles on the arista of the three-jointed antennae, and (4) the distinctive

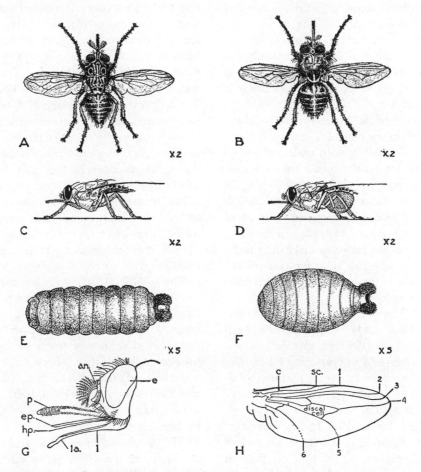

Figure 15-19. Tsetse flies. A. *Glossina palpalis,* male. B. *G. morsitans,* female, C. *G. palpalis,* lateral view, before feeding. D. *G. palpalis,* lateral view, after blood meal. E. Larva of *G. palpalis.* F. Puparium of *G. pallidipes.* G. Head and mouth parts of *G. palpalis.* H. Wing of *G. palpalis,* showing venation.

an., antenna; c, costal vein; sc., subcostal vein; e, eye; ep., epipharynx; hp., hypopharynx; l, labium; la., labella; p, palps; 1–6, longitudinal veins. (A–D and F redrawn from Austen, 1911. G redrawn from Surcouf and González-Rincones. H adapted from Hegner, Root, Augustine, Huff: Parasitology, 1938. Courtesy of D. Appleton-Century Company.)

venation of the light-brown wings. *G. palpalis* is a blackish-brown fly with pale lateral markings on its abdomen. *G. morsitans* is a gray fly with brown transverse bands on its yellowish-orange third to sixth abdominal segments. The mouth parts are the labium-piercing type, the whole proboscis entering the wound.

Habits. The various species occupy a wide range of habitats. There are two general classes: (1) the riverine species, such as *G. palpalis,* which frequent hot, damp areas on the borders of streams, rivers, and lakes in West and Central Africa, and (2) the bush species, such as *G. morsitans,* which are found in wooded and bush country that provides moderate shade in East Africa. The fly belts are irregular zones of varying dimensions surrounded by localities that are practically fly-free. For the bush species, ridge-top glades and thickets in valleys or along the slopes of hills are good habitats.

The life span of the male is half that of the female, which in the case of *G. palpalis* is about 13 weeks (in captivity). Both male and female flies are day biters of animals and humans. Vision, body heat, and to a lesser extent smell are the primary factors in directing the flies to their hosts. *G. palpalis* is attracted by black or blue cloth, particularly if flapping in the wind. The effective flight range is short; it is probably less than one-half mile for *G. morsitans,* but *G. palpalis* is capable of crossing barriers more than 3 miles wide.

Life Cycle. The breeding grounds of the riverine species are sandy beaches and loose soil near water; those of the bush species, loose soil near fallen trees or low-branching limbs. The female produces single, large, mature, third-stage larvae at intervals of about 10 days. *G. palpalis* yields a total of nine larvae. The yellow, knobbed larva (Fig. 15-19), nearly as long as the abdomen of the fly, has a pair of dark protuberances, tumid lips, on the last segment. It burrows to a depth of 2 inches in the ground and immediately pupates. The adult fly emerges in about 5 weeks.

Pathogenicity. The bite of the fly is of minor consequence. Persons may become sensitive to the saliva.

Vectors of Disease. Tsetse flies are important vectors of trypanosomiasis of humans and domesticated animals. At least seven species are vectors of trypanosomal infections of domesticated animals. The vectors of *Trypanosoma rhodesiense,* the causative agent of Rhodesian trypanosomiasis, are *G. morsitans, G. swynnertoni,* and *G. pallidipes.* The chief vectors of *T. gambiense,* the agent of Gambian sleeping sickness, are the riverine *G. palpalis, G. palpalis fuscipes,* and in certain districts *G. tachinoides.*

Control. The control of the riverine species comprises reduction of their habitats and breeding places in areas frequented by people and the destruction of the adult flies. An unsuitable environment may be created by (1) clearing trees and bush from stretches of river bank at least 800 yards in length by 50 to 150 yards in width in the vicinity of water holes and crossings, (2) the erection of barrier clearings to prevent the passage of flies along the river courses, and (3) more extensive clearance of river systems by selective removal of shrubs and trees, starting upstream. As the fly reproduces, the number of flies may be reduced slowly by hand-catching, trapping, and insecticides in the lightly foliated small rivers and water holes. Frame and cloth traps, impregnated with pyrethroid concentrates and placed at intervals along river courses, have been effective in reducing tsetse populations.

The woodland tsetse flies are more difficult to eradicate. Methods of control are (1) barrier clearance to isolate blocks of infested country by removing the upper canopy of trees, (2) clearance of tracts for agricultural purposes, (3) selective bush clearance in crucial areas, (4) trapping of flies, (5) the use of insecticides such as Dieldrin, BHC, and DDT to eliminate residual flies by aerial spraying or by herding cattle, sprayed twice a week with DDT, in infested bush areas, and (6) the destruction of the wild game animals upon which the flies feed. The destruction of game, a controversial subject, is only suitable to isolated fly belts of manageable size. It is less effective in reducing the versatile *G. pallidipes* than in reducing *G. morsitans* and *G. swynnertoni.* The areas are susceptible to reinfestation, and discriminative clearance, especially if it is accompanied by human settlements, is preferable because of its permanence.

Nonbloodsucking Flies

The nonbloodsucking flies have mouth parts adapted for sucking liquids or minute particles. They live under filthy conditions, the larval stage usually being passed in decaying material. They affect human health by the mechanical transmission of disease-producing organisms and by the parasitic activities of their larvae. The invasion of mammalian tissues by dipterous larvae is known as *myiasis*.

Myiasis. Clinically, myiasis may be classified as cutaneous, atrial, wound, intestinal, and urinary. Larvae are able to burrow through either necrotic or healthy tissue with their chitinous mandibular hooks, aided by secondary bacterial infection and possibly by their preteolytic secretions. Some migrate in tortuous channels, producing a type of larva migrans creeping eruption *(Hypoderma)*. When the larvae mature they migrate out of the host in an effort to reach soil and to pupate. The larvae deposited in the atria either remain there or migrate to the sinuses and adjacent tissues. The larvae of several species of flies have been found in the urine. Urethral infections with *Fannia, Musca,* and *Eristalis* cause dysuria, hematuria, and pyuria, presumed to be due to the invasion of larvae deposited upon the genitalia. Intestinal myiasis is largely accidental through ingestion in food. Larvae that are able to live in the intestinal tract may cause nausea, vomiting, and diarrhea.

Classification of Myiasis-producing Flies. A satisfactory classification is to group the myiasis-producing flies by their ovi- or larvipositing habits as (1) specific, (2) semispecific, and (3) accidental. The specific flies deposit their eggs or larvae in or near the tissues of obligate hosts, and the larvae inevitably become parasites by invading the skin or atria. These flies may deposit their eggs or larvae in the habitat, on the hairs or body, or in the wounds and diseased tissues of the host. The semispecific flies usually deposit their eggs or larvae in decaying flesh or vegetable matter and, less frequently, as facultative parasites in diseased tissues or neglected wounds, although a few species have acquired a purely parasitic habit. The accidental myiasis-producing flies of diverse genera and habits deposit their larvae in excrement or decaying organic material and at times in food. A person becomes infested by the accidental ingestion of the eggs or larvae or by the contamination of external wounds or atria.

Human infection with flesh fly larvae is largely confined to infants and small children, particularly those with nasal discharges, who sleep unscreened, out of doors. The deposited larvae are able to penetrate the tender skin of infants and produce furunculous lesions. Extensive superficial lesions of the cheek, neck, eyes, arms, and chest of infants have been reported. Drunkards who have vomited and are lying in a stupor are favorites of these flies. The genera and families of myiasis-producing flies of medical and veterinary importance are listed below with their clinical types. They are designated as (1) specific and (2) semispecific; the location of deposition of eggs or larvae, as (A) hairs and body of host, (B) external habitat of host, and (C) wounds of host. In addition, flies of the families ANTHOMYIDAE, MUSCIDAE, and SYRPHIDAE occasionally produce an accidental myiasis. Also the adult nonmyiasis-producing flies of the family OSCINIDAE attack human eyes.

Family CALLIPHORIDAE
    Genus *Auchmeromyia* (1 B) bloodsucking (Congo floor maggot)
        Calliphora (2 C) wounds, eye
        Chrysomyia (1 C) atrial, wounds
        Cochliomyia (2 C) atrial, cutaneous, wounds
        Cordylobia (1 B) cutaneous
        Phormia (2 C) wounds
Family OESTRIDAE
    Genus *Dermatobia* (1 B) cutaneous (arthropod transmitted)

Gasterophilus	(1 A)	atrial, intestinal, cutaneous
Hypoderma	(1 A)	cutaneous
Oestrus	(1 A)	atrial, eye
Rhinoestrus	(1 A)	atrial, eye
Family SARCOPHAGIDAE		
Genus *Sarcophaga*	(2 C)	wounds
Wohlfahrtia	(1 C)	atrial, cutaneous, wounds

Morphology of Larva. The mature third-stage larva (Fig. 15-20) of the nonbloodsucking fly usually has a broad truncated posterior, a narrow anterior with hooklike processes and paired papillae, and a spinose area on each segment. Certain structures are useful for identifying genera and species: (1) shape and ornamentation, (2) structure of the anterior end, the cephalopharyngeal skeleton, (3) the small fanlike, branched anterior spiracles on the second segment, and (4) most important of all, the posterior spiracles on the last abdominal segment. The shape of these openings varies from species to species, as does the completeness and thickness of the peritreme. In addition, identification of certain species may be made by rearing the adult fly from the larva.

Treatment. Cutaneous and subcutaneous myiasis require the surgical removal of the larvae after local anesthesia. The eggs and maggots may be washed from hair, skin, and wounds with soap and water. Urinary myiasis usually terminates spontaneously, although cystoscopic treatment is sometimes necessary. Purgation with sodium sulfate or anthelmintics may be used for gastrointestinal myiasis.

Control. Diverse methods are employed to reduce the number of myiasis-producing flies. Prevention in humans necessitates the control of infestations in animals by larvicides and other measures. Destruction of carcasses and the disposal of offal reduces the breeding grounds of certain species. Fly traps are effective under special circumstances. The screening of susceptible domesticated animals, treatment of wounds, and repellents are useful. Persons, especially infants, with catarrhal or suppurative lesions should not sleep in the open. Control of the African floor maggot consists of the application of insecticides and raising sleeping mats to platforms off the floor.

Vectors of Disease. Filth flies are mechanical vectors of pathogenic organisms, especially those of enteric diseases. Pathogenic viruses, bacteria, protozoa, and helminthic eggs may be carried on their bodies, legs, and mouth parts, or even may pass unharmed through their intestinal tracts. Several species, especially the common house fly, have been incriminated on experimental and epidemiologic evidence as vectors of typhoid, salmonellosis, cholera, bacillary and amebic dysenteries, tuberculosis, plague, tularemia, anthrax, yaws, conjunctivitis, undulant fever, trypanosomiasis, leishmaniasis, and spirochetal diseases.

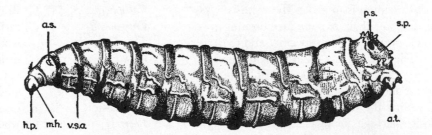

Figure 15-20. Mature larva of a muscid fly.
a.s., anterior spiracles; a.t., anal tubercle; h.p., head papillae; m.h., mouth hooks; p.s., posterior spiracles; s.p., stigmal plate; v.s.a., ventral spinose area. (Redrawn from Hegner, Root, Augustine, Huff: Parasitology, 1938. Courtesy of D. Appleton-Century Company.)

Musca domestica (House Fly)

The common house fly *M. domestica* infests human habitations throughout the world. The eggs are laid in lots of about 100 in manure or refuse. The entire life cycle occupies 7 to 10 days, and the adult fly lives about a month (Fig. 15-21). Its larvae are responsible for an occasional intestinal and genitourinary myiasis. The fly, however, is a mechanical vector of pathogenic bacteria, protozoa, and helminthic eggs and larvae, especially of enteric disease organisms. The extent of disease transmission by flies under natural conditions is difficult to determine. Control is a community measure, since flies travel considerable distances, but screening and trapping protect the individual home. Adequate control involves the elimination of breeding places by the disposal or chemical treatment of animal excrement, garbage, and decaying vegetation, and residual spraying of the interiors of houses and barns with appropriate insecticides. Pyrethroid-coated fiberglass strips can be hung in barns. On chicken farms, biologic control in

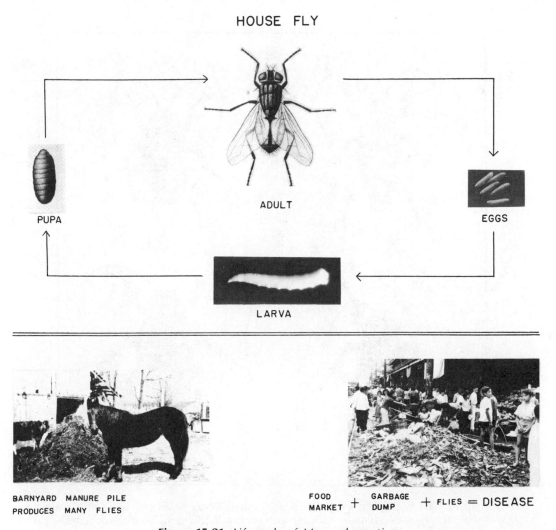

Figure 15-21. Life cycle of *Musca domestica.*

the form of feeding juvenile hormone to chickens has been used to inhibit development of larvae in the chicken manure. In addition, in this setting, the release of a microhymenopteran parasite, *Spalangia endius,* has been effective.

ORDER ORTHOPTERA (COCKROACHES)

Cockroaches of the family BLATTIDAE are important household pests and may be mechanical vectors of pathogenic organisms as well as intermediate hosts of helminthic parasites.

They are large, swift-running, omnivorous, terrestrial insects with long antennae, biting mouth parts, narrow hardened forewings, membranous hindwings, and legs approximately equal in length.

In North America, north of Mexico, there are several species of cockroach of economic importance that infest buildings (Fig. 15-22). The oriental cockroach, *Blatta orientalis,* a dark-brown insect about 2.5 cm in length, has spread from the Far East throughout the world. The smaller, light-brown German cockroach or Croton bug, *Blattella germanica,* about 1.3 cm in length, and the large reddish-brown American cockroaches, *Periplaneta*

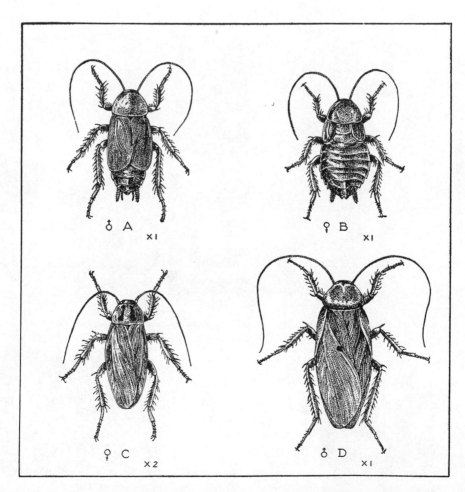

Figure 15-22. The cockroach. A. Oriental cockroach, *Blatta orientalis,* male. B. Oriental cockroach, *B. orientalis,* female. C. German cockroach, *Blattella germanica,* female. D. American cockroach, *Periplaneta americana,* male. (Redrawn from Laing, 1938.)

americana, about 3.8 cm in length, have well-developed wings. *Periplaneta fuligniosa* is common in the southern United States. The brown-banded *Supella supellectilium,* the common household cockroach of Hawaii, has become, in the past two decades, increasingly prevalent in the United States.

Habits. The oriental and German cockroaches frequent homes and food-handling establishments, while the American and Australian species prefer ships, warehouses, sugar refineries, sewage systems, and hothouses. Cockroaches are nocturnal, shun bright sunlight, and seek concealment during the day in crevices and basements. They are omnivorous, with a partiality for starchy foods. They may infest buildings through their introduction in food supplies or by migrating along plumbing installations. *B. germanica,* the most resistant species, has been used for testing insecticides.

Life Cycle. The eggs are deposited at random in oothecas, so-called egg cases. The incubation period at 25 C varies from 26 to 69 days for the several species. Development is by incomplete metamorphosis. The nymph passes through 13 molts to reach the adult stage. The length of the life cycle is 2 to 21 months according to the species. The life span of the adult is slightly more than 40 days (Fig. 15-23).

Pathogenicity. The omnivorous habits of these pests cause damage to books, leather, and woolen goods, while the roachy odor from the glandular secretions spoils food and, when eaten, may cause asthma in some persons. Its dual contact with filth and food suggests the mechanical transmission of pathogenic organisms. The oriental, German, and American cockroaches have been incriminated as intermediate hosts of the cestode *Hymenolepis diminuta,* the German of the nematode *Gongylonema pulchrum,* and the American of the acanthocephalid, *Moniliformis moniliformis.*

Control. Their wary habits make methods of control difficult. Cleanliness in kitchens and the protection of stored foods are primary essentials. Repair of cracks and tight-fitting plumbing installations in the walls are preventive measures. Hercon Insectape impregnated with Baygon, Dursban, or Diazinon placed in

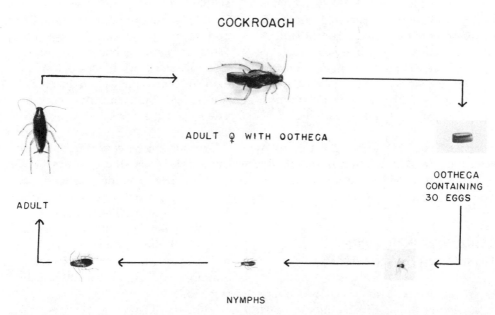

COCKROACH

ADULT ♀ WITH OOTHECA

OOTHECA
CONTAINING
30 EGGS

ADULT

NYMPHS

Figure 15-23. Life cycle of *Blattella germanica* (the cockroach).

strategic locations is generally effective for up to a year. Half (0.5) percent resmethrin in conjunction with boric acid dust is quite effective for months. Control in sewers is by two foggings 1 month apart, then at 2-month intervals, with 0.15 percent bioresmethrin or 0.10 percent cismethrin. Dusts containing insecticide are usually more effective than sprays, and are spread in cracks and across lines of traffic of the insects.

ORDER COLEOPTERA (BEETLES)

A few families of beetles contain species that are injurious to humans by the action of vesicating or blistering fluids, or by being intermediate hosts of helminthic parasites. The blister beetles of the family MELOIDAE produce cantharidin, a volatile vesicating substance. The commercial preparation, obtained from the Spanish fly, *Lytta vesicatoria,* is used as a rubefacient, diuretic, and aphrodisiac. When cantharidin comes in contact with the skin, mucous membranes, or conjunctiva by crushing the beetle or by the discharge of its body fluids, it causes a painful, burning blister. Species of rove beetles of the family STAPHYLINIDAE produce another vesicating substance. Rare instances of the canthariasis of the digestive tract, urinary system, and nasal passages, due to the incidental invasion of vesicating beetles, have been reported.

Larval and adult beetles serve as intermediate hosts for rare helminthic parasites of humanity.

Treatment. The skin lesions are treated by soothing lotions and at times by antiseptics. Purgation with sodium sulfate is recommended for intestinal canthariasis.

ORDER HYMENOPTERA (BEES, WASPS, AND ANTS)

Bees, wasps, and ants, the venenating insects, possess membranous wings, mouth parts adapted for chewing, licking, or sucking plants, and an ovipositor modified for piercing, sawing, or stinging. The stinger has a barbed sheath, a pair of serrated lancets, and a pair of lateral palps. The venom, secreted by paired glands, is forced down the canal formed by the sheath and lancets. During the act of stinging, the ovipositor is cast off by the honeybee and some wasps, but it is retained by other species. The exact nature of the venom is unknown, but it contains toxic proteins: histamine, acetylcholine, and phospholipases.

The sting of bees, wasps, and hornets causes pain, edema, and local inflammation. Ordinarily, the symptoms disappear after a few hours, but at times there may be marked swelling and inflammation, depending upon the location and number of the stings. Supersensitive persons manifest mild to severe systemic reactions, depending upon the degree of sensitiveness and the rapidity of absorption of the venom. A number of cases of severe systemic manifestations, in some instances with fatal terminations, have been reported. Such individuals manifest symptoms of anaphylactic shock with respiratory and cardiac impairment, general edema, and urticaria. Among 50 patients who died of stings, death was attributed to respiratory tract angioedema in 35, anaphylactic shock in 6, vascular reactions in 6, and nervous system reactions in 3. Thirteen were known to be allergic. Twenty-nine patients died within 6 hours from one sting. In a small number, death was delayed for more than 96 hours. Thirty-eight died of only one or two stings. Supersensitive persons should avoid, as far as possible, exposure to these insects.

The stinging ants of the temperate zones cause little injury, but the large tropical species give rise to considerable pain and inflammation and, if the stings are numerous, may even endanger life. The foraging ants of India and Africa bite viciously with their mandibles. The small fire ant of the genus *Solenopsis,* which is spreading in the southern United States, causes a fiery sting and pruritic vesicles (Fig. 15-24).

Treatment. The stings of bees, wasps, and ants are treated locally with analgesic-corticosteroid lotion. The stingers of bees should be

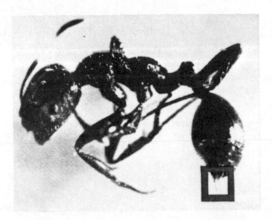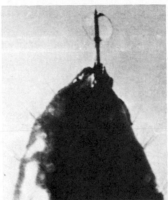

Figure 15-24. Fire ant *(Solenopsis saevissima richteri)*. Note posterior stinging apparatus with drop of venom. (Courtesy of Medical World News.)

removed from the wound and an ice pack applied. Hypersensitive persons who experience severe reactions from a bee sting and manifest symptoms of anaphylactic shock with respiratory and cardiac impairment, edema, and urticaria should be treated with epinephrine and 30 mg Prednisone along with a quick-acting antihistaminic, to be repeated in 15 to 30 minutes if necessary. Allergic persons may be desensitized by injections of extracts of bee venom or of whole bees, which are group specific for bees and wasps. Polyvalent, whole-body extract antigens of honeybee, bumble-bee, wasp, yellow jacket, hornet, red ant, and fire ant are reported to produce comprehensive protection against the stings of HYMENOPTERA. A kit containing epinephrine and an antihistamine for injection should be carried by known hypersensitive persons.

Control. Baits prepared from amidinohydrazones in granular soybean oil have proven very effective. Mounds in yards may be drenched with 7 to 14 gm of malathion or carbaryl in 7.5 liters of water.

ORDER LEPIDOPTERA (CATERPILLARS, MOTHS, AND BUTTERFLIES)

In the United States the common form of caterpillar dermatitis is caused in the eastern part by the brown-tail tussock moth, *Nygmia*

phaeorrhoea, and in the eastern and central sections by the silkworm moth, *Automeris io.*

The poisonous hairs are of two types, the venom being secreted (1) by a single gland cell at the base of the hair (tussock moth and puss caterpillar), and (2) by cells lining the lower part of the sharp chitinized spines (flannel moths). Caterpillars that fall on exposed portions of the body cause excruciating pain. The exact composition of the poison is unknown, but it is probably proteic or linked with a protein. Poisoning is acquired by contact with caterpillars or their nests, or by windblown hairs settling upon the exposed body or upon drying underclothing. The severity of the dermatitis depends upon the species of caterpillar, the site and extent of the exposure, and the sensitiveness of the victim. There is an early burning or prickling sensation with numbness and pronounced itching, followed by a vesicular edematous erythema. Windblown hairs may produce an irritating ophthalmia and a serious inflammation of the respiratory tract. Allergic reactions may occur in sensitive persons. Prevention requires the avoidance of localities frequented by poisonous caterpillars and the destruction, where possible, of the caterpillars and their nests by insecticidal sprays of DDT or Chlordane, or the application of creosote to the egg masses.

Several species of moth larvae serve as intermediate hosts of the tapeworm *Hymenolepis diminuta.*

Treatment. Calamine lotion, lime water, or zinc oxide may be applied to the cutaneous lesions. Systemic reactions in supersensitive persons are treated with epinephrine.

REFERENCES

Goldman: Tungiasis in travelers from Africa. JAMA Vol. 236: 1386, 1976.

Lichtenstein, et al: Insect allergy—the state of the art. J Allergy Clin Immunol 64: 5–12. 1979.

Pence: Stinging insect allergy. Primary Care 6: 587–596, 1979.

Quraiski: Biochemical insect control—its impact on economy, environment, and natural selection. New York, Wiley, 1977.

Shama, et al and Beaucher and Farnham: Gypsy-moth caterpillar dermatitis. N Engl J Med 306: 1300–1301 and 1301–1302, 1982.

16

Class Arachnida—Ticks, Mites, Spiders, Scorpions

The arachnids differ from the insects in the absence of wings, antennae, and compound eyes; the presence of four pairs of legs in the adult stage; and the fusion of the head and thorax into a cephalothorax in spiders and scorpions. The head, thorax, and abdomen are fused into a single body region in ticks and mites. The ARANEIDA (spiders) and SCORPIONIDA (scorpions) are injurious to humans by their bites and stings; the degenerate wormlike PENTASTOMIDA are rare parasites of humans; the ACARINA (ticks and mites) are of special importance as vectors of human diseases.

ORDER ACARINA (TICKS AND MITES)

The order ACARINA, ticks and mites, includes many parasites and vectors of diseases of humans and lower animals. The mouth parts and their base, the capitulum, are attached to the anterior portion of the body by a movable hinge. The sexes are separate.

Parasitic Ticks

The tick differs from the mite in its larger size, hairless or short-haired leathery body, exposed armed hypostome, and the presence of a pair of spiracles near the coxae of the fourth pair of legs. About 300 species are bloodsucking ectoparasites of mammals, birds, reptiles, and amphibians, and nearly all are capable of biting human beings.

Classification. Ticks are divided into the ARGASIDAE, or soft ticks, and the IXODIDAE, or hard ticks. The argasid ticks are more primitive, are less constantly parasitic, produce fewer progeny, and infest the habitat of the host. The ixodid ticks are more specialized, more highly parasitic, produce more progeny, and infest the host itself.

Family Ixoidae

The hard ticks, so-called because of the horny scutum, have a cosmopolitan distribution. The sexes are usually dissimilar. There is a hard dorsal scutum on the anterior dorsal surface in the female but covering the entire dorsum in the male; the capitulum is visible dorsally at the anterior end.

Morphology. The reddish or mahogany-brown cephalothorax and abdomen are fused into an oval or elliptical body with four pairs of six-segmented legs that arise from the plates of the basal coxae (Fig. 16-1). The false head, or capitulum, projects from the anterior end in the hard ticks and is concealed in the soft ticks. In the hard ticks it consists of a basal plate, or basis capituli, of taxonomic value, and the mouth parts comprising hypostome, chelicerae, and pedipalps. The median hypostome with its transverse rows of recurved, filelike teeth anchors the parasite to the host. The dorsally paired, chitinous, shaftlike chelicerae act as cutting organs to permit the insertion of the hypostome. The paired, four-jointed pedipalps do not penetrate the tissues but serve as supports. The eyes, when present, are on or near the anterior lateral margin of the scutum. Coxal glands between the first two coxae secrete a tenacious fluid during feeding and copulation by some of the soft ticks.

Life Cycle. Both sexes are bloodsuckers. The female hard tick, *Dermacentor,* increases greatly in size after an engorgement of blood for 5 to 13 days. It then drops off the host to deposit, in 14 to 41 days, 2000 to 8000 small, oval, brown eggs and dies in 3 to 36 days after oviposition (Fig. 16-2). The soft ticks lay 100 to 200 eggs in several batches following successive blood meals. After 2 to 7 weeks, larvae with three pairs of legs emerge from the eggs. These active "seed" ticks attach themselves to small animals for a blood meal, then drop off and molt into nymphs with four pairs of legs but without a genital pore. Hard ticks have a single nymphal stage, but soft ticks may have several. Nymphs may hibernate unfed over the winter and then, after one or more blood meals, molt into adults on the ground. The life cycle is usually completed in 1 or 2 years, occasionally in 3. The adults may hibernate unfed, and then the fertilized female, after a blood meal, deposits her eggs. The same or different species of mammal may serve as hosts for the various stages. Various modifications of the cycle such as change of host, length of time on the host, number of molts, and frequency of oviposition occur in different species.

During their larval, nymphal, and adult stages, ticks are intermittent parasites of animals and spend most of their existence on the ground. Some species *(Boophilus),* however,

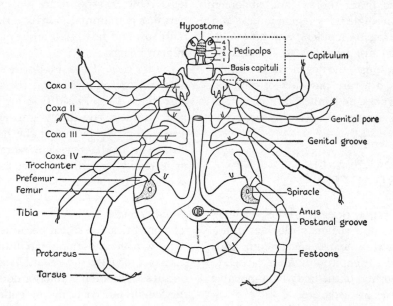

Figure 16-1. Ventral view of male *Dermacentor andersoni,* showing anatomic structures.

spend most of their lives on animals. Favorable environmental conditions include abundant vegetation, moisture, and numerous animal hosts. Ticks are susceptible to sunlight, desiccation, and excessive rainfall, but are resistant to cold. Ticks are long-lived; the soft tick, *Ornithodoros turicata*, survives more than 25 years and undergoes starvation for 5 years. The larval and nymphal ticks feed on small animals, and the adult ticks on medium to large ones, attaching themselves when the animals come in contact with infested vegetation.

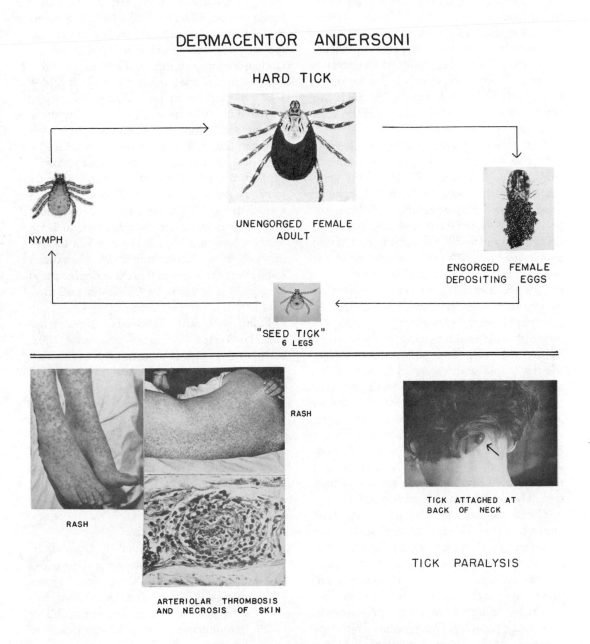

DERMACENTOR ANDERSONI

HARD TICK

NYMPH

UNENGORGED FEMALE
ADULT

ENGORGED FEMALE
DEPOSITING EGGS

"SEED TICK"
6 LEGS

RASH

RASH

ARTERIOLAR THROMBOSIS
AND NECROSIS OF SKIN

TICK ATTACHED AT
BACK OF NECK

TICK PARALYSIS

Figure 16-2. Life cycle of *Dermacentor andersoni*.

Pathogenicity. Ticks harm humans and lower animals by (1) the mechanical injury of their bites, (2) the production of tick paralysis, and (3) the transmission of bacterial, viral, rickettsial, spirochetal, and protozoan diseases.

After the chelicerae have cut the skin, the toothed hypostome anchors the tick during the blood meal. Its insertion produces an inflammatory reaction of the perivascular tissues of the corium, with local hyperemia, edema, hemorrhage, and thickening of the stratum corneum. The wound may become necrotic or secondarily infected. If the capitulum is broken off in the skin during removal of the tick it may cause a festering wound.

Tick paralysis occurs in sheep, cattle, dogs, cats, and occasionally in humans. About 12 ixodid ticks, and even soft ticks of the genus *Ornithodoros,* have been implicated. The disease is usually associated with species of *Dermacentor* and *Amblyomma* in North America, and of *Ixodes* in Australia and South Africa. The paralysis is sometimes severe in domesticated animals. The disease manifests itself as a progressive, ascending, flaccid motor paralysis that is due to a neuromuscular blockade at the presynaptic level, with electrodiagnostic evidence of peripheral nerve involvement caused by the tick toxin. The toxin is elaborated by the tick's ovaries and secreted by the salivary glands. The pathology comprises small hemorrhagic foci, diffuse hyperemia, and focal agranulocytic infiltration around the nerve cells in the brain and cord. The lower motor neurons of the spinal cord and cranial nerves are chiefly involved. There is destruction of the myelin sheath and perivascular infiltration. The cerebrospinal fluid is normal.

The disease has a rapid onset, with malaise, vague body pains, lassitude, cephalgia, irritability, and slight or no fever. In a few hours an ascending flaccid paralysis ensues with muscular incoordination, ataxia, dysphagia, and muscular paralysis, usually bilateral but sometimes localized. Sensory signs are very rare in tick paralysis. Death occurs from respiratory paralysis, although most affected persons recover. Children are usually affected; occasionally aged adults are affected. Chil-

dren under 2 years of age succumb rapidly. The paralysis subsides after the removal of the tick.

Other types of human disease associated with exposure to ticks are a systemic illness with skin lesions, erythema chronicum migrans (ECM), and, with arthritis, so-called Lyme disease. The former, ECM, is characterized by chronic annular erythematous skin lesions, fever, and constitutional symptoms, including aseptic meningitis. This has been recognized in Europe and in the United States. Lyme disease, or Lyme arthritis, also begins with a skin lesion as in ECM, but goes on to involve the joints. Although direct proof is lacking that tick bites cause these diseases, there are very strong epidemiologic data to support the hypothesis that the diseases are somehow related to bites of *Ixodes* ticks. A spirochete, which has been found in the gut of *I. dammini* ticks, and to which Lyme arthritis patients have antibody is suspected in the etiology of Lyme disease and ECM. The species implicated are *I. dammini* in New England and Wisconsin, *I. pacificus* in California and Oregon, and *I. ricinus* in Europe.

Vectors of Disease. Ticks have been recognized as vectors of disease ever since 1893, when Smith and Kilbourne discovered that *Boophilus annulatus* was the transmitting agent of Texas fever in cattle. In some species the causative organisms pass not only through the metamorphic stages of the tick, but also through the eggs, to succeeding generations. The diseases transmitted among domesticated animals cause heavy financial loss. An incomplete list of the vector ticks for the various human diseases is given below.

A. Rickettsial diseases
    1. American spotted fever *(Rickettsia rickettsii).* Mainly *Dermacentor andersoni* and *D. variabilis* in North America. Various species of *Ixodes* and *Ornithodoros* can serve as vectors from Mexico to Brazil.
    2. Boutonneuse fever or African tick fever *(R. conorii);* Russian tick typhus *(R. siberica),* and Queensland tick typhus *(R. australis).* All are transmitted by ixodid

ticks, such as *Rhipicephalus sanguineus, D. Reticulatus, I. hexagonus, D. marginatus, D. nuttalli,* and *I. holocyclus*

3. Q fever *(Coxiella burnetii). D. andersoni,* species of *Amblyomma, R. sanguineus,* and *Ornithodoros moubata* are involved in the transmission to wild mammals and domestic livestock. But human infection is acquired mainly by contact with domestic animals.

B. Viral diseases
1. Colorado tick fever. *D. andersoni*
2. Hemorrhagic fevers (Crimean-Congo). Various species of *Hyalomma*
3. Louping ill. *I. ricinus*
4. Kyasunur Forest disease. *Haemaphysalis spinigera*
5. Powasson eacephalitis. Various species of *Ixodes;* also *D. andersoni*
6. Russian spring-summer encephalitis. Mainly *I. persulcatus*

C. Bacterial and spirochetal diseases
1. Relapsing fever (tick-borne). Various species of *Ornithodoros*
2. Tularemic *(Francisella tularensis). Amblyomma americanum;* various species of *Dermacentor, I. ricinus,* and *R. sanguineus.*

D. Protozoal diseases
1. Babesiosis *(Babesia microti). I. dammini*

E. Possible systemic diseases
1. Lyme arthritis and ECM. *I. dammini, I. ricinus,* and *I. pacificus.*

Family Argasidae

The soft ticks are primarily ectoparasites of birds, less commonly of mammals and humans. They have a cosmopolitan distribution but are more abundant in warm climates. The sexes are similar; there is no dorsal plate, the capitulum is not visible dorsally, the spiracles lie in front of the third pair of unspurred coxae, and the tarsi bear no pads or pulvilli. They are nocturnal feeders and seldom travel far from their local habitat. *Argus persicus,* a natural parasite of fowl and a vector of avian disease in many tropical and semitropical countries, occasionally bites humans, producing painful wounds that are subject to secondary infection. *Ornithodoros moubata* (Fig. 16-3) of Africa, an oval, yellowish-brown, tuberculated, leathery tick, 8 to 9 mm, is the best known parasitic species of this genus. This tick inhabits the cracks in the floors of native huts and bites its victims at night. The bites of both nymphs and adults produce hard red wheals that remain painful for 24 hours. It is an important vector of endemic relapsing fever. Several other species of *Ornithodoros* are vectors of local types of relapsing fever throughout the world.

Treatment. The painless bite of the tick seldom calls for treatment. The ticks may be removed from the skin by gentle traction after applying chloroform, ether, alcohol, gasoline, kerosene, glycerol, ethyl chloride, or a glowing

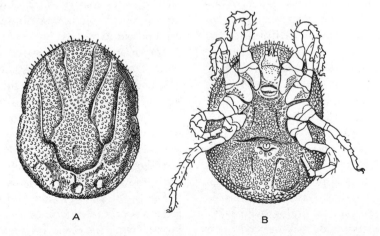

A   B

Figure 16-3. *Ornithodoros moubata.* A. Dorsal view, female. B. Ventral view, female.

match or cigarette to the tick. Care should be taken not to break off the capitulum in the wound. Early removal is indicated in order to prevent tick paralysis. Paralysis, if present, soon subsides after the removal of the tick. In endemic areas of rickettsial and spirochetal diseases, careful search for ticks should be made on persons exposed to tick-infested areas, and care should be taken not to contaminate the hands with the fluid secretions of the tick during its removal.

Control. Argasid ticks are best combated by destroying their nests or lairs. Infested native huts should be burned, or the floors and walls should be plastered to eliminate the crevices and then sprayed with BHC or the less effective DDT. More than one application is required, since these insecticides are ineffective against the eggs. Rodent-proofing of buildings is desirable. Inhabitants should avoid sleeping on the floor.

Ixodid ticks may be eliminated by exterminating their rodent hosts and destroying their habitats. The infested grounds, houses, and animals may be sprayed with Diazinon, DDT, Chlordane, Dieldrin, or BHC. BHC and Diazinon have the most rapid immobilizing action but less residual toxicity than the others, which give good control within a few days and prevent reinfestation for a month or more. Sprays and 5 to 10 percent dusts are equally effective. Suspensions and emulsions are preferable to oil solutions. Effectiveness depends upon the amount and the thoroughness of distribution. It is advisable to start spraying in the spring, but a subsequent treatment at the peak of population in the summer is necessary. Ticks may be brought into houses on clothing or animals, and the dog tick, *R. sanguineus,* may pass its entire life cycle indoors. It is difficult to eliminate ticks from houses. DDT, Chlordane, and Diazinon, when applied as liquid sprays to floors and walls, are effective for several weeks; more than one application may be required. It is preferable to prevent house infestation by the removal of infested clothing and the treatment of dogs with DDT or BHC. Those traversing tick-infested areas should use tick-proof clothing, and, after re-moving the clothing, a search should be made for ticks on their bodies. Repellents applied to the skin provide little protection, but clothing treated with diethyltoluamide gives protection for from several days to a week. Indalone is a better tick repellent than dimethyl phthalate and Rutgers 612, but all give fairly good protection.

Parasitic Mites

The term *mite* is usually applied to members of the order ACARINA other than the ticks. Mites are much smaller than ticks and do not have a leathery covering. Spiracles are present on the idiosoma of some mites, and the hypostome is unarmed. The parasitic species infest plants and animals, and some cause direct injury to people or transmit human diseases. The parasitic mites are chiefly ectoparasites, but a few are endoparasites. Most species have a cosmopolitan distribution. Some species use insects as a means of transportation and a source of food. General rather than specific host specificity seems to be the rule.

Life Cycle. The eggs are deposited in the soil or on the skin of the host. The six-legged larvae, which feed on blood or plant juices, metamorphose into eight-legged nymphs, and finally into eight-legged adults.

Family Trombiculidae (Red Bugs and Chiggers)

The larvae of the trombiculid mites, known as harvest mites, red bugs, or chiggers, are annoying pests to picnickers, hunters, berry pickers, and campers.

Morphology. The orange-red or brilliantly spotted adult mites are usually scavengers. The body is partly covered with minute hairs and has four pairs of legs (Fig. 16-4).

Habits. Chiggers inhabit moist grassy or brushy terrain frequented by domesticated animals or wild rodents or birds. As larvae they feed on surface tissue cells of mammals, birds, reptiles, and amphibians.

Life Cycle. The eggs are laid in clusters on the moist ground rich in humus. The hatched larvae (Fig. 16-4) feed on animals and then drop to the ground to become nymphs and, finally, adults. The life cycle covers 50 to 70 days, and the adult females live more than a year.

Pathogenicity. The North American chigger or red bug, *Trombicula alfreddugèsi,* infests grasses and bushes, whence it attacks animals and people. The larva crawls actively up the legs and attaches itself to the skin by the capitulum. Its bite, typical of other chiggers, causes itching, increasing to a maximum on the second day. Then the swelling subsides, and a light pinkish color surrounds the punc-

TROMBICULA ALFREDDUGESI

CHIGGER

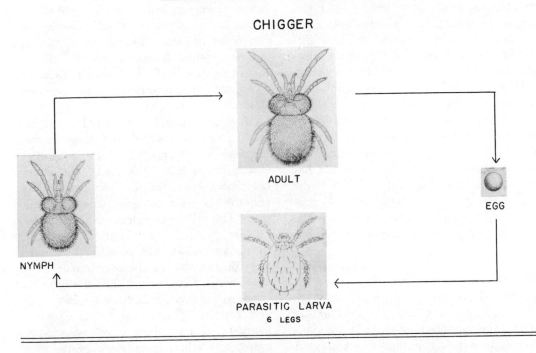

ADULT

EGG

NYMPH

PARASITIC LARVA
6 LEGS

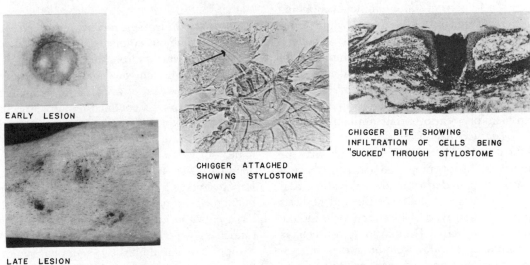

EARLY LESION

LATE LESION

CHIGGER ATTACHED
SHOWING STYLOSTOME

CHIGGER BITE SHOWING
INFILTRATION OF CELLS BEING
"SUCKED" THROUGH STYLOSTOME

Figure 16-4. Life cycle of *Trombicula alfreddugesi.*

ture; this gradually turns to a deep red on the third day. The patient suffers severe discomfort with attendant loss of sleep. Severe infestations may produce fever and secondary infection from scratching.

T. autumnalis, the harvest mite of Europe, and allied species in other parts of the world, are also annoying pests.

Vectors of Disease. Tsutsugamushi disease, or scrub typhus, is characterized by an initial ulcer at the site of the bite, remittent fever, lymphadenitis, splenomegaly, and a bright-red eruption. Chloramphenicol and the tetracyclines are curative. The chief vectors belong to the subgenus *Leptotrombidium.* The larval mites are parasites of mice, voles, rats, and shrews in Japan, and field rats in Taiwan and Indonesia. Humans act as an incidental host, the larvae attaching themselves to field workers. The organism, *Rickettsia tsutsugamushi,* has been isolated from the salivary glands of the larval mites. It can be transmitted from generation to generation, so that the larvae of the second generation are capable of infecting humans.

Several species of the house-breeding mite genus *Dermatophagoides* are responsible for "house-dust" allergy.

Treatment. For the irritating dermatitis caused by chiggers, a hot soap and water bath is followed by the application to the affected skin of a 10 percent sulfur ointment containing 1 percent phenol. Palliative treatment includes the application of alcohol, ammonia, baking soda, alcoholic iodine, camphor, or a saturated solution of salicylic acid in alcohol with a little sweet oil. Pyogenic infections are treated with 30 percent ammoniated mercury ointment or an appropriate antibiotic.

Control. Control of mites in their habitats is difficult. (1) The breeding grounds may be destroyed by burning and clearing the tall grasses and underbrush, by cultivation, and by sheep grazing, and (2) the rodent hosts may be destroyed. Chlordane or Lindane sprays are effective. Ground sprays with chlorpyriphos or ultralow-volume sprays of propoxur can also be used. Persons may be protected by boots and closely woven clothing with tight-fitting edges or, better, by clothing impregnated with repellents such as a mixture of equal parts of diethyltoluamide and benzyl benzoate with an emulsifier.

Family Sarcoptidae (Scabies)

The itch and mange mites of the family SARCOPTIDAE are of medical and veterinary importance. Species of the genus *Sarcoptes* cause itch or mange by burrowing into the skins of mammals. *S. scabiei* is the only species that commonly produces human disease, although domestic animal species occasionally infest humans temporarily. This mite has a cosmopolitan distribution, especially among the poorer classes.

Morphology. *S. scabiei* is a small, oval, dorsally convex, ventrally flattened, eyeless mite, the male measuring 200 to 250 μ, and the female 330 to 450 μ (Fig. 16-5). The anterior notothorax bears the first two pairs of legs, and the posterior notogaster the second two pairs. The first pairs of legs terminate in long tubular processes each with a bell-shaped sucker and claws. The posterior legs end in long bristles, except the fourth pair in the male, which have suckers. The dorsal surface is ridged transversely and bears spines, scales, and bristles. The mouth parts consist of toothed chelicerae, three-jointed conical pedipalps, and labial palps fused to the hypostome.

Life Cycle (Fig. 16-5). The mites live in slightly serpiginous cutaneous burrows. When activated by warmth from the skin the female, usually at night, burrows into the skin, progressing at the rate of about 2 to 3 mm per day. The burrow is confined to the corneous layer of the skin. The male excavates lateral pockets or branches in the burrows. The female, during her life span of 4 to 5 weeks, deposits up to 40 to 50 eggs in the burrow. Larvae emerge from the eggs usually in 3 days but sometimes not for 10 days. The hexapod larva either forms a lateral branch or a new tunnel, in which it becomes an eight-legged nymph. The female has two nymphal stages, the male only a single one. The life cycle is completed in 8 to 15 days. The female may survive off the host for 2 to 3 days at room temperature. Scabies is transmitted by personal contact, especially by persons sleeping together, and less frequently by towels, clothing, and bed linen. Infectivity is low, and the infection tends to run a limited course in healthy persons of clean habits. Infection is common in slum sections, jails, and armies.

Pathogenicity. The preferential sites are the interdigital spaces, the flexor surfaces of the wrists and forearms, elbows, axillae, back, inguinal region, and genitalia. The lesions appear as slightly reddish elevated tracts in the skin. Minute vesicular swellings, possibly produced by the irritating fecal deposits or excretions, form beneath the gallery a short distance behind the mite. The intense itching, aggravated by warmth and perspiration,

SARCOPTES SCABIEI

SCABIES OR ITCH MITE

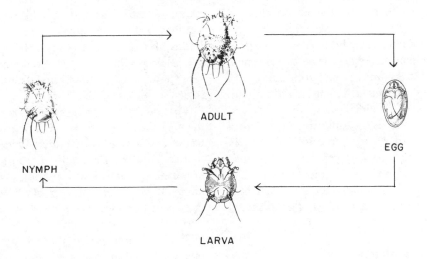

NYMPH   ADULT   EGG   LARVA

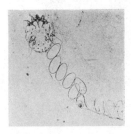

SKIN BURROW CONTAINING ADULT FEMALE AND EGGS

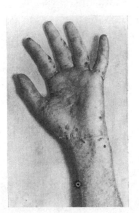

LESIONS ON HAND AND WRIST

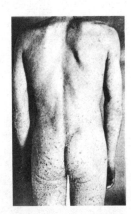

TYPICAL SCABIES RASH

Figure 16-5. Life cycle of *Sarcoptes scabiei.*

causes scratching, which spreads the infestation, irritates the lesions, and induces secondary bacterial infection. As a result, multiple papular, vesicular, and pustular lesions may be produced. At first, clinical manifestations may be mild, but after some weeks the skin becomes sensitized, resulting in an itching, widespread, erythematous eruption.

Diagnosis. The type of lesion and an itching rash are suggestive. Conclusive evidence is obtained by removing the mite from its burrow with a needle. The mites are not always easy to find, since the number of females, in spite of the high rate of reproduction, is small.

Treatment. The most satisfactory treatment of scabies is the application of Kwell, a 1 percent gamma benzene hexachloride ointment, after a hot, soapy bath. A second application is seldom necessary, since the ointment kills both mites and eggs. Crotaminton, 10 percent, is preferred in infants, children with large areas of denuded skin, and pregnant women, because of possible toxicity.* Benzyl benzoate, 12 to 25 percent, applied topically as directed in the package insert is effective.

Control. Prevention of scabies requires the treatment of infected individuals, the sterilization of garments and bedding, and personal cleanliness.

Family Demodicidae

Species of the genus *Demodex* (Fig. 16-6) are parasites of the sebaceous glands and hair follicles of mammals. They produce mange in dogs and tubercles in the skin of hogs and

---

*Another preparation if toxicity from skin absorption is a worry is a pyrethrin with piperonyl (such as RID); see p. 254.

cattle. *D. folliculorum* is a cosmopolitan parasite of the hair follicles and sebaceous glands of humans, including the senior author. It is a wormlike mite with a short capitulum and long, tapering abdomen. It rarely causes discomfort. Its presence, often unnoticed, may manifest itself in acne, blackheads, or localized keratitis, particularly in women using facial cream instead of soap and water. Treatment is rarely required.

Mites of Incidental Importance to Human Beings

The chicken mite, *Dermanyssus gallinae,* a serious pest of poultry, sometimes attacks humans. Its bite causes an itching dermatitis in poultry farmers, usually on the backs of the hands and on the forearms. The virus of St. Louis encephalitis and western equine encephalomyelitis has been isolated from naturally infected chicken mites.

The rat mite, *Ornithonyssus bacoti,* is prevalent in warm countries, including the United States and Canada. Its bite produces a papulovesicular dermatitis with urticaria in workers in stores, factories, warehouses, and stockyards. It serves as a vector of *Rickettsia typhi,* the agent of endemic typhus, from rat to rat, and is a suspected vector of Q fever. R. W. Williams demonstrated that *Ornithonyssus bacoti,* the tropical rat mite, transmits *Litomosoides,* the rodent filaria. *Allodermanyssus sanguineus,* an ectoparasite of mice, causes a dermatitis by its bite and is the vector of *R. akari,* the agent of rickettsialpox. These mites may be controlled by destruction of their hosts and the use of malathion or other insecticides.

Species of the genus *Pediculoides* produce dermatitis among workers in the grain-pro-

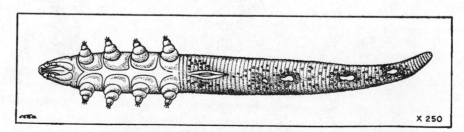

Figure 16-6. Schematic representation of female *Demodex folliculorum.*

ducing countries of the world. The North American grain-itch mite, *P. ventricosus,* feeds upon the larvae of insects that infest grains, straw, or hay. Threshers, grain handlers, and persons sleeping on straw mattresses are subject to infestation. The mites do not penetrate, but burrow superficially in the skin over the entire body, producing petechiae and erythema followed by wheals, vesicles, and pustules.

The food mites of the family TYROGLYPHIDAE feed on cheeses, cereals, and dried vegetable products, and a few on hairs, feathers, and insects. Although not bloodsuckers, they produce a temporary pruritus by penetrating the superficial epidermis. Species of *Glyciphagus* that infest sugar and species of *Tyroglyphus* that infest cheese, cereals, flour, grains, and stored food are considered responsible for "grocer's itch." *T. siro,* or a similar species, causes "vanillism" in workers handling vanilla pods; a subspecies of *T. longior,* "copra itch" in persons handling copra; and *Rhizoglyphus parasiticus,* "coolie itch" on tea plantations in India. It is doubtful whether these mites cause other than transitory intestinal symptoms, although they are found in the feces. When inhaled they produced a pneumonitis with associated eosinophilia that is known as *acariasis.*

Treatment. Various soothing lotions may be used for the cutaneous lesions caused by chicken, rat, and mouse mites. For grain and food mites, local applications of mild antiseptics relieve the annoying pruritus and prevent secondary infection. Menthol-phenol paste or soothing lotions afford relief for tyroglyphic infestations, but the affected parts should be thoroughly cleansed and Kwell ointment also applied. Pneumonitis due to mites has been treated with Stibophen or diethylcarbamazinc, although specific effectiveness of these agents is questionable.

ORDER ARANEIDA (SPIDERS)

Many species of spiders use venom to paralyze their prey. Humans rarely suffer, since the common spiders are seldom able to penetrate the skin or, if successful, produce only a mild local erythema. A few species, however, cause serious symptoms.

The unsegmented body consists of a cephalothorax, with four pairs of legs, which are separated by a slender constriction from the hairy sacculated abdomen. The mouth parts include a pair of poison jaws, or chelicerae, through the tips of which venom from paired glands in the cephalothorax is discharged.

Life Cycle. Spiders spin their webs in all manner of recesses or out-of-the-way places, both inside and outside human habitations. They trap flies and other insects in the web, paralyze them with venom, and suck the body juices. Spiders develop by gradual metamorphosis. The eggs are laid in masses, usually encased in a cocoon in which the young remain for long periods. The spiderlings pass through eight to nine molts before becoming mature adults.

Spiders Injurious to Human Beings

Many species throughout the world produce systemic poisoning by their bites. The large, hairy, ferocious-looking tarantulas, the "banana spiders," although sometimes capable of killing small animals, inflict only slight, or at most painful, injury to humans. The small spiders of the genus *Latrodectus* (Fig. 16-7), however, possess a potent venom that may produce serious symptoms. Various species of this genus are found in Europe, Australia, New Zealand, the Philippines, Africa, the West Indies, and South and North America.

Latrodectus mactans. The black widow, *L. mactans,* sometimes called the hourglass, shoe-button, or po-ko-moo spider, is the most dangerous species in the United States, where cases of spider bite with death have been reported. It ranges from southern Canada to Chile and is most abundant in the far western and southern sections. The female, 13 mm, considerably larger than the male, 6 mm, has a dark brown or black thorax and legs, and a jet-black abdomen with a characteristic orange-red spot in the form of an hourglass on the ventral surface. The spider infests lumber heaps, rail fences, stumps, undersides of privy seats, outbuildings, cracks in basements, and even houses. It avoids strong light and usually

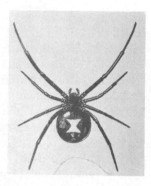 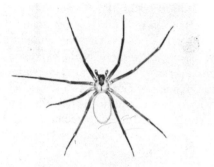

Figure 16-7. Spiders poisonous for human beings. Natural size. Left: *Latrodectus mactans* (black widow spider), ventral view. Note "hourglass" on abdomen. Right: *Loxosceles reclusa* (brown spider), dorsal view. Note "violin" on cephalothorax.

bites only when disturbed. During the summer the female lays several masses of 100 to 600 eggs in a cocoon attached to her web. The young spiderlings hatch in 2 to 4 weeks and become adults the next spring.

PATHOGENICITY. The nonhemolytic venom of *L. mactans* is probably a toxalbumin that acts as a peripheral neurotoxin. The symptoms vary with the location and the amount of venom. The bite is accompanied by a sharp, smarting pain. The site, most frequently on the buttocks or genitalia of males, shows a bluish-red spot with a white areola and sometimes an urticarial rash. Systemic symptoms follow a uniform course, corresponding to the stages of lymphatic absorption, vascular dissemination, and elimination of the toxin. At first there are throbbing, lancinating pains, and numbness in the affected part. Then pains of increasing intensity spread over the abdomen, chest, back, and extremities with rigidity and spasticity of the muscles, which may simulate the acute abdomen of perforated gastric ulcer or appendicitis.

The patient becomes dizzy, weak, thirsty, and nauseated and shows symptoms of shock. Elimination of the toxin is characterized by recovery from shock, diminished muscular pains, and residual fever and toxic nephritis. The mortality is low and occurs chiefly among children. Death may result from respiratory or circulatory failure.

TREATMENT. The following treatment for the bite of the black widow spider, *L. mactans*,

is representative for all poisonous species, except for specific antivenin. Local treatment is usually ineffective, although the following has been used. If the patient is seen soon after the bite, apply a constriction band proximal to the bite and then loosen it for 90 seconds every 15 minutes. Incision and suction are of little value if begun more than 30 minutes after the bite. Methocarbamol (1 gm in 10 ml saline), 10 ml intravenously followed by 10 ml in an intravenous drip of 5 percent dextrose solution, will usually control the muscle spasm and pain. Intravenous administration of 10 ml of 10 percent calcium gluconate is also effective. Cortisone has been reported to give some relief. The intramuscular injection of *L. mactans* antivenin, if available, usually gives relief within 30 minutes.* The injection may be repeated in 1 to 2 hours, if necessary.

CONTROL. DDT, Chlordane, and Dieldrin have been used with some success in outdoor privies, a favorite habitat of *L. mactans*. Children should be taught to be careful in localities frequented by this spider.

Necrotic Arachnidism

The bites of the small brown spider *Loxosceles laeta* of South America and *L. reclusa* of the United States produce necrotic cutaneous lesions (Fig. 16-8). Within an hour after the bite a painful edema, erythema, and even coma

---

* Antivenin *(L. mactans)* Lyovac, Merck Sharp and Dohme, West Point, Pa.

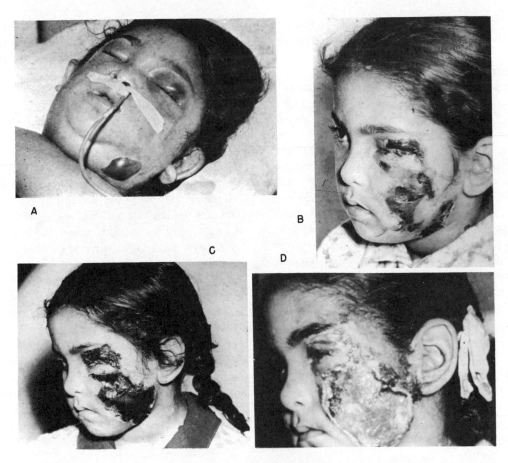

Figure 16-8. Severe necrotic arachnidism (bite of *Loxosceles laeta.*) A. 8 hours. B. 6 days. C. 23 days. D. 40 days. (Courtesy of Dept. of Parasitology, School of Medicine, University of Chile.)

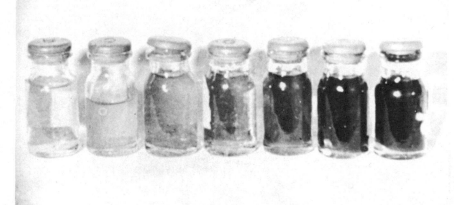

Figure 16-9. Urine from patient bitten by *Loxosceles.* Note increasing amount of hemoglobinuria. (Courtesy of Dept. of Parasitology, School of Medicine, University of Chile.)

develop, and soon large areas of the skin are involved. As the edema subsides gangrene develops, and later, with the detachment of the eschar, deep ulcerations remain (Fig. 16-8). Occasionally, the toxin of *Loxosceles* causes a systemic involvement characterized by hematuria (Fig. 16-9), anemia, high fever, convulsions, coma, and cyanosis, which may terminate fatally. The early administration of hydrocortisone, 200 to 400 mg intravenously, followed by prednisone, 40 to 60 mg orally daily for 4 to 7 days, is effective. The injection of small amounts of venom causes a minimal lesion; hence evaluation of therapy is difficult. Extensive plastic surgery is often required. Lindane and Chlordane sprays are toxic to those spiders. Recovery from loxoscelism gives a solid immunity.

Chiracanthium mildei may produce mild necrotizing lesions.

ORDER SCORPIONIDA (SCORPIONS)

Scorpions are elongated terrestrial arachnids with large pedipalps terminating in stout claws, a nonsegmented cephalothorax with four pairs of legs, and an elongated abdomen. The caudal extremity bears a hooked stinger for the discharge of venom (Fig. 16-10)

Scorpions, nocturnal in their activities, lie under rocks, logs, boards, or other protective coverings. They may invade human habitations, especially during the rainy season in the tropics. They seize their prey, usually spiders and insects, in their claws and by a backward-downward thrust of the taillike abdomen insert the stinger with the paralyzing venom. They are viviparous, and the young are carried for some time on the back of the female. There are numerous species of scorpions throughout the world.

The small species either are not able to penetrate human skin or will merely cause minor stings. The large venomous scorpions are species of *Buthus* in northern Africa and southern Europe, and *Centruroides* in Mexico and Arizona. Humans are usually stung when their bare hands or feet unexpectedly come in contact with scorpions concealed in clothing, shoes, or other hiding places. Serious and even fatal systemic reactions, especially in young children, have been reported in India, Egypt,

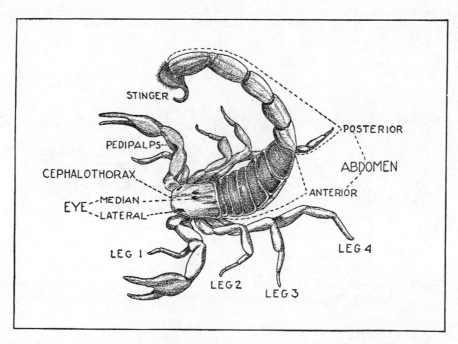

Figure 16-10. Schematic representation of scorpion with arched abdomen.

and Israel. Scorpion venom is a toxalbumin that produces paralysis, convulsions, and pulmonary disorders. The local symptoms are extremely painful. Systemically, there is a radiating burning sensation and a rapid onset of general numbness, muscular twitching, and itching. In severe cases there are muscular spasms and convulsions resembling strychnine poisoning and symptoms of shock. Fatal cases show accelerated respiration, pulmonary edema, hypotension, and myocardial damage at autopsy.

Treatment. A tourniquet should be applied immediately and the venom removed by suction from wounds made by the stingers of the large scorpions. Pain may be relieved by local applications of ice packs, ethyl chloride spray, ammonia, analgesics, or injections of novocaine or epinephrine in the vicinity of the wound. Systemic treatment is designed to combat shock and pulmonary edema. Corticosteroids have been reported to be useful. In severe cases, antivenin, if available, should be given.

Control. Attempts to reduce the scorpion population have not proved particularly successful. For houses and their vicinity, the spraying with 0.5 percent Dieldrin or a mixture of 10 percent DDT, 2 percent Chlordane, and 0.2 percent pyrethrum in a light oil base has been recommended.

ORDER PENTASTOMIDA (TONGUE WORM)

The species of medical interest in these degenerate wormlike anthropods belong to the genera *Linguatula* and *Armillifer*.

The adult and nymphal stages of *L. serrata* (Fig. 16-11) are found in the nose, paranasal sinuses, and body cavities of dogs, birds, and reptiles and encapsulated nymphs in herbivorous animals. Human infection with the adult is rare, but a number of larval infections have been reported in Europe, Africa, and North, South, and Central America. The females lay eggs that are passed in the respiratory mucus. The eggs, when ingested by a mammalian host, hatch into four-legged larvae that pass through the intestinal wall to the liver, lungs, spleen, mesenteric glands, eye, and other organs and then transform into nymphs and become encapsulated. Halzoun, or parasitic

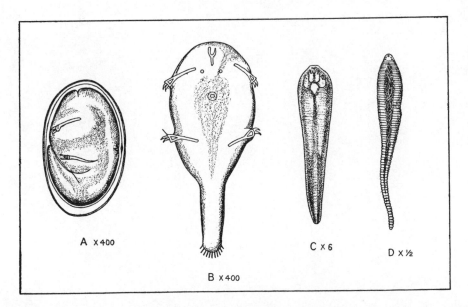

Figure 16-11. *Linguatula serrata.* A. Embryonate ovum. B. Acariform embryo. C. Nymph. D. adult. (A and B redrawn from Leuckart, 1860. C. adapted from Darling and Clark, 1912. D adapted from various sources.)

pharyngitis, is an unusual manifestation of human infection. It has been described from Lebanon as an attack of pharyngeal pain, coughing, and sneezing that comes on within minutes or a half hour after ingestion of raw liver or poorly cooked visceral lymph nodes of sheep or goats. The viscera of these herbivores contain *Linguatula* nymphs, and the symptoms result from direct irritation or possible sensitization to the organisms as they attach to the upper respiratory mucous membranes. Affected individuals sometimes notice a 5 to 10 mm "white worm" that is coughed up or extracted from the throat.

  A. armillatus of Africa, *A. moniliformis* of Asia, and possibly other species of this genus have been found in humans. They are distinguished from *L. serrata* by their cylindrical ringed bodies, resembling a string of beads. The adult is a parasite of pythons and other snakes. The nymphs are found in primates and various wild and domesticated mammals. Human infection with the larvae and nymphs is fairly common in Africa, particularly in the Repub-

lic of the Congo. The nymphs are found in the liver, intestinal mucosa, peritoneal cavity, lungs, and conjunctiva. They usually come to notice as 3 to 6 mm, rectilinear calcifications within pleural or peritoneal cavities on radiographs. But infection is usually asymptomatic. Boiling or filtering drinking water should prevent infection by eliminating infective eggs.

REFERENCES

Hoogstraal: Changing patterns of tickborne diseases in modern society. Ann Rev Entomol 26: 75–99, 1981.

Khalil and Schacher: *Linguatula serrata* in relation to halzoun and the marrara syndrome. Am J Trop Med Hyg 14: 736–746, 1965.

Orkin and Maibach: This scabies pandemic. N Engl J Med 298: 496–498, 1978.

Self, et al: Pentastomiasis in Africans. Trop Geogr Med 27: 1–13, 1975.

Steere and Malawista: Cases of Lyme disease in the Untied States: Locations correlated with the distribution of *Ixodes dammini*. Ann Intern Med 91: 730–733, 1979.

Wharton: House dust mites. J Med Entomology. 12: 577–621, 1976.

TECHNICAL METHODS

17

Diagnosis of Parasitic Diseases

I. **Include parasitic diseases in differential diagnosis.**

   A patient from Colombia with myocarditis had Chagas' disease.

II. **Where has the patient been?**

   A patient with amebic liver abscess, missed in diagnosis, had spent some months in Pakistan.

III. **How well trained is the technician? Can you rely on the report?**

   The "peculiar red blood cells" were laden with *Plasmodium malariae*. The baby also had an enlarged spleen and had received four blood transfusions.

It must be remembered that inhabitants of the tropics may have not only parasitic and the so-called tropical diseases, but also any of the numerous cosmopolitan diseases. Thus, a young missionary from Africa with a high fever, considerable weight loss, an enlarged liver, and a high alkaline phosphatase level had widespread carcinomatosis, and not malaria or African sleeping sickness. A Puerto Rican youth with a slight fever and weight loss was suffering from tuberculosis, and the few *Schistosoma mansoni* eggs in his stool did not point to his chief problem. Not infrequently, the finding of a few helminth eggs or protozoan cysts is given so much diagnostic prominence that the real cause of the patient's illness is overlooked.

Many parasitic infections are asymptomatic or produce only mild symptoms. Hence, one must develop a high index of suspicion. Routine blood and stool examinations will uncover many unsuspected infections. It is obvious that a busy clinician will not do his own laboratory examinations, but he should know their pitfalls and accuracy. Most important, the physician should know what specimen to collect, the occasional value of purged stools in amebiasis, the uselessness of stool examination in enterobiasis, and the necessity for repeated stool examination in amebiasis and schistosomiasis.

Recently, several instances of fatal overwhelming infections with *Strongyloides* have been reported. One patient had several hospital admissions with chief complaints of diarrhea, dysentery, and abdominal pain. Operations were performed several times, yet no stools were examined for eggs or parasites. With a toothpick, glass slide, feces the size of a small rice grain, and a microscope, a suspicious medical student or intern could have made the diagnosis. The patient also had a significant eosinophilia.

Eosinophilia is often given excessive importance in the medical mind as indication of a parasitic infection. Infections with parasitic worms rather than protozoa may have associated eosinophilia, especially if there is tissue invasion by the worm. But there can be considerable variation from patient to patient. Eosinophilia is usually more marked in recent than in chronic infections. But eosinophilia may be due to other conditions; numerous other diseases have been irregularly associated with eosinophilia:

Parasitic Diseases
  Nematoda
    Trichinosis
    Visceral larva migrans } may be
      (Toxocara)   } very high
    Filariasis
    Strongyloidiasis
    Ascariasis } only in first few months
    Hookworm }
  Trematoda
    Schistosomiasis
    Paragonomiasis
    Fascioliasis
    Chlonorchiasis
  Cestoda
    Echinococcus }
    Cysticercosis } occasionally
    Hymenolepis }
Bacterial Infections
  Scarlet fever (late)
  Brucellosis (chronic)
Allergic Conditions
  Asthma
  Hay fever
  Drug reactions
  Bronchopulmonary aspergillosis
  Urticaria, or hives

Malignancy
  Eosinophilic leukemia
  Hodgkin's disease
  Carcinomas of bowel, uterus, lung, etc.
Miscellaneous
  Hypereosinophilic syndrome
  Eosinophilic gastroenteritis
  Chronic eosinophilic pneumonia
  Agammaglobulinemia plus pneumocystis
    infection
Some Skin Diseases
  Eczema
  Dermatitis herpetiformis
Collagen-Vascular Disease
  Periarteritis nodosa
  Dermatomyositis
  Rheumatoid arthritis

The geographic distribution of parasitic infections is varied, and knowledge of their distribution is of great value in knowing what to look for in a patient. The patient with urologic problems who had been living in New Jersey all of her life, with no history of foreign travel, could not have had *S. haematobium*. It is true she was experiencing urinary discomfort and passing red blood cells in her urine. Desquamated epithelial cells were mistaken for the terminal-spined *S. haematobium* eggs. On the other hand, a Yemeni gentleman who had lived in Portland, Maine, from 1919 to 1944 was found to have far-advanced liver damage with marked ascites. He had lived in Yemen until he was 14 and then spent 5 years in the British Navy before taking up residence in Portland. Eleven consecutive daily stools were examined before live schistosome eggs were found in his stool. His early Arabian habitat, fortunately, encouraged the medical resident to continue stool examinations.

Although the geographic distribution of parasites aids us in diagnosis by directing our attention toward certain possibilities, the world is so vast and careful surveys so limited that one may be the first to find the initial case from a region. A number of years ago a missionary, Miss B. from Angola, appeared at the New York City Tropical Clinic with extensive skin lesions (see Figure 5-6). Scrapings of the lesions revealed *Onchocerca* microfilariae. Miss B. then asked us if by any chance this parasite could be responsible for the gradual loss of sight of her fellow missionary who had accompanied her and was in the waiting room. Poor Miss M.'s vision was 20/400, and in spite of repeated visits to ophthalmologists in Canada and the United States, nothing had been achieved. It was onchocerciasis; a nodule containing numerous adult worms was removed from her head, and she was treated with Hetrazan with considerable improvement in her vision. The area where these two missionaries served was in a supposedly *Onchocerca*-free area. At least the parasite had not been reported there. This solved the eye difficulties of a number of the missionaries, as a skin-snip survey of the area showed the parasite to be quite prevalent. New and even more extensive distribution of parasites is being reported: a focus of leishmaniasis in the Dominican Republic, *S. japonicum* in Thailand, and visceral larva migrans and *Naegleria* from many areas.

Parasitic infections may have relatively long incubation periods or may be present for a long time before producing symptoms, and this must be recognized in history taking. We have seen a primary attack of malaria delayed 3 years by chemoprophylaxis, an onchocerca nodule develop 4 months after exposure, echinococcosis 9 years after last exposure, and schistosomiasis 25 years after the patient left the endemic area.

Food habits, lack of shoes, swimming or other exposure to fresh water, and insect bites are helpful in ruling out—or in—parasitic infections. The aunt who visited her farmer-nephew in El Salvador and gave a history of many mosquito bites and a nephew who was experiencing chills and fever had reason to be sick and to have a good supply of *Plasmodium vivax* in her blood. Her first diagnosis was influenza.

The clinical picture of parasitic infections is varied, as would be expected from the many mechanisms by which they injure humans. Tissue invasion and destruction may produce fever, headache, pain, chills, nausea, and vomiting. Pressure of growing parasites give

rise to pain and, in the brain, to various motor and sensory abnormalities. Parasites may obstruct the intestine, bile ducts, lymph channels, and capillaries of the brain, and cause serious and bizarre symptoms. Extensive anemia may be produced by red cell destruction, hemorrhage, ingestion or action on the hemopoietic tissues.

To the physician, the usual site of the parasite in the host is necessary information, but we must not forget the parasitic peregrinations that lead to exotic signs and symptoms. Several years ago, an upstate New York physician called long-distance and asked about the treatment of schistosomiasis. We gave him the desired information, thinking that he had a Puerto Rican under his care. On asking whether his patient was from that island, we learned that the patient was an elderly woman who had resided in New York State all of her life except for a short excursion to Hawaii several years before. On the removal of her gallbladder a small mass was noted on the upper intestinal wall, which on sectioning contained a parasite they diagnosed as *Schistosoma*. Her stool was negative for eggs. As this patient had never visited a recognized endemic area of schistosomiasis, we requested a section of the material for study and suggested that antimony therapy for schistosomiasis be withheld. Careful study of the sections gave the diagnosis of *Fasciola* (see Figure 12-9). This wayward worm was causing its host no recognizable symptoms, and because of its encysted position, no eggs found their way into the patient's stool. *Fasciola* is not uncommon in Hawaii, a delicious metacercarial-infected watercress salad being the source of infection.

DIRECT IDENTIFICATION OF PARASITES

The successful identification of parasites requires experience in the differential characteristics of the various species of parasite, their cysts, eggs, and larvae, as well as familiarity with the pseudoparasitic forms and artifacts that may be mistaken for parasites.

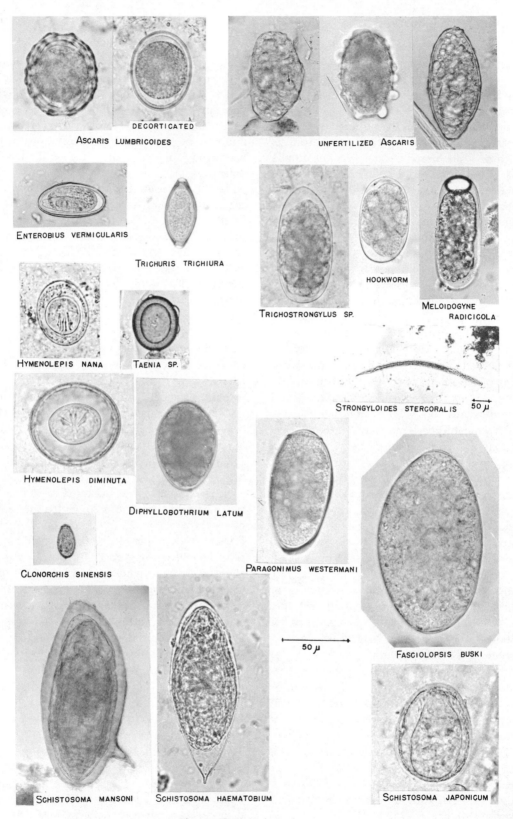

Figure 17-1. Helminth eggs.

306

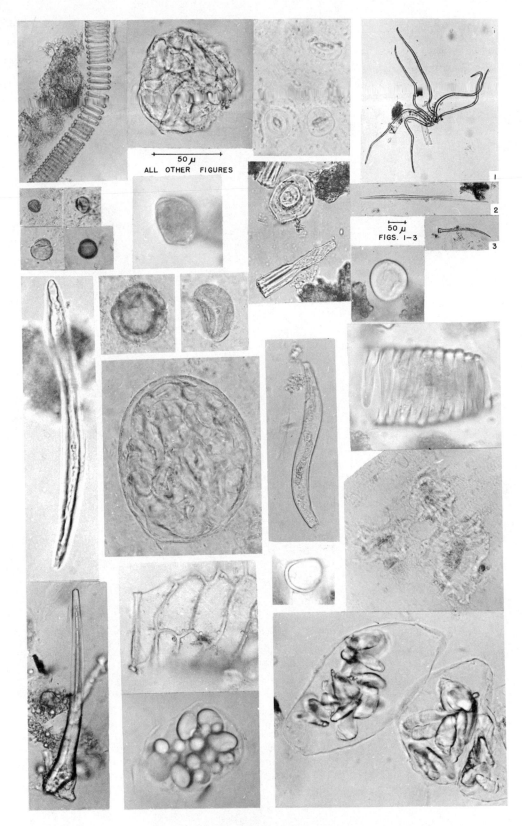

50 μ
ALL OTHER FIGURES

50 μ
FIGS. 1-3

Figure 17-2. Fecal vegetable artifacts.

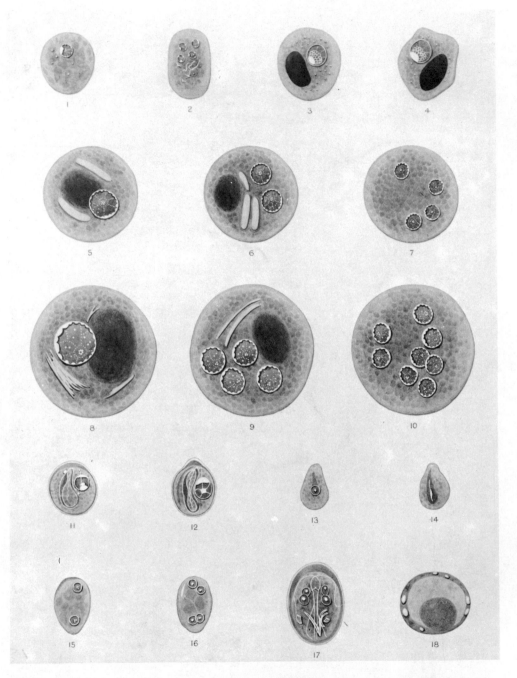

Figure 17-3. Cysts of intestinal protozoa treated with iodine (× 2000). 1 and 2. *Endolimax nana.* 3 and 4. *Iodamoeba bütschlii.* 5, 6, and 7. *Entamoeba histolytica.* 8, 9, and 10, *Entamoeba coli.* 11 and 12. *Chilomastix mesnili.* 13 and 14. *Embadomonas intestinalis.* 15 and 16. *Enteromonas hominis.* 17. *Giardia lamblia.* 18. *Blastocystis hominis,* an unusual protozoan.

Pseudoparasites. In the feces, a variety of objects may be mistaken for intestinal protozoa and helminthic eggs, and free-living nonparasitic or nonpathogenic animals may be confused with the pathogenic. The free-living protozoa, known as *coprozoic* species, either reach the feces after its passage from the human body or are swallowed and pass unchanged through the alimentary tract. A safe rule to follow is that motile trophozoites in old feces, or in specimens kept warm and moist, belong to coprozoic species. A single, egglike artifact in the stool of a patient with pernicious anemia is given undue prominence in the diagnosis of a diphyllobothriasis anemia. Blood platelets above or with superimposed red blood cells in patients with fever become malaria parasites. A patient with fever of undiagnosed lymphoma origin was given unwarranted hope by an intern for this reason. All diagnosis by the enthusiastic and partially tutored should be checked by experts. Stools that have lain around the patient's home for a day or two, insecurely covered, may present bizarre and wonderful artifacts that crawl or are wafted into the specimen. Fly maggots and other arthropods are common.

Some of the animal and plant cells and artifacts that may be mistaken for intestinal protozoa or helminthic eggs by the inexperienced observer are shown in Figure 17-2. The intestinal yeasts and fungi furnish perhaps the greatest source of confusion. *Blastocystis hominis* (Fig. 17-3, #18), a harmless intestinal commensal, 10 to 15 μ, is frequently mistaken for protozoan cysts because of its spherical central mass, thick outer protoplasm, and thin cell membrane. Vegetable cells may be differentiated by their thick cellulose walls and striations, and pollen grains by their capsular markings, micropyles, and coloring. Epithelial and squamous cells, leukocytes, and particularly large endothelial macrophages may be mistaken for protozoa. Air bubbles, oil and fat globules, mucus, and starch granules have been mistaken for protozoan cysts. Plant hairs resemble larvae.

Parasites. The intestinal and luminal protozoa are identified by the morphology of their trophozoites and cysts, and those of the blood and tissues by their characteristic intra- and extracellular forms. Helminthic parasites are identified by the morphology of the adult, egg, and larva (Fig. 17-1).

IMMUNOLOGIC METHODS OF DIAGNOSIS

Various serodiagnostic procedures, including skin test antigens, are available from private and governmental clinical laboratories. Reagents and test kits* can be purchased commercially. Although serologic tests for parasitic infections can be very useful at times, their limitations must be recognized. Because of the complex and often overlapping antigenic composition of parasites, especially helminths, antibodies may cross-react with more than one parasite. The lack of well-standardized reagents and test procedures makes the interpretation of results difficult. The different types of tests available for a single parasitic infection adds to the confusion. Finally, the serologic tests do not differentiate parasitic infection from disease and hence are not always useful in decisions concerning clinical management of an individual patient.

The antigens that evoke the production of antibodies are somatic components of parasite structures and metabolic products of secretion and excretion. Depending upon the antigenic nature of the parasite and its location in the body, a host reaction is initiated involving various subpopulations of T- and B-lymphocytes, macrophages and inflammatory cells. Antibodies of various subclasses, IgM, A, G, and E are generated. Then, depending upon where and how long the parasite persists or whether or not reinfection occurs, the immune response may be modulated, i.e., either enhanced or turned off. These dynamic events will determine the levels and types of specific immunoglobulins produced, as well as cellular reactivity to parasite antigens as revealed by

---

* Some of the companies include Hyland, Difco, Cordis, and Cooke Engineering in the United States; Wellcome in England; and Behringwerke in Germany.

skin tests. Parasites that invade the tissues produce the most pronounced immune response. Ectoparasites and worms in the intestinal tract are less likely to evoke an antibody response.

An initial response in IgM antibodies, as occurs in response to other antigens, is seen in the early phase of some parasitic infections, with a later shift to IgG antibody. Helminthic parasites, especially those that invade tissues, are more likely than protozoa to provoke IgE antibody responses. Antibody-specific mediated release of mast cell products after exposure to certain parasite antigens can be demonstrated in vitro by histamine release and in vivo as an immediately reacting skin test.

Types of Serologic Tests. Further technical details about the different serologic tests can be obtained from standard texts on laboratory methods. A very brief characterization of the main tests used in parasite diagnosis is listed here.

COMPLEMENT FIXATION (CF). The test serum is allowed to react overnight with the antigen in presence of complement. The presence and amount of specifically reactive antibody is inversely proportional to the amount of complement that has not been "fixed" in the antigen-antibody reaction. This is determined by the degree of hemolysis resulting after addition of a second antigen-antibody system of sensitized sheep red cells the next day. The test is rather complicated and requires well-standardized reagents and experience.

INDIRECT HEMAGGLUTINATION (IHA). Red blood cells that have been coated with antigen are allowed to react with test serum. The red cells agglutinate in the presence of specific antibody. The test is relatively simple to perform and requires only a few hours.

FLOCCULATION OR AGGLUTINATION. Inert particles, such as bentonite or latex, or the organism itself (usually formalin-fixed), are exposed to the test serum. Agglutination indicates the presence of a specific antibody. This is a simple and rapid test, but it requires careful controls for nonspecific agglutination. 2-mercaptoethanol treatment of serum is often useful to eliminate nonspecific agglutination produced by IgM antibodies.

INDIRECT FLUORESCENT ANTIBODY (IFA). A microscopically visible parasite fixed on a slide is stained with the test serum, then washed and stained again with anti–human globulin that has been conjugated with fluorescein. When the preparation is examined in a fluorescence microscope the presence of specific antibody in test serum is indicated by characteristic fluorescent color in those parts of the parasite with which antibody combined. The test is rapid but requires the parasite, good reagents, and special equipment. The final reading is a subjective determination.

GEL DIFFUSION (OUCHTERLONY) AND COUNTERCURRENT ELECTROPHORESIS (CEP). The test serum is placed in a hole or well adjacent to the antigen and both are allowed to diffuse toward each other through agar. The formation of precipitates or bands between the wells indicates a specific reaction. In CEP an electric current is applied to the agar slab to hasten diffusion. The test requires concentrated antigens and takes several days before results are available; moreover, it is not very sensitive. However, positive reactions are generally specific.

ENZYME-LINKED IMMUNOSORBENT ASSAY (ELISA). The test serum is allowed to react with an antigen that has been absorbed to surfaces of plastic wells. The next reagent added is an enzyme that has been conjugated to an anti–human IgG antibody. If specific antibody was present in the original test serum it also reacts with the anti–human IgG to hold the enzyme in the well. This is demonstrated by addition of a suitable substrate to generate a visible color reaction with the enzyme that can be quantified by optical methods. The test requires considerable expertise for standardization, but thereafter it is much less demanding and can even be read visually.

SABIN-FELDMAN DYE TEST. This test is intended specifically for toxoplasmosis; the test serum is allowed to react with viable parasites in the presence of an accessory factor from fresh normal serum. The presence of specific antibody is detected by the failure of the trophozoites to stain when methylene blue dye is added. The test is surprisingly specific but has the disadvantages of requiring manipulation of infectious organisms each time it is done.

CIRCUMOVAL PRECIPITIN TEST (COP). The test serum is added to schistosome eggs, and a positive reaction requires the development of fingerlike precipitates around the eggs over 2 to 24 hours. This same principle, i.e., the development of precipitates around larval stages of nematodes, was the basis for the earliest tests for antibodies to parasites. Such tests are mainly of research or historical interest now because they are cumbersome to do and difficult to quantify.

Interpretation of Serologic Tests. For most infectious diseases, serologic diagnosis requires the development or rise in antibody levels in two blood samples over the course of an active illness. In the case of parasites, however, infection has usually been present for some time before symptoms develop, so a rise in antibody titer cannot always be demonstrated. In few instances, e.g., invasive amebiasis and trichinosis, does the presence of antibody, even in high titer, indicate probable disease due to a parasitic infection. The sharing of antigens among parasites and the consequent development of cross-reacting antibodies, especially with helminthic infections, makes the interpretation of positive tests for antibody more difficult. In addition, the persistence of antibodies from a previous but clinically inactive infection may confound the interpretation of serologic tests done for a completely unrelated disease. Finally, appropriate epidemiologic and clinical information must be correlated with the results of serologic tests so that diagnoses are reasonable and consistent with the clinical picture and not based solely upon the laboratory test. For example, a serologic test for kala azar on a patient with hepatosplenomegaly and fever who has not been out of the United States is ridiculous and will only confuse the issue if it is done and comes back positive.

A practice that has tended to give serologic tests for parasitic infections more credibility than they deserve perhaps is their widespread use in large-scale epidemiologic surveys. For community studies in which the prevalence of a particular infection is sought it is not critical that a serologic or skin test be completely specific; a 5 or 10 percent rate of error may be entirely acceptable. The errors can be false positives as well as false negatives. However, in dealing with an individual patient who presents as a diagnostic problem the specificity of serologic tests is a more critical issue; falsely positive or falsely negative results can lead to serious errors in the management of patients. Laboratories that offer a serologic test for the diagnosis of parasitic infection should be responsible for defining the specificity of the test. This should be done with adequate numbers of different clinical varieties of proven cases, as well as with known negative cases and cases with other infections, including those that may give cross reactions. In the early stages of defining specificity of a new test the laboratory should do them "blindly", i.e., without knowledge of the diagnosis.

For any given serologic test, antibody must be present at or above a certain diagnostic level before the test is considered positive. This minimum level is obtained by testing many sera from normal uninfected individuals to determine the range of nonspecific reactions below the diagnostic titer. However, a test result above this diagnostic titer does not necessarily signify that the patient is suffering from clinical disease because of the parasite. It simply means that the patient has been infected and that antibodies are present in the serum. With a few parasites the presence of a moderate or high level of antibodies is very suggestive not only of recent infection, within the last year or two, but also of probable recent disease. Antibodies to *E. histolytica* at a diagnostic level are compatible with active or recent extraintestinal amebiasis or severe amebic dysentery. A positive bentonite flocculation test for trichinosis is also indicative of active or recent trichinella infection. One of the tests for toxoplasmosis, namely IgM antibodies for the parasite demonstrable by the IFA test, is frequently positive during infection and up to a year after active infection. In this case, however, falsely positive reactions may occur in those situations in which rheumatoid factor or antibodies to IgG are present.

Another consideration that the physician must face with regard to serodiagnosis of parasitic infections is its relative usefulness in comparison to other diagnostic procedures. For some infections, such as malaria, ascariasis, and filariasis, direct demonstration of the parasite, eggs, or a microfilaria is far simpler and more definitive than a positive serologic test. Hence, except for some unusual circumstances in these infections there is no need for a serologic test. This would usually be the case for schistosomiasis, too, since treatment for the infection would not be justified without finding eggs in the stool or urine or adult worms in some tissue specimen. On the other hand, a serologic test can be very helpful in some situations in which the parasite is inaccessible or difficult to demonstrate. For example, it is not unusual for the stool to be negative for amebae in cases of amebic liver abscess, so the finding of a high–titer amebic serology in a patient with otherwise unexplained fever and an enlarged liver will virtually clinch the diagnosis. Similarly, a positive Casoni skin test as well as a high level of antibodies to echinococcus antigen in a former sheepherder with radiographic signs of a liver mass is very useful evidence for a diagnosis of hydatid disease. In summary, serologic tests are no panacea for diagnosis of parasitic diseases. As for other infectious diseases, they are only an additional laboratory test that must be correlated with the history and other clinical findings. Sometimes the serology adds crucial information; commonly it may be of little help compared to other clinical laboratory tests and at times it actually may be misleading. It must be remembered, too, that laboratories are not infallible; there may be technical and even administrative errors, such as issuing the wrong report. Results of laboratory tests must always be interpreted in light of the overall clinical picture.

Skin tests can be helpful in diagnosis of parasitic infections, but they are available for relatively few entities. The Casoni skin test (immediate reaction) for echinococcosis, in which the antigen is hydatid cyst fluid, is not as specific as tests for antibody, but nonspecific reactions can be reduced if a properly prepared and standardized antigen is available. A positive delayed hypersensitivity skin reaction to leishmanial antigen is often used as confirmatory evidence of cutaneous leishmaniasis. This test can be used also to evaluate the immunologic reactivity of the host to the parasite antigen, rather than as a diagnostic aid. An immediate-type skin reaction to trichinella larval antigen frequently was used earlier, but it may not even be available now because the bentonite flocculation test with serum is superior. This skin test was useful in diagnosis when a conversion from negative to positive could be demonstrated. Skin tests for diagnosis of some parasitic infections such as paragonomiasis and gnathostomiasis have been used in research studies but are not generally available in the United States.

FUTURE TRENDS IN IMMUNODIAGNOSIS

With the greater interest and emphasis on immunology in recent years, changes and improvements are occurring in serologic tests for the diagnosis of parasitic infections. Various components of parasite antigens are being identified and purified. More sensitive tests, such as the ELISA, are being developed. With these new developments it must be remembered that more sensitive tests that use the same old antigens will simply give the old results in a new format and possibly accentuate problems of cross reactions. Highly purified antigens may be less reactive than crude antigens, so new techniques must be evaluated carefully. Use of stage-specific antigens, such as the larval antigen recently reported in the ELISA test for toxocara infection, is one example of a real advance in serodiagnosis. Another example is the identification of one component of hydatid cyst fluid, band 5, which appears to be the most specific insofar as human infections are concerned and to which antibodies disappear after successful surgical treatment.

Antibody response to specific antigenic components and/or an IgM antibody response may be used to establish the timing of parasitic infection. The IgM response to toxoplasma organisms by the IFA test is already used as an indicator for currently or recently active toxoplasmosis. An IgM response to a polysaccharide antigen of the schistosome gut has now been shown to be characteristic of recent but not chronic schistosomal infections of human beings. The demonstration of an antigen in the circulation or in body fluids, instead of measuring serum antibody, would probably be one of the most reliable indicators of an ongoing, active parasitic infection. If the test for antigen could also be quantified, it would reflect the intensity of the infection. This principle is used in diagnosing cryptococcal meningitis by detecting and determining the titer of antigen in the spinal fluid. Detection of schistosomal antigens has been reported in the urine of human cases, but methods have not been sufficiently accepted and developed for general application as yet. The demonstration of circulating antigen in the blood has been reported in animals experimentally infected with schistosomiasis and toxoplasmosis.

The area of immunodiagnosis that has actually lagged rather than advanced is the development of diagnostic skin tests. This is unfortunate because it is a method that can be applied directly by the physician, and the results are available within a few minutes, or at most 2 days in the case of delayed skin reactions. One of the inhibiting factors for greater interest in skin tests is the mass of regulatory requirements, both administrative and scientific, that must be met before any new drug or injectable substance can be tested in humans.

In Table 17-1, parasitic infections are listed in categories based on the current applicability of serologic tests for their diagnosis. It should be emphasized that for some of the

TABLE 17-1
CATEGORIES OF SERODIAGNOSIS FOR PARASITIC INFECTIONS IN THE INDIVIDUAL PATIENT*

I. Infections for which serodiagnosis is clinically most useful
   Amebiasis
   Toxoplasmosis
   Trichinosis
   Echinococcosis
   American trypanosomiasis (Chagas')
   Toxocariasis (with species specific antigen)
II. Infections for which serodiagnosis looks promising but needs more evaluation
   Cysticercosis
   Babesiosis (B. microti)
   Leishmaniasis
   Strongyloidiasis
III. Infections for which serodiagnosis is of marginal or dubious clinical significance
   Filariasis†
   Malaria
   Schistosomiasis
   Toxocariasis (without specific antigen)
   Ascariasis
   Pneumocystosis
IV. Infections for which serodiagnosis is not available or has not been evaluated
   Giardiasis (experimental, not evaluated)
   Trichomoniasis (not available at CDC, experimental)
   Paragonomiasis (available but not evaluated)
   African trypanosomiasis (available but not evaluated)

* Serologic tests for these infections offered by CDC, with the exception of trichomoniasis. The arrangement in these categories is the interpretation of clinical usefulness by the authors of this book.
† In patent infections, search for microfilariae in blood or skin is recommended because serology is not reliable. However, in tropical eosinophilia due to filarial infection, but with no circulating microfilariae, the test is useful because antibody levels are high.

infections, current serologic tests may be reasonably specific and reliable, but they are not considered useful in the usual clinical context by the authors—e.g., schistosomiasis, ascariasis, and malaria. For others, such as babesiosis and cysticercosis, test results appear promising, but they have not been sufficiently or critically evaluated. The infections listed are those for which tests are done at the Center for Disease Control (CDC), Atlanta, Georgia, where quality control and standardization of tests are excellent. Except in emergency situations, serums must be submitted to CDC through State Health departments.

REFERENCES

Ash and Orihel: Atlas of human parasitology. Chicago, Am Soc Clin Pathol. 1980.

Kagan: Chapter 78 In Rose and Friedman (ed); Manual of Clinical Immunology, 2nd Ed. Washington, D.C. Am. Soc. for Microbiol. 1980.

18

Technical Diagnostic Methods

In a small textbook it is only possible to describe a few simple technical methods that are most practical and commonly used.

The identification of parasites depends upon the proper preparation of material for their microscopic study both in the living state and in stained preparations. The warm stage is an aid in examining the vegetative forms of protozoa. It is advantageous to know the approximate size of the various parasites, but individual variation precludes the differentiation of species by size alone. Whenever practical, material should be examined in the fresh state and in as natural a medium as possible. Fixed material is more convenient to transport, does not deteriorate, and can be examined at leisure, but the immediate examination of fresh material is often essential.

COLLECTION OF MATERIAL FOR EXAMINATION

Feces should be collected in a clean, dry container free from urine. Feces from patients receiving barium, bismuth, oil, or antibiotics are unsatisfactory for the identification of protozoa. Feces should be examined *before* administration of barium or bismuth or not until 1 week after their use. A formed specimen may be examined for protozoan cysts, but a liquid specimen, either diarrheic or after a saline purge (see p. 35 *E. histolytica* diagnosis), is more satisfactory for identification of trophozoites. A liquid or semiliquid specimen should be examined immediately, or it must be preserved. Thin fecal smears or small bulk specimens of liquid stools may be preserved with the MIF fixative stain (see p. 317) or polyvinyl alcohol in Schaudinn's solution (p. 318) for later examination. Adult *Ascaris,* pieces of *D. latum* strobila, and proglottides of *T. saginata* and *T. solium* may be passed in the feces. Adult pinworms may be seen on the outside of the stool or, occasionally, in a diarrheic specimen.

Except for those of hookworm, which deteriorate more rapidly, most helminth eggs are identifiable for days after the passage of the stool.

At times duodenal contents will reveal *Giardia, Strongyloides* larvae, and *Clonorchis* eggs when they are undetected in the feces. Specimens obtained by duodenal drainage, or by the "string test" (see Chapter 3) should be allowed to settle or be centrifuged, and the sediment examined in a direct smear. *Giardia* trophozoites lose their motility and disintegrate quickly so duodenal material should be examined without delay.

The sigmoidoscope not only is useful for visualization of the lower bowel but also is of value for biopsies or collecting aspirated material for microscopic examination or cultures for amebiasis, balantidiasis, schistosomiasis or shigellosis. Liquid material from sigmoidoscopy should be placed in a very small amount of normal saline in a small tube; the sediment should be examined. Cotton-tipped swabs are useless for obtaining specimens of ameba trophozoites. Perianal swabs are used for the collection of eggs of *Enterobius* and *Taenia*. The most effective of these techniques is the Graham Scotch tape swab. In this technique, a strip of ¾-inch *transparent* Scotch tape (the *translucent* variety is not satisfactory) is attached to the underside of a microscope slide, brought over the edge to the top—extending three-fourths the length of the slide—then the end turned under for a tab. This slide is then attached to a tongue depressor at 1 inch from its end (see Figure 6-12). After use, the Scotch tape is smoothed onto the slide, and examined under low power and reduced light. The preparation may be cleared by placing a drop of toluol between the slide and tape. A drop of iodine in xylol, which gives a stained background for the eggs, as well as clearing, is preferred by some workers. Eggs and, occasionally, whole pinworms may be detected this way.

PRIVATE AND PUBLIC LABORATORY FACILITIES

Examination of specimens for parasites may be done in private or hospital laboratories.

Public health departments of the larger cities offer laboratory service, and all state health departments have such service available. They supply specimen containers and mailing tubes, which are available through the local health department. State and city health departments supply physicians with a list of laboratory services available to them, and instructions for collecting and mailing specimens. Special serologic tests may be available at the National Centers for Disease Control of the U.S. Public Health Service, Atlanta, Ga. Often, investigators who are developing a new laboratory diagnostic test welcome serum from patients with the suspected disease.

PREPARATION OF SPECIMENS FROM FECES FOR EXAMINATION

Adult Helminths

Adult worms recovered from the feces are washed in warm sodium chloride solution with prolonged shaking to promote relaxation, and then are examined fresh or are killed by fixing solutions for preservation in toto or for sectioning. For large nematodes, 5 to 10 percent formalin at 80 C with a small amount of glycerol makes a good fixative and preservative. Specimens may be left in the formalin or stored in 70 percent alcohol plus 5 percent glycerol after transfer through graded alcohols. Small nematodes may be fixed in warm 70 percent alcohol and preserved in the same solution. Trematodes and the proglottides of cestodes may be examined by pressing them between slides or after relaxation by chilling in a refrigerator.

Proglottides may be cleared somewhat by mounting in 5 percent acetic acid to dissolve the calcareous corpuscles or by the gradual addition of glycerine. They may also be cleared after a brief preservation in 70 percent alcohol by immersion in carbolxylol (75 percent carbolic acid, 25 percent xylol), or dehydration in 95 percent alcohol, 100 percent alcohol, and immersion in oil of wintergreen.

If the uterus of the proglottid is empty of eggs, making identification difficult, a method for demonstration of the branches of the uterus is to inject India Iuk into the central uterine stem using a 1- to 2-ml hypodermic syringe with a ³/₄-inch, 25-gauge needle. After injection, wash off excess ink on the surface and press the proglottid between slides. This is very satisfactory with fresh or relaxed proglottides but may also be used on proglottides that have been brought into the laboratory already fixed in alcohol.

Search for the small scolices, scarcely larger than a pinhead, is a tedious but necessary task in checking the results of anthelmintic treatment of tapeworms. All posttreatment stools should be collected and washed through a 20-mesh screen. Rectal snips should be pressed between two slides and examined microscopically for *Schistosoma* eggs.

Cysts and Eggs in Unconcentrated Feces

The examination for protozoan trophozoites and cysts and for helminth eggs and larvae may be made with fresh material or with fixed stained preparations. In fluid and semifluid feces, select the bloody mucus or tiny specks of tissue, and in formed feces, scrape material from the surface in several parts of the fecal mass.

Unstained Preparations. A small quantity of the selected fresh material is placed on a warm slide with a toothpick, applicator, or platinum wire, thoroughly emulsified in one or two drops of warm physiologic sodium chloride solution, and mounted with a coverglass. A satisfactory preparation should have a slightly opaque density but should be sufficiently thin to allow newspaper print to be legible through it. Examine first with the low-power, 10x objective and then study suspicious objects or selected fields with the high-power, 40x objective. Trophozoites and cysts of protozoa and helminth eggs and larvae appear in their natural shapes and colors. It is advantageous in searching for motile trophozoites to use a warm stage. For helminth eggs, success de-

pends upon freeing the eggs from fecal debris. At least three films should be examined before negative results are reported. Concentration methods are necessary in light infections.

Iodine and Supravital Staining. The treatment of fresh coverglass mounts with iodine or supravital staining aids in the differentiation of protozoa. The iodine mount, which may be made on the same slide as the plain mount, is useful for the examination of cysts and eggs, but the trophozoites are killed. The chromatin material of amebic cysts stands out in relief against the yellow-brown cytoplasm, the nuclear structures are differentiated, and the glycogen masses stain a mahogany brown (see Figure 17-2). Lugol's iodine solutions (see below) of various strengths have been used. Equal quantities of 1 percent isotonic eosin solution and 0.2 percent brilliant cresyl blue added to a coverglass preparation of feces provide a satisfactory vital stain, the active trophozoites appearing as clear, translucent, shiny, pale, blue-green objects against a pink background.

Fixation and Staining. The merthiolate-iodine-formaldehyde (MIF) fixative stain is a valuable asset in preserving specimens of feces containing intestinal protozoa and helminth eggs intact for later laboratory examination. It is useful in preserving specimens in survey studies, in mailing fecal material to the laboratory, and in collecting large samples for teaching purposes or for concentration procedures. The ordinary loss and deterioration of organisms in stools that are allowed to stand may be prevented by placing the fecal specimens in the fixative within 5 minutes after passage. The fixative stain consists of two solutions, which are combined immediately before the preservation of the feces.

Merthiolate-formaldehyde
  Tincture of merthiolate
    No. 99, Lilly (1:1,000)   200 ml
  Formaldehyde, U.S.P.   25 ml
  Glycerol   5 ml
  Distilled water   250 ml

Lugol's iodine

Iodine	5 gm
Potassium iodide	10 gm
Distilled water	100 ml

For bulk feces the solutions are mixed in the proportion of 9.4 ml MIF and 0.6 ml Lugol's for each gram of feces, and in proportionate volumes for lesser amounts. The fecal material is added with an applicator and mixed thoroughly. The preserved material will keep for at least a year in tight-fitting bottles. Screwtop vials are convenient. The Lugol's solution should not be more than 3 weeks old; if it is more than 1 week old, increase amount used by 25 percent, and more than 2 weeks old by 50 percent. For examination, remove a drop of the surface layer of the sedimented feces to a glass slide, mix the particles of feces, and apply a coverglass. The staining reaction comprises an initial iodine staining phase and a subsequent eosin stage that gradually replaces the iodine. Trophozoites stain immediately, but cysts respond more slowly. For flotation concentration, the supernatant fluid in the vial containing the bulk preparation is replaced with a brine solution, and the usual procedure is followed. For fresh fecal specimens brought to the laboratory, a drop of distilled water is placed on a slide and an equal amount of MIF solution is added, a small fleck of feces is thoroughly mixed, and the preparation is mounted with a coverglass for examination.

Permanent and Preserved Mounts. Permanent mounts permit species differentiation through detailed study of structures and ensure material for demonstration or reference. This method requires fixation and staining. The method of choice is wet fixation, which causes less distortion of the parasites than dry fixation. The thin, moist, undried smear on a coverglass or slide is immersed in the fixing solution. Material that contains no albuminous matter should be mixed with serum or smeared upon a slide coated with egg albumin in order to make it adhere. Schaudinn's sublimate solution and its various modifications are satisfactory fixatives. They are described in standard laboratory textbooks.

POLYVINYL ALCOHOL FIXATION. Polyvinyl alcohol added to Schaudinn's solution is a good fixative, adhesive, and preservative for protozoa in dysenteric feces and other liquid material. The powdered polyvinyl alcohol should be added with continuous stirring to the solution at 75 C. It remains satisfactory for use for several months. Prepared PVA-Schaudinn's* solution is available commercially.

Schaudinn's fluid (two parts saturated aqueous solution of HgCl$_2$ to one part 95 percent ethyl alcohol)	93.5 ml
Glycerol	1.5 ml
Glacial acetic acid	5.0 ml
Polyvinyl alcohol, powdered	5.0 gm

1. One part of the fecal suspension may be mixed with three parts of the fixing solution in a vial. Smears may be prepared immediately or months later by spreading a drop or two of the mixture on a slide.
2. Dry thoroughly at 37 C overnight.
3. Relatively thin rectangular smears should be made to prevent wrinkling.
4. The films may be stained by the long or rapid Heidenhain iron-hematoxylin procedures. Before staining, the dried films should be placed in 70 percent alcohol containing iodine to remove the mercuric chloride.

PERMANENT STAINS. There are many methods of staining fecal smears. Those that produce the best results are usually the longest and most complicated. The iron-hematoxylin method, with its numerous modifications to increase the rapidity of the process, is the classic method of staining protozoa in fixed preparations. Both the long and rapid methods are described in standard laboratory textbooks.

Lawless' permanent mount stain provides a rapid method of staining trophozoites and cysts, the protozoa appearing blue to purplish.

* *Delcote, Inc. 76 S. Virginia Ave., Penn Grove, N.J. 08069.*

The fixative stain remains stable for 6 months if kept in tightly stoppered brown bottles.

Saturated solution of mercuric	
chloride in water	594 ml
Alcohol, 95 percent	296 ml
Glacial acetic acid	50 ml
Acetone	50 ml
Formaldehyde, U.S.P.	10 ml
Acid fuchsin	1.25 gm
Fast green FCF	0.50 gm

1. Transfer staining solution with pipet in sufficient quantity to cover the moist fecal film.
2. Heat over flame to steaming, but do not boil.
3. Wash gently in tap water and drain.
4. Pass through 50 and 70 percent alcohols, 30 seconds each, and through 95 and 100 percent, 15 seconds each.
5. Clear in xylol for 1 minute and mount in a synthetic mounting medium, such as Permount.

Wheatley's modification of Gomori's trichrome stain gives a rapid method for staining of intestinal protozoa:

Chromotrope 2R	0.6 gm
Light green SF	0.3 gm
Phosphotungsic acid	0.7 gm
Glacial acetic acid	1 ml
Distilled water	100 ml

The acetic acid is added to the dry ingredients and allowed to stand 15 to 30 minutes; then distilled water is added. Good stain is purple in color.

1. Place thin, moist fecal smear in Schaudinn's fixative for 10 minutes.
2. 70 percent alcohol with iodine (amber color) 2 minutes
3. 70 percent alcohol, two changes, 2 minutes each
4. 50 percent alcohol, 2 minutes
5. Rinse in tap water

6. Stain 8 to 15 minutes
7. 90 percent alcohol with 1 percent acetic acid—10 to 20 seconds
8. 100 percent alcohol, rinsed twice
9. Xylol, 1 minute or dip until clear
10. Mount with synthetic mounting medium.

Concentration Methods for Protozoan Cysts and Helminth Eggs and Larvae

Concentration methods fall into two main classes: (1) sedimentation and (2) flotation, each with a number of techniques. In both types a preliminary straining of the feces through wire mesh or cheesecloth, to remove bulky material and coarse particles, is advisable.

Sedimentation. Sedimentation is less efficient than flotation for the concentration of protozoan cysts and many eggs but is more satisfactory for schistosomal and operculated eggs. Simple sedimentation in tall glass cylinders with settling, decantation, and replacement with wash water, although time-consuming, causes no distortion of the eggs and, if prolonged, permits the hatching of miracidia. Centrifugal concentration, either with water or chemicals, is more efficient than simple sedimentation.

For simple sedimentation, emulsify feces with water, and strain through wire gauze into conical sedimentation glasses (conical beer glasses are satisfactory and economical). Allow to stand approximately 30 minutes or until the line of separation between sediment and supernate is clear; pour off supernate; add fresh water with sufficient force to mix contents of glass; allow to stand, and repeat process until supernate appears relatively clean (usually about three times). With a Pasteur pipet, remove some of the sediment for examination. For schistosome eggs, the whole stool should be used, and the process should be completed within 1 to 1½ hours or eggs will hatch. This simple sedimentation technique is also excellent as the first step for the preservation of eggs and protozoan cysts. After the last sedimentation, pour off the supernate and replace with at least an equal volume of 10 percent formalin, hot for *Ascaris* and hookworm eggs, either hot or cold for other eggs and cysts.

Formalin-Ether Concentration. This is a sedimentation technique that concentrates helminth eggs, larvae, and protozoan cysts. The procedure is rapid and has the advantage of removing lipid and colloidal material to yield a clear sediment. In addition, the presence of formalin preserves eggs, larvae, and cysts so the material can be examined hours or even days later.

1. The fecal specimen is first comminuted with sufficient water so that at least 10 to 12 ml of strained suspension can be recovered, which will yield 0.5 to 1.0 ml of centrifuged sediment.
2. The suspension is strained through two layers of gauze or a stainless steel-wire screen to remove particulate material.
3. The suspension is then washed twice by centrifugation in a 15 ml conical centrifuge tube (2 minutes at 2000 rpm), with the supernate being poured off.
4. After the second centrifugation, the fecal sediment is thoroughly mixed with 10 ml of 10 percent formalin. At this point, the suspension can be held indefinitely, if necessary.
5. The final step is to add about 3 ml ether to the 10 ml formalinized suspension, stopper with a rubber or cork stopper, and shake vigorously. Careful release of the pent-up aerosol of ether after shaking by loosening the stopper is necessary before a final centrifugation for 2 minutes. The plug of debris plus ether that forms at the top of the tube is rimmed with an applicator stick, and this as well as the entire supernate is poured off, leaving only sediment in a small volume of formalin that drains back from the sides of the tube. Debris on the sides of the tube is cleaned off with a cotton swab.
6. A drop of the concentrated sediment is mixed with a drop of 2 percent aqueous iodine for examination under a coverslip.

Flotation. The flotation techniques for the concentration of cysts and eggs are based on the differences in specific gravity of certain chemical solutions (1.12 to 1.21) and of helminth eggs and larvae and protozoan cysts (1.05 to 1.15). Sugar, sodium chloride, or zinc sulfate solutions are chiefly employed. The eggs and cysts float to the surface in the heavier solutions, while fecal material sinks gradually to the bottom. Flotation is superior to sedimentation for concentrating cysts and eggs other than operculated, schistosomal, and infertile *Ascaris* eggs. Zinc sulfate flotation is used most frequently and is preferable to sugar, sodium chloride, or brine flotation. The optimal time for examination of specimens from chemical solutions is 5 to 20 minutes, since the cysts tend to disintegrate after 30 minutes.

ZINC SULFATE CENTRIFUGAL FLOTATION TECHNIQUE. This valuable method of concentrating cysts and eggs employs a zinc sulfate solution of specific gravity 1.18, which is made by dissolving 331 gm of granular $ZnSO_4$, technical grade, in 1000 ml of water and adjusting to exact specific gravity using a hydrometer. Filter through glass wool. For formolized feces, a solution of higher specific gravity, 1.20, should be used. It is considered about 80 percent effective in detecting eggs and cysts in light infections. It destroys trophozoites but does not impair the morphology of cysts for an hour, although immediate examination is advisable.

1. A fine suspension is made by comminuting 1 gm of freshly passed feces in about 10 ml of lukewarm tapwater.
2. In order to remove the coarse particles, the suspension is strained through one layer of wet cheesecloth in a funnel into a small test tube, 100 by 13 mm. This step may be omitted without material loss.
3. The suspension is centrifuged for 1 minute at 2300 rpm. The supernatant fluid is poured off; about 2 ml of water is added; the sediment is broken up by shaking or tapping; and additional water is added to fill the tube.
4. The washing and centrifuging is repeated

until the supernatant fluid is fairly clear. Usually it is necessary to do this three times.

5. The last supernatant fluid is poured off, about 2 ml of zinc sulfate of specific gravity 1.18 is added, the sediment is broken up, and sufficient additional zinc sulfate to fill the tube to the rim is added.

6. A coverglass is placed over the top of the tube, which is centrifuged again for 1 minute at 2300 rpm.

7. The coverglass is removed and mounted on a clean slide in a drop of Lugol's iodine solution for microscopic examination.

Methods of Counting Eggs

In surveys of infected populations, as well as in individual cases, it is sometimes desirable to estimate the intensity of infection by counting the number of eggs in the feces. Even though many variables affect concentration of eggs in the stool, such as daily variation in output, effects of host on egg production, consistency of stool, etc., egg counts provide a reasonable estimate of the numbers of adult worms present. Egg counts before treatment may help determine whether treatment is needed, and counts after treatment assess its success.

Beaver Direct Smear Method. This is a crude but useful semiquantitative method based upon the assumption that an ideal fecal smear contains 1 to 2 mg of stool. If greater precision is desired, the amount of stool per smear can be calibrated with a photoelectric light meter. An estimated 1 to 2 mg of stool in a standard smear is covered by a 22 by 22 mm coverslip, and all eggs in the entire preparation are counted. The number of eggs per gram is obtained by multiplying the total count times 667 if the standard smear has 1.5 mg feces (1000 mg divided by 1.5); the factor is 500 if the smear has 2 mg feces, etc. Obviously, results are subject to large variation if the total egg count per coverslip is low, e.g., only one or two eggs.

Stoll's Egg-counting Technique. The technique is a dilution method in which 4 ml of feces (determined by displacement) is suspended in 60 ml of N/10 sodium hydroxide, and the total number of eggs are counted in a standard volume of suspension. A special displacement flask, graduated at 56 and 60 ml, as well as pipettes for 0.075 and 0.150 ml are needed to perform the count as originally described. Glass beads are also added to the suspension, after bringing it to 60 ml volume, so the suspension can be shaken from time to time for complete disintegration of the fecal material. However, there is nothing indispensable or magic about the Stoll flask and pipette; if this equipment is not available, a suspension of feces can be prepared and sampled with conventional laboratory equipment. The basic concept is to count all eggs in a known volume of a known concentration of fecal suspension in N/10 NaOH, and to calculate the number present per gram of feces. The 4 gm of feces in 60 ml (6.6 percent) is an optimal dilution; a greater concentration is too difficult to suspend in N/10 NaOH. Regardless of whether a Stoll flask or other equipment is used for the preparation of the suspension, a sample of 0.075 ml is a convenient volume to cover with a 22 by 40 mm coverslip for counting. A larger than normal slide (1½ by 3 inches) also makes the counting easier.

COMPUTATIONS. To compute the number of worms present:

1. Assume 100 gm human (adult) feces daily.
2. Therefore, the total number of eggs passed per day is obtained by multiplying the egg count per gram by 100.
3. The number of female worms present is obtained by dividing the total number of eggs passed per day by the number of eggs produced by a female worm per day.
4. The total number of worms can be estimated by assuming an equal number of males.
5. Female *Necator* pass about 9000 eggs per day; female *Ascaris* pass about 200,000 eggs per day, and female *Trichuris* pass about 5,000 eggs per day.

Kato Thick Smear Technique. 50 mg fresh feces are pressed between a microscope slide and a wettable cellophane cover slip, 22 by 30 mm, previously soaked in a solution of 100 ml pure glycerine and 100 ml of water for 24 hours. After the fecal film has cleared, eggs on the entire film are counted.

TECHNICAL METHODS FOR EXAMINATION OF PARASITES FROM BLOOD

Preparation of Blood Films
The preparation of good blood films is important for the differentiation of parasites, especially the protozoa.

Fresh Wet Film. The fresh wet film is useful for the detection of trypanosomes and microfilariae.

Thin Dry Film. The stained thin dry film permits the study of the morphology of the parasite and the condition of the blood corpuscles. It provides a more reliable morphologic differentiation of protozoan parasites and their relation to the blood cells than does the thick film. The technique of making the thin film, either on a coverglass or slide, is the same as in hematologic studies.

Thick Dry Film. The dehemoglobinized thick film, which yields a much higher concentration of parasites than the thin film, is useful when parasites are few or thin films are negative. It is of particular value for the detection of plasmodia in malarial surveys and in patients with chronic infections or under antimalarial therapy. It is also of value in detecting trypanosomes, leishmaniae, and microfilariae. The thick film is not a thick drop, but a smear spread at a thickness of 50 μ or less, so that it is sufficiently transparent for microscopic examination when the hemoglobin is removed.

The technique of preparing the thick film is as follows:

1. One large drop or several small drops of blood the size of a dime are placed on one end of a clean glass slide. Before the drop dries, it should be "puddled," or stirred with the corner of another slide or a needle to defibrinate the blood. This defibrination of the drop makes it less likely to flake off during staining.

2. Allow the thick film to dry thoroughly, protected from dust and insects (roaches and flies eat the film and leave confusing deposits), for 1½ hours in an incubator at 37 C or overnight at room temperature, so that it will adhere to the slide. Drying can be speeded up by using a warm air stream from a hair dryer. A thin film can also be made on the unused portion of the same slide.

3. *Only the thin smear* can be fixed with methyl alcohol and dried. The thick film is *not* fixed. The slide with the dried thick film (or the combined thick and thin) is placed in the 50 ml diluted Giemsa stain (see below) with the thick portion dependent. Hemoglobin in the thick drop is laked in the buffered water, leaving stainable elements on the slide. After 45 minutes of staining, the smear is carefully rinsed with tap or buffered water and dried.

Giemsa Stain for Blood Protozoa. This aqueous stain uses a small amount of concentrated stock stain that is diluted 1 ml with 49 ml of buffered water, pH 7.0 to 7.2. Thin smears must first be fixed in absolute methyl alcohol for 10 to 15 seconds and allowed to dry before being stained.

STOCK STAIN.

Powdered Giemsa stain	1.0 gm
Glycerin (C.P.)	66.0 ml
Methyl alcohol, absolute	66.0 ml

The powdered stain and glycerin are ground together. The mixture is placed in a water bath at 55 to 60 C to dissolve the stain in glycerin. After cooling, the methyl alcohol is added, allowed to stand for 2 to 3 weeks, filtered, and stored in several small brown bottles for protection from light and humidity. The stain will improve with age.

PREPARATION OF BUFFERED WATER. A buffer solution of desired pH can be made from mixing the two phosphate buffers described below. The separate buffers can be kept indefinitely in separate pyrex glass-stoppered bottles, and they should be filtered before making the buffered water mixture.

M/15 Na_2HPO_4 (disodium phosphate, anhydrous)   9.5 gm/liter

M/15 $NaH_2PO_4 \cdot H_2O$ (sodium acid phosphate)   9.2 gm/liter

FORMULA FOR 1 LITER BUFFERED WATER

Final pH	M/15 Na_2HPO_4	M/15 NaH_2PO_4 H_2O	Distilled Water
6.8	49.6 ml	50.4 ml	900 ml
7.0	61.1 ml	38.9 ml	900 ml
7.2	72.0 ml	28.0 ml	900 ml
7.4	80.3 ml	19.7 ml	900 ml

STAINING PROCEDURE. Smears are first fixed in absolute methyl alcohol. One ml of stock Giemsa is mixed with 50 ml of buffered water, pH 7.0 or 7.2, and the smear is allowed to stain for 45 minutes in the diluted stain that has been freshly prepared. The smear is washed in tap water and dried. If smears come out too red, use a more alkaline buffer; if too dark, use a more acid buffer.

Techniques for Concentration of Microfilariae

Knott Procedure

1. Draw 1 ml of blood from the vein and immediately expel this blood into a centrifuge tube containing 9 ml of 2 percent formalin solution.
2. The blood and formalin solution are thoroughly mixed by inverting the tube and shaking it. The solution kills the microfilariae, which die in a stretched-out attitude; it also lakes the red blood cells.
3. a. Allow the tube to stand for 12 to 24 hours; the sediment will collect in the tip.
   or
   b. Centrifuge the material for 5 to 10 minutes to throw the microfilariae and other solid blood constituents to the tip of the tube.

4. Decant the supernatant fluid.
5. With a long capillary pipet draw up the sediment from the bottom of the tube and spread it over a glass slide, uniformly covering an area approximately 2 by 5 cm.
6. Examination
   a. If one wishes an immediate diagnosis, the slide can be examined wet for microfilariae.
   or
   b. Allow the slide to dry overnight and stain with Giemsa for 45 minutes (1 part concentrated Giemsa to 50 parts buffered water, pH 7.2). Destain 10 to 15 minutes in water, pH approximately 7.2. Allow to dry and examine.

Membrane Filtration

1. One to five ml of anticoagulated blood is passed through a Nucleopore filter* of 3 μm or 5 μm pore size, held in a Swinney adapter. Use of an interlocking-type syringe is recommended.
2. Wash the membrane by passing 5 to 10 ml of distilled water through it to hemolyze red cells and wash out some of the white cell debris. A small amount of air can be passed through the membrane before removal to expell all liquid.
3. Undo the adapter. Pick out the filter and place it on a glass slide, keeping filtered material on the outside; i.e., do not invert the filter on the slide.
4. The filter can be examined wet for microfilariae, or it can be allowed to dry and stained with Giemsa.

TECHNICAL METHODS FOR EXAMINATION OF PARASITES FROM TISSUES AND BODY FLUIDS

Protozoa helminths, particularly larvae, may be found in various organs and tissues of the body, as well as in the blood.

* Nucleopore Corporation, Pleasanton, Calif. 94566.

Bone marrow and hepatic puncture is useful in the diagnosis of visceral leishmaniasis. Liver biopsy may reveal *Toxocara* larvae and schistosomal eggs.

The lymph nodes may be examined directly, cultured, or inoculated into animals for the diagnosis of trypanosomiasis, leishmaniasis, toxoplasmosis, and filariasis, either by puncture or by biopsy.

Material for examination may be obtained from mucocutaneous lesions by scraping, aspiration, or biopsy. Scrapings or sections may be taken from the dermal lesions of post–kala-azar leishmaniasis. Material may be obtained from the ulcer or nodule of oriental sore by puncturing the indurated margin of the lesion with a sterile hypodermic needle or by passing a sterile capillary tube through an incision into the tissues at the base of the ulcer and aspirating gently. Stained films or cultures are made from the aspirated material. Similar methods are used for the early lesions of American leishmaniasis. However, for the advanced mucosal lesions, biopsy of the infected tissues is necessary.

The migratory larvae of *Ancylostoma braziliense, A. caninum, Strongyloides sterocoralis,* or *Gnathostoma spinigerum* may be found in skin sections.

Onchocerca volvulus may be found in subcutaneous nodules or skin snips. *Dracunculus medinensis* may be removed from its subcutaneous canal by traction or surgical incision. *Loa loa* may be removed surgically from its migratory tract, often about the head and eye, and, rarely, *Gonglyonema pulchrum* may be located in the subcutaneous tissue of the buccal mucosa.

Rectal snips for schistosomiasis may be made through a proctoscope, and a piece of rectal mucosa from the region of Houston's valve, 2 by 2 by 1 mm, may be extracted with cutting forceps. The material is examined microscopically by compression between slides. Viable eggs have active flame cells. Several stool examinations should first be done.

Diphyllobothriid spargana are obtained from the skin and subcutaneous and deeper tissues. The cysticerci of *Taenia solium* may be found in muscles and subcutaneous tissues by biopsy or by roentgen rays. The hydatid cysts of *Echinococcus granulosus,* usually in the liver, lungs and other organs, very rarely may be present in the muscles.

Cerebrospinal Fluid. The cerebrospinal fluid is examined after centrifuging for trypanosomes, toxoplasma, and, rarely, trichinae or other helminth larvae. In suspected *Naegleria* infection, search for active motile amebas. If cells are present, they should be stained for a differential count.

Sputum. The eggs of *Paragonimus westermani* are commonly found in the brown-flecked sputum and in the stool of infected persons. Occasionally, the larvae of *S. stercoralis,* and, more rarely, those of *A. lumbricoides* and the hookworms may be coughed up during their pulmonary migration. In pulmonary echinococcosis, the contents of the hydatid cyst may be evacuated in the sputum.

A small amount of sputum is transferred to a slide with a toothpick and examined under a coverglass. The sputum may be mixed with an equal amount of 3 percent sodium hydroxide and, after standing, centrifuged. The sediment is examined microscopically.

The identification of parasites in the cerebrospinal, pleural, pericardial, peritoneal, hydrocele, and joint fluids, the urine, and the sputum is usually confined to the microscopic examination of the centrifuged sediment in wet coverglass preparations or in stained films. The physiologic character of the various fluids may modify the procedure.

Staining of Parasites from Tissues. The methods of staining smears containing parasites from tissues and body fluids are similar to those used for blood films.

CULTURAL METHOD FOR PROTOZOA

Entamoeba histolytica. E. histolytica grows readily under partial anaerobiosis in nutrient mediums containing bacteria and rice flour, although strains may show growth idiosyncrasies. The other intestinal amebas may grow, at least for a few generations, on such noncellular mediums. Boeck and Drbohlav's diphasic medium, as modified by Dobell and Laidlaw, and Cleveland and Collier's medium are commonly used for diagnosis.

Leishmania and Trypanosomes. The best single-culture medium for leishmania and *T. cruzi* is the diphasic Novy, MacNeal, and Nicolle (N.N.N.) medium. Thirty percent defibrinated rabbit blood is preferable in the agar slant, and antibiotics (penicillin and streptomycin, or gentamycin) should be included in the fluid overlay to prevent bacterial contamination. For recovery of the African trypanosomes, inoculation of mice or young rats is better than culture.

Cellular Media. *T. cruzi* and *Toxoplasma* may be isolated by inoculation of cell cultures. Although *P. falciparum* malaria parasites can be grown in human red blood cells for research purposes, this technique is less sensitive than direct smear to demonstrate organisms for making a diagnosis.

REFERENCES

Section VIII. In Lennette (ed): Parasites. in Manual of Clin. Microbiol. 3rd Ed., pp. 669–759. Wash D.C., Am. Soc. for Microbiol. 1980.

Section E: Clin. Microbiol. (Parasites), in CRC—in Seligson (ed): Handbook Series in Clinical Lab Science, Vol II. Cleveland, C.R.C. Press. 1977, pp. 73–248.

Chapter 51—Medical Parasitology In Henry (ed): Clinical Diag. and Management by Laboratory Methods. Vol. II, 16th Ed., Philadelphia, W. B. Saunders Co., 1979, pp. 1731–1813

19

Treatment of Parasitic Diseases

READ THE DIRECTIONS IN THE DRUG PACKAGE!

Treatment of the infected patient includes medical and surgical measures, a hygienic regimen to build up general resistance, and the use of specific chemotherapeutic agents. General medical treatment, largely supportive and symptomatic, is designed to maintain or increase the resistance of the patient. It includes rest in bed during the acute stages, reduction of fever, maintenance of fluid balance, opiates, diphenoxalate (Lomotil), and sedatives to reduce intestinal peristalsis and give repose, a bland nutritive diet of proper vitamin content, and treatment of complications and intercurrent diseases. Iron may be necessary for anemic patients. In certain parasitic diseases, surgery may be indicated, ranging from the minor extraction of the capitulum of a tick to the major removal of a hydatid cyst.

The physician should be familiar with the parasiticidal action and toxic properties of the common chemotherapeutic agents, in order to be able to select appropriate drugs. Before treatment starts, the parasite should be identified, its location in the host determined, the intensity of the infection estimated, and the amount of damage approximated. Successful chemotherapy depends upon the use of a drug that has a minimal toxic effect on the host and a maximal action on the parasite. Success depends also upon its administration and dosage, auxiliary therapeutic preparation and aftercare of the patient, and additional procedures to prevent reinfection. The physical condition of the patient and the impairment of vital organs by other diseases may contraindicate the use of certain drugs. Some drugs should not be given during pregnancy.

Prepurgation with sodium sulfate tends to eliminate the mucus and fecal debris that protect the parasite, but sometimes the increased peristalsis may accelerate the passage of the drug through the intestinal tract. Postpurgation aids in the removal of killed or anesthesized worms from the intestine. Fleet's phosphosoda is an acceptable and effective agent. Contraindications for purgation are signs of intestinal obstruction, appendicitis, debilitation, and pregnancy. Drugs are administered orally, intravenously, and/or intramuscularly, depending upon the nature of the drug and the condition of the patient. In addition, some may be used in enemas or applied to local lesions.

The dosage for children can be calculated in proportion to the weight of the child or by certain empirical rules, although children usually tolerate proportionately greater amounts than adults. Clark's rule is to multiply the average adult dose by the weight of the child in pounds and divide by 150. Fried's rule for infants is to divide the age in months by 150 and multiply by the adult dose.

The first problem is who should be treated? The patient with a hookworm infection with 10 worms? One with an asymptomatic *Giardia* infection? A patient passing an occasional *S. mansoni* egg? In general, if we have a safe, effective chemotherapeutic agent, all infected individuals should be treated. A few hookworms may consume little blood, but they consume it 365 days a year, including Sundays and holidays, for as long as 14 years. Until a parasite is shown to be beneficial to humanity, there is no reason to give it housing and hospitality and to permit it to continue its asexual or sexual orgy. In underdeveloped areas, where reinfection is certain and cost may be prohibitive, usually only patients with heavy infections or whose health is threatened are treated.

The object of therapy is to cure the patient, which involves the elimination of the parasite. In infections with such parasites as hookworm and *Schistosoma*, elimination of 95 percent of the parasites may lead to the disappearance of the patient's signs and symptoms. In parasitic infections where there is a multiplication of the parasite in the host, as in amebiasis and malaria, elimination of the parasite must be complete. As we reduce the host's parasite load, careful laboratory search, using proper techniques on adequate specimens at proper intervals, must be made. It may be necessary to wait weeks or months for the parasite to reappear in diagnosable numbers.

Patients with multiple parasitic infections present interesting therapeutic problems, especially as to the order in which the several infections should be treated. If one of the infections is especially painful or threatens life, it should be treated first—and vigorously. The order of treatment of patients with more than one chronic infection depends upon several factors. In general, short oral courses of therapy are given before long courses of therapy involving injection. Many patients defect before the completion of long series of injections and hence do not have the benefit of needed shorter oral therapy for other parasites. Often, several drugs may be given concurrently. One must take care, however, that their side effects and toxicities are not additive.

In some situations, when clinical diagnosis cannot be made and when laboratory tests are unavailable or equivocal, chemotherapy can be a reasonable diagnostic measure. This type of therapeutic trial is especially justified with life-threatening illnesses, such as suspected falciparum malaria or amebic liver abscess.

An extensive discussion of antiparasitic drugs, dosages, side effects, and toxicity is presented in Goodman and Gilman's *The Pharmacological Basis of Therapeutics* (New York, Macmillan).

READ THE DIRECTIONS ON THE DRUG PACKAGE!

A number of chemotherapeutic agents that are not readily available commercially or are not approved by the Food and Drug Administration for use in the United States are available through:

Parasitic Diseases Drug Service
Parasitic Diseases Branch
Bureau of Epidemiology
Centers for Disease Control
Atlanta, Ga. 30333
Telephone: (404) 329-3670

Among these drugs, which are indicated in the text by a raised circle, are:

Antimony sodium dimercaptosuccinate
  (Astiban)
Antimony sodium gluconate (Pentostam)
Bayer 2502 or nifurtimax (Lampit)
Bithionol
Dehydroemetine
Diloxanide furoate (Furamide)
Metrifonate (Bilarcil)
Melarsoprol (Mel B, Arsobal)
Niclosamide
Niridazole (Ambilhar)
Oxamniquine
Pentamidine isethionate
Praziquantel

Suramin (Antrypol or Germanin)
Tryparsamide

Parenteral chloroquine and parenteral quinine, although commercially available in the
United States, are sometimes difficult to obtain quickly. They are also available through
this excellent service. Information on dosage,
contraindications, and side effects of the various drugs are included with the drugs.

REFERENCE

The Medical Letter: Drugs for parasitic infections.
    24: 5–12, 1982.

Index

329